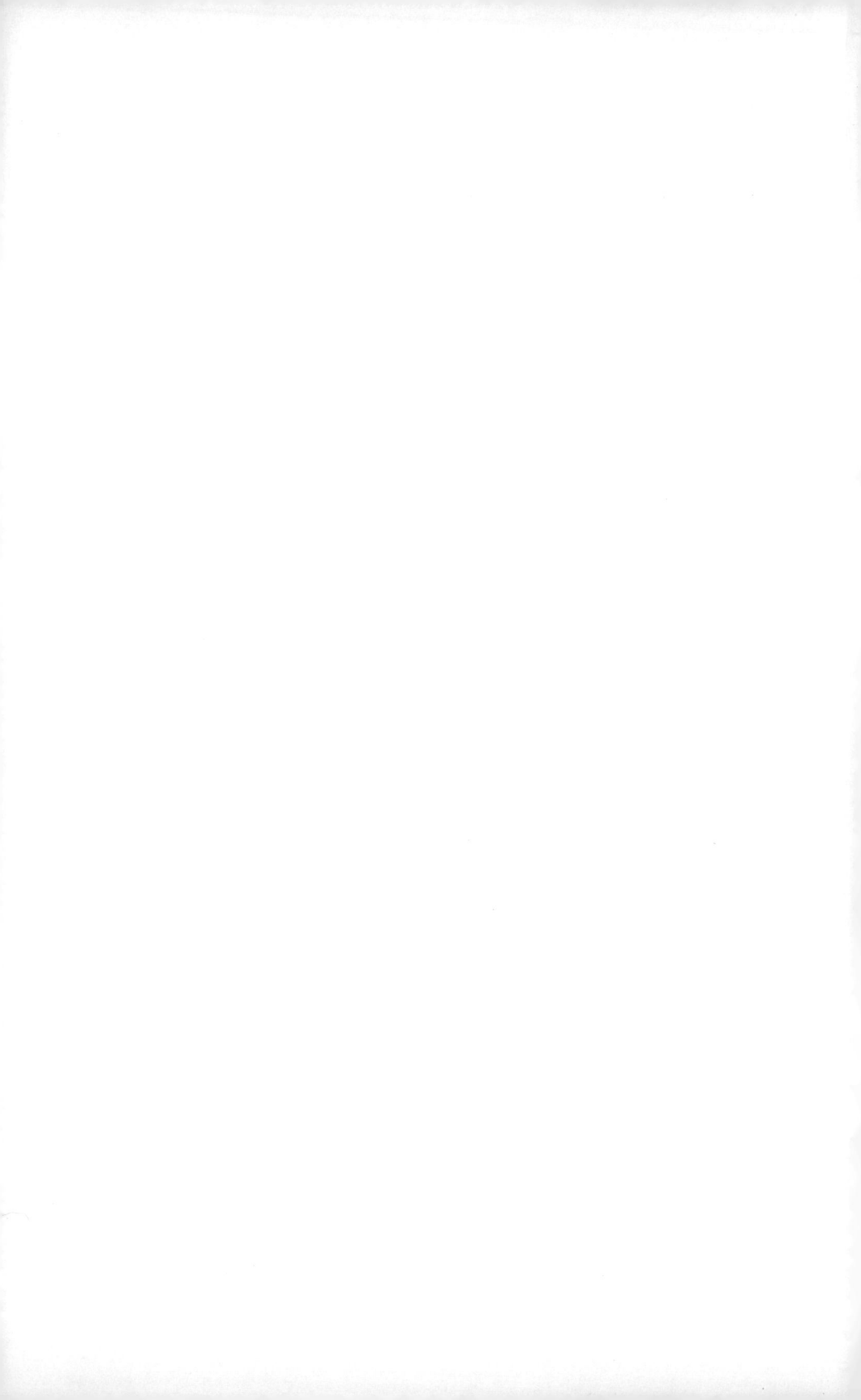

The Impact of Parenthood on the Therapeutic Relationship

This volume covers the range of reactions that both patients and clients have to the circumstance of a child entering the therapist's family. Through research, the authors show these reactions can be extremely powerful, and when fully explored can be used to advance the therapy and the development of the patient. Rich clinical illustrations are provided throughout the text. In addition, the reader is offered many therapeutic strategies for working with patient–therapist reactions as they unfold. Many practical issues arise in conjunction with this life transition. Examples include announcing a pregnancy or an imminent adoption, planning parental leave and covering the patient's needs during the hiatus. In this second edition, therapists who are members of LGBT families and single parent families are described in terms of their special needs, challenges and resources. This updated edition also contains a new chapter on special problems that can arise during pregnancy.

April E. Fallon, PhD, is a faculty member of Fielding Graduate University and clinical professor at Drexel University College of Medicine. She has published books and articles on the adoptive parent, group psychotherapy, therapist pregnancy and body image. She has taught and supervised psychiatric residents and graduate students in clinical psychology for 30 years.

Virginia Brabender, PhD, ABPP, is a professor within Widener University's Institute for Graduate Clinical Psychology. She has published books and articles on the adoptive parent, group psychotherapy and psychological assessment. She has taught and supervised graduate students in clinical psychology for over 30 years. She is on the editorial board of the *International Journal for Group Psychotherapy* and the *Journal of Personality Assessment*.

The Impact of Parenthood on the Therapeutic Relationship

Awaiting the Therapist's Baby

Second Edition

April E. Fallon and Virginia Brabender

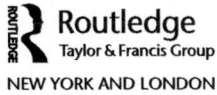

Routledge
Taylor & Francis Group

NEW YORK AND LONDON

Second edition published 2018
by Routledge
711 Third Avenue, New York, NY 10017

and by Routledge
2 Park Square, Milton Park, Abingdon, Oxon, OX14 4RN

Routledge is an imprint of the Taylor & Francis Group, an informa business

© 2018 Taylor & Francis

The right of April E. Fallon and Virginia Brabender to be identified as authors of this work has been asserted by them in accordance with sections 77 and 78 of the Copyright, Designs and Patents Act 1988.

First edition published by Routledge 2015

Library of Congress Cataloging-in-Publication Data
A catalog record for this book has been requested

ISBN: 978-1-138-11961-1 (hbk)
ISBN: 978-1-315-65224-5 (ebk)

Typeset in Minion
by Apex CoVantage, LLC

We dedicate this book to the mothers in our lives who have mentored us in our transition to motherhood. April pays tribute to Elizabeth Fallon, Elizabeth Englemann Goers and Marie Englemann. Virginia honors Toni Whitmore, cousin and inspirational predecessor in motherhood.

Contents

Acknowledgments

We are grateful for the many individuals who have helped us with this endeavor. There were many therapists, men and women too many to mention by name, who completed our questionnaires and interviews and shared their personal experiences with us at a point in their lives when time was very precious and juggling professional and personal lives was often a struggle.

Our initial efforts at developing questions, interviewing and collecting vignettes were aided by Dr. Nadine Anderson, a post-doctoral student and two spirited graduate students, Lori Maiers and Keeley Rollins—now full-fledged psychologists. They were also central in networking to find therapists with the appropriate life experiences who would willingly share their experiences. Some of this research was also financially supported by a Provost Grant from Widener University. Many colleagues and friends brought our attention to relevant literature, provided us with particularly poignant and personal clinical material, and/or contributed editorial comments. In particular we wish to thank Joan Cooper, Gloria Crespo, Francine Deutche, Ted Fallon, Tammy Feldman, Rachel Ginzberg, Mikal Hicks-Black, Stuart Lipner, Corinne Masur, Farid Nader, Sam Osherson and David Ramirez for their special efforts.

We want to thank the editorial staff at Lawrence Erlbaum, specifically Susan Milmoe, who carefully edited our first edition; and Meira Bienstock, Marta Moldvai, George Zimmar and Elizabeth Graber at Taylor & Francis, who shepherded us through the process of the second edition. Very special thanks goes to Judith Schoenholtz-Read, who has written the foreword. She carefully read the entire first edition and then in record time reviewed the second edition, each time expediently producing a thoughtful piece that would enable us to keep our timetable. We also want to thank the special secretarial efforts of Kim D'Letto, Carol Bricklin and Helen Pokropski for the first edition. Hailey Bourgeau and Jane Holloway aided us in our research updates for the second edition.

Lastly, we wish to acknowledge the importance of our families in this work. Our children Emile, Jacob, Gabi and Marianna provided us with the firsthand life experience that became the subject matter of this book. Our husbands, Rao and Arthur, both willing participants in the initial life transition and co-parenting, gave us their enthusiastic emotional support to complete the project over two editions.

Foreword

Getting pregnant, being pregnant and giving birth is a major life event for any mother or father. Adopting a baby and awaiting her or his arrival is a life-changing experience. Yet, it is surprising that many aspects of the process are untold. Where do we go to find the stories of pregnancy and adoption? What literature has captured the passionate, sometimes frightening fantasies and the profound physiological changes that occur in women and their partners during pregnancy and while awaiting the adoptive child to arrive? Where are the stories of spouses, lovers, children, parents and colleagues, all affected by the many and diverse changes taking place in the expectant parents?

Carolyn Heilbrun, in *Writing a Woman's Life* (1988), laments the literary void. She explains that women's biographies have been incomplete, and that vital female experiences have been omitted. The price our culture pays for the silencing of women's intimate bodily experiences is costly in psychological terms. Heilbrun wrote:

> What matters is that lives do not serve as models; only stories do that. And it is a hard thing to make up stories to live by. We can only retell and live by the stories we have read or heard. We live our lives through texts. They may be read, or chanted, or experienced electronically, or come to us, like the murmurings of our mothers, telling us what conventions demand. Whatever their form or medium, these stories have formed us all; they are what we must use to make new fictions, new narratives.
>
> (1988, p. 37)

The meanings and interpretations of female bodily experiences during pregnancy are uniquely individual, yet women tend to seek to understand them through the external messages powerfully embedded in our culture. Images of pregnancy as a period of confinement, a time of vulnerability, are still with us. Within my lifetime, pregnant teachers were not allowed into their classrooms, flight attendants could not work, nurses had to take leave from their profession, to name a few examples. Pregnancy was something women had to endure behind closed doors. Many popular movies promoted and still promote the pain and danger associated with childbirth, and disconnect women from the complex physiological changes they experience. Little attention is paid to the importance of sexuality as it relates to pregnancy. In a fashion-centered world, women's relationships are often threatened by bodies that swell and sometimes never return to their pubescent form. Different families, ethnic and religious groups celebrate and ritualize the period of pregnancy and childbirth with ceremonies that focus on the gender of the child, where the women's body is a vessel for the lineage and provides continuity for traditional values. As Judith Daniluk states, sexuality is shaped by "unique biological, psychological and social realities" (1998, p. 19), and so is pregnancy.

In this second edition, April Fallon and Virginia Brabender have eloquently crafted a complex and scholarly map to help guide expectant therapists, both women and men, their supervisors, colleagues and students. The clinical vignettes highlight the rich variety of unique personal experiences and frame these in the broader therapeutic context, as they play out during the therapist's "expectant state," or period waiting for the child to arrive. The authors address diverse therapist experiences by including therapists who are women in conventional heterosexual relationships, women who are pregnant by in vitro fertilization, women who are single mothers or cohabiting in lesbian relationships, fathers who are in conventional relationships or in gay relationships, as well as mothers and fathers who are adopting children. Fallon and Brabender take on a challenging task to attend to the cultural shifts in family constellations, and they are highly sensitive to elaborating the psychological, physiological and broad cultural responses to the "expectant period" (from conception to birth) in the professional and personal life of the therapist. Through analytic and family systems frameworks, the deeply personal stories are applied to therapeutic issues and techniques to provide guidance about how to handle difficult therapeutic issues and practical concerns that inevitably arise. The authors' talent in combining the analytic framework with research and personal experience provides tools to ensure the expectant therapist will sensitively deal with the complexity of their "expectant state."

This book is skillfully organized to reveal how expectancy and pregnancy create complex relationships and contexts. It breaks new ground in exploring the unique issues faced by the therapist who is adopting and LGBT therapists who are expecting a child. The relationships are given voice, understood and communicated to enable the therapeutic process to flourish. Attention to patients' diagnoses and their developmental stages adds to the context for professional decision making and responsiveness. The structure acknowledges the influences of the clinical setting, whether it is a private practice or community/ hospital clinic. Specifically, how the therapist's pregnancy or the adoption impacts clients with different diagnoses—ranging from the seriously mentally ill to patients with personality disorders to those with less profound distress—provides techniques to help the therapist frame interventions and work with powerful and often frightening fantasies that are sometimes awakened both in the patient and the therapist. Difficult themes of envy, jealousy and hate and related problems associated with patients' acting out are identified as they occur in therapeutic relationships.

By focusing on the mutual dance of interactions, the authors present dilemmas related to the central issue of therapist transparency and decisions about self-disclosure with sensitivity and clarity. Information on practical topics is also offered, including how to schedule appointments during the pregnancy, what to say when taking leave, returning to or terminating practice, and how to handle being sick. For adoptive parents, advice is given on how to make clinical decisions amidst the uncertainty that often accompanies the adoptive process. Throughout the book, research is provided to support the presentation.

This is an optimistic and brave perspective. Fallon and Brabender offer an invaluable tool with an abundance of guidance not to be found elsewhere in dealing with many unusual issues facing the expectant parent. Intimate waters are navigated in the pregnancy or expectancy period. The human aspect of therapeutic work so easily neglected comes alive through a therapeutic metaphor— the fetus within the therapist's womb can represent new life for all in the relationship—parent and child, therapist and patient.

Judith Schoenholtz-Read, Ed.D.
Fielding Graduate University
Santa Barbara, California

References

Daniluk, J.C. (1998) *Women's sexuality across the lifespan: Challenging myths, creating meanings*. New York: Guilford.

Heilbrun, C.G. (1988) *Writing a woman's life*. New York: Ballantine.

CHAPTER 1

Introduction

Parenthood is a transformational experience, both personally and professionally. Awaiting a child, whether through pregnancy, assisted reproductive technology or adoption, can be a wonderful time in the lives of men and women.
Expectant parents feel the joy of having what is perhaps a long-term dream
realized. They experience the excitement of fantasizing about who this new little
person will turn out to be. They feel satisfaction in engaging in the preliminary
steps of embracing the parental role. For example, a pregnant woman might
find fulfillment in watching her diet, knowing that this is a fledgling means by
which she can nurture her child. A foster couple planning on adopting a child
placed in their home might find fulfilling the opportunity to form long-term
plans for their forever child-to-be. Yet, expectant parenting[1] brings enormous
anxiety and stress for multiple reasons. Traversing this developmental milestone
requires revising personal and professional identities; quelling and reorganizing
internal conflicts; developing a relationship, first with the fantasy of the child,
and ultimately with the child himself or herself; adjusting other relationships;
and handling the concomitant changes in self-esteem that occur as a result of all
of these. These demands are stressful, and depression and anxiety are common
manifestations of this anxiety and stress.

A Sociocultural Profile of Today's Expectant and New Parents

The mental health practitioner who is an expectant parent, a new parent or both
is likely to be affected by an array of sociocultural forces related to work, gender
roles, economics and education. We see two forces as having particular importance for the mental health professional: lessened role specialization and family
structure.

Roles

For a number of decades in American culture, the traditional family held sway.
This family was characterized by a mother who saw herself as having primary

responsibility for childcare and a father who saw himself as the breadwinner, the person who would bring resources into the home. The children were generally the couple's own biological offspring. Multiple factors led to the erosion of the traditional family. A major factor was that women were being educated beyond high school in increasing numbers. This shift meant that women could have a more significant role in bringing resources into the family and would be likely to have an interest in doing so—that is, in engaging in activities for which their education prepared them. Today, relative to the 1950s, many more women work outside the home. For example, in 1950, 12.6% of married mothers with children under 17 worked outside the home for pay. In 1994, this figure increased to 69%, and 58% of wives with children 1 year old or younger were in the workforce (Hochschild, 1997). These numbers continued to rise until 1999 and then slowly dipped again. In 2012, 80% of women who were married in a heterosexual relationship worked outside the home, and black and Hispanic women were even more likely to do so (Cohn, Livingston, & Wang, 2014).

At the same time, fathers are staying home to provide childcare in increasing numbers. According to a Pew survey, in 2012, 16% of all stay-at-home parents are fathers (Livingston, 2014). This same survey reveals that whereas mothers state their primary motive is to be available to their children, 23% of all fathers say they are providing childcare because they are unable to obtain employment. Twenty-one percent of fathers do identify the wish to care for children as primary. Even if fathers are not providing full-time childcare, evidence exists that they are spending increased amounts of time with their children by engaging in both routine and enrichment activities (Ferree, 2010; Sayer, Bianchi, & Robinson, 2004). They are also spending a greater proportion of time engaging in housekeeping, an activity traditionally assigned to women (Bianchi, Milkie, & Robinson, 2012). However, this finding is more pronounced in countries in which women are more likely to be engaged in full-time employment and where gender views are more egalitarian (Cooke & Baxter, 2010).

These sociocultural shifts signify that the role specialization that was so pronounced in the mid-twentieth century has loosened up considerably. Both men and women are responsible for work and for childcare. This circumstance has a multiplicity of consequences, both positive and negative. A major advantage of this reduced role rigidity is that both men and women can derive the fulfillments of both spheres—work and family. Sharing responsibilities in the two realms, particularly if the collaboration is effective, can diminish the pressure on each partner to satisfy the needs of the family and of the workplace. Children, too, can be the beneficiaries of the father's greater involvement in caregiving. Evidence exists that with infants and toddlers, mothers and fathers play with their children differently. For example, whereas mothers are likely to be more verbal, instructional (for example, labeling colors and shapes), and engage in pretend play, fathers are more likely to engage in physical play that emphasizes excitement and uncertainty (Parke, 2002, 2013). However, it must be emphasized that these differences are relatively subtle, and both mothers and fathers generally exhibit the gamut of interactions with their children.

Lessened role specialization can increase the psychological burden of parents, in that it leads both mothers and fathers to question whether sufficient time is spent either at work or at home. The refrain from working parents is: "When I am working, I feel that I should be at home, and when at home, I should be at work." The joint involvement of both partners in both arenas can be a source of conflict, as each looks to the other to fulfill household and childcare responsibilities. Also, despite lessened role specialization, in most countries the woman's work status is more likely to be affected by the entry of the child, unless the woman makes much more money than the man (Roy, Schumm, & Britt, 2014). The mother may resent the fact that the father can pursue his career uninterruptedly ("Why am I the one making all of the sacrifices?"). Such a reaction will be particularly acute when the relationship, up until the arrival of the child, has been egalitarian and lacking in behaviors corresponding to gender role stereotypes. The mother's partner, in turn, may feel guilt and resentment as a reaction to that guilt. In this way, tensions rise.

Although the effects of multiple roles are seen in their fullness once the child has entered the family, they nonetheless can be present even during the period of expectancy. Women increasingly tend to work well into the third trimester of their pregnancies (Laughlin, 2011), a trend more pronounced in older mothers and in mothers who are more educated. Managing the demands of the job and those of the pregnancy enables them to get a taste of the opposite pulls when the demands of attending to the pregnancy conflict with the demands of the workplace. Students and trainees, in particular, may find meeting the challenges of both arenas daunting, in that missing days of academic time or taking a hiatus from a placement can limit the student's ability for success. For both students and professionals, as their child's arrival grows nigh, the need to plan for childcare, particularly if the return to work or school occurs soon after the arrival of the child, becomes a major investment of time and energy. In some cases, the progressing pregnancy requires that the workplace make accommodations. Recently, the news featured the case of *Young v. United Parcel Service*, in which a woman sued her employer for putting her on unpaid leave when she informed the company that she could not lift packages of a certain weight (Sneed, 2015). She was told that she did not qualify for light duty work. Ultimately, she took her case to the Supreme Court and won under the Pregnancy Discrimination Act. This case highlights the vivid way in which conflicts between family needs and work needs can emerge during the expectancy period. It also underscores a point we make later in this text about the importance of family dynamics and workplace culture in the intensity level these conflicts reach.

Family Structure

Non-traditional or alternative family structures are burgeoning. Examples are families forged through adoption, families created through assisted reproductive technologies, families in which the parents are both female or both male, single parent families and cohabitating parents. Prospective parents in these and other non-traditional families face their own distinctive sets of challenges. For example, lesbian prospective parents oftentimes struggle with one individual being the biological parent and the other unrelated to the child by blood (Aizley, 2006). How each parent is going to relate to the child and what responsibilities each member of the couple will carry are issues that the couple is likely to begin to face well before the child enters the family. Prospective adoptive parents might face the issue of uncertainty as to when the child will enter the family. They also may confront the absence of any paid family leave that biological parents typically receive. On the other hand, non-traditional families can offer resources that traditional families sometimes lack. For example, gay men who are parenting a young child show a particularly strong commitment to the equal sharing of childcare and household work (Johnson & O'Connor, 2002).

Mental Health Professionals as Expectant Parents and New Parents

As faculty and supervisors, we both have had repeated experiences of having anxious students and trainees in psychology, psychiatry and social work, as well as young professionals, enter our offices eager to discuss their plans to begin building their families and the implications of these plans. They expressed concern about how this life event would affect the continuation of their training both in the classroom and in the field. How would they be able to manage the demands of pregnancy or adoption? How would they be able to cope with the rigors of fertility treatment? How would they manage the responsibilities of raising a child while still fulfilling their responsibilities as a student and as a new professional? How would their patients respond? Would their supervisors understand their needs for special considerations? If they received such considerations, would their peers resent it?

Listening to the fears and concerns of our students and junior colleagues invariably whisks us back to an earlier point in our own careers when each of us dealt with the circumstances of pregnancy. At that point, we were both fairly established, having functioned as psychologists for over 10 years. But just like our students, we both faced myriad special issues. For example, each of us ran a long-term psychotherapy group and needed to decide whether to have an interval in which the group did not meet or to hire a substitute therapist. We also wondered whether our professional images would be altered in the male-dominated psychiatric institutions in which we practiced, and what the consequences of the shift might be. Would motherhood lead others to imbue us with particular attributes (for example, nurturing or unavailable), and would these attributions affect how they worked with us? However, these issues paled in relation to the most basic issue: would the combination of motherhood and professional activity ensure the compromising of our careers and the emotional shortchanging of our children and family life? Like all aspiring parents with demanding careers, we had difficulty imagining how we could do justice to both realms.

Nearly a decade later, each of us aspired to become parents again, this time through adoption. In so doing, we embraced a process that is far less certain than pregnancy. We each were adopting internationally—April from Pakistan and Virginia from Honduras. Although our daughters are now young adults, we remember well the challenges of this process. As all prospective adoptive parents learn, the time frame for when a child will be assigned and the waiting period following assignment are quite unpredictable. We knew that a significant interruption in our professional lives would occur, but we did not know when. We also had some anxiety about how accommodating our workplaces would be with respect to our adopted children's needs to adjust to a new environment. In addition to the complexities of adoption, we were expanding our families. We knew our enlarged responsibilities would create even greater tension between home and career. Again, we found ourselves questioning: could we manage?

Two Levels to Negotiate

The process of becoming a parent—be it through pregnancy, adoption or some other means—presents the therapist with much that is new. There are two levels that must be successfully negotiated by the mental health professional so that this life circumstance can be a catalyst to one's work: the feelings engendered in the therapist and those around him or her by this expectant state, and the practical decisions that the life change requires. These two levels are deeply entwined, for each expectant parent must traverse his or her own and others' attributions, and these in turn affect the practical decisions to be made. With regard to the first, the therapist must brook the spectrum of feelings, fantasies, conflicts and impulses that are activated within both the self and other by the upcoming life change. Moreover, this negotiation is necessary regardless of theoretical orientation. For example, if a therapist using a behavioral regimen is attempting to have a patient proceed through a desensitization hierarchy for a phobia, but the patient is consumed with feelings of envy toward the therapist because of her pregnancy, or with feelings of disappointment because the therapist is about to embark upon a paternity leave, the therapist will be forced to reckon with the envy or disappointment in order for the patient to participate fully in the desensitization procedure.

The second level the therapist must address is the series of professional practicalities and decisions that expectant parenthood and the entrance of the child into a family present. The moment the pregnancy is confirmed or an adoption assignment is made, the therapist can choose to reveal it to professional associates or to withhold the information until a later time. The prospective parent must decide whether to accept new patients and responsibilities or abridge current activities. Many other decisions present themselves as the arrival of the child nears. The therapist's ability to navigate his or her own vast sea of feelings and those of others will inform that therapist's decisions. Consider the following vignette:

Vignette 1.1
Mark, a social work trainee, had never been out as a gay man to his supervisor at work—a remote, conservative figure. However, his and his partner's plan to adopt a child was reaching fruition, and he was going to need to ask for a change in his work schedule. He realized that his anxiety about his

supervisor's possible shock and dismay led him to procrastinate having the needed exchange. He also recognized that the procrastination could limit the supervisor's ability to accommodate his needs, at least in the short run.

The quality of the expectant parent's professional decisions will undoubtedly affect his or her sense of well-being while waiting for the child, and once the child arrives. In this example, Mark would be prone to worry about his supervisor's reaction until he confronted the problem directly. As Waldman (2003) notes, the therapist's expectant state can pose situations that are relatively unfamiliar, especially to new therapists. In some cases, long-term professional consequences can ensue from the decisions an expectant parent-therapist makes during this transitional period, as in the following vignette:

Vignette 1.2
Emily, a psychiatric resident, dreaded the upcoming interruption of her treatment of a very disturbed client, Harriet, which was going to occur once she went into labor. Although she had discussed the pregnancy with Harriet in general terms, she avoided talking about the particulars. In fact, she neglected to even think about a plan for Harriet until her labor was imminent. During her absence, Harriet made a number of self-destructive gestures. In retrospect, Emily realized that a more carefully wrought plan would have afforded Harriet greater protection. She also believed that more careful forecasting of and planning for the maternity leave might have strengthened Harriet's capacity for trust.

As therapists await their child and adjust to the child's entrance into the family, the necessity of making good clinical judgments with consistency requires that these parents-to-be have access to abundant resources to help them through this period. Of particular benefit are any tools that will aid in anticipating their own likely reactions while awaiting the child and once the child arrives, as well as the reactions of others. For example, a therapist who knows that sexual acting-out is a common response in certain types of clients to therapists' pregnancies is likely to respond to nascent manifestations of such acting-out efficiently and effectively. Resources also enable the therapist to appreciate the diversity of possible solutions to the problems that present when the client knows that the therapist is anticipating the arrival of a child. For example, the imminent arrival of a child introduces a wide range of issues concerning the complex topic of therapist self-disclosure (Knox & Hill, 2003). Many therapists have thought about the issue of how to communicate with patients about the birth of the baby and about the advantages and disadvantages of providing various types of information, such as the gender and health status of the child.

Today, various kinds of resources are available to the therapist in formulating an approach to the consequences of his or her expectant parent status for his or her work. Certainly, a rich source of information and support are colleagues who faced this life-altering event at some earlier point. Supervisors who have dealt with a transition to parenthood while pursuing their careers can be especially helpful in providing supervisees with a safe forum in exploring reactions engendered by novel experiences in the treatment, such as the patient being privy to personal information about the therapist (Ulman, 2001). The supervisor's empathy for some of the difficulties the expectant and new parents face is likely to be a much-valued resource.

Another potentially valuable resource is the growing literature on the psychological ramifications of expectant and new parenting in general (e.g., Roy, Schumm, & Britt, 2014), and for the mental health professional specifically. Certainly, if one is in a professional environment where role models are lacking, the literature on this topic becomes an important but admittedly less vivid substitute. Beyond this circumstance, however, the expectant parent can consult the literature to delve more deeply into some aspect of his or her experience, sometimes in concert with others in one's professional environment who are interested in this topic. In the section that follows, we offer a brief overview of the available literature for the expectant and new parenting situations we explore in this text.

The Literature on the Expectant Therapist

Our conceptualization of the expectancy and new therapist literature encompasses two broad and related categories: the method of building a family and the parenting structure. The *methods of building a family* encompass pregnancy, adoption, stepparenting, foster parenting and assisted reproductive technology. Some of these methods are not mutually exclusive. For example, a woman could use assisted reproductive technology to become pregnant. Some forms of assisted reproductive technology are seen as a form of adoption, albeit one that has complex ethical dimensions, as when a fertilized egg from another couple is implanted in the prospective mother's womb (Moore, 2007). *Parenting structure* concerns who is doing the parenting (future or present), and the ways in which co-parents are connected to one another. Up until the recent past, the primary parental unit was the heterosexual couple parenting in the context of marriage. Yet, decreasingly this form dominates the family landscape (Parke, 2013). Today's parenting structures include gay, lesbian and queer parents; married or not; cohabiting individuals; stepparents; and single parents. All of these individuals may be mental health professionals and experience issues at the intersection of the parenting/professional aspects of their lives. However, the particular form these issues take depends upon both the way of building the family and the parenting structure itself.

Of all expectancy situations, the pregnant therapist has received the most attention. We have identified myriad articles, a handful of dissertations and one prior book written on this topic. Early attempts to cover this topic dealt primarily with the pregnancy's ramifications for long-term individual therapy. Then, beginning in the late 1980s, an examination of pregnant therapist/patient phenomena occurred in terms of modalities, time frames and theoretical perspectives. This literature is composed of anecdotal accounts and empirical studies. The latter are listed in Table 1.1.

Table 1.1 Research Studies on the Pregnant Therapist (1975–2016)

Author	Year	Participants	Methodology	Type of Therapy	Salient Finding
Berman	1975	9 psychiatrists, one-third of whom were in analytic training	Interviews and a checklist yielding retrospective** data for period of pregnancy and 6-month control period	Insight-oriented therapy with neurotic (two-thirds) and borderline (one-third) adults on outpatient basis	Acting out, particularly in the form of dropping out of therapy, was common during the therapist's pregnancy.
Baum & Herring	1975	An unspecified number of individuals who had completed a psychiatric residency; some were analytically trained	Semi-structured interviews focusing primarily on reactions of staff and supervisors to the resident's pregnancy	Unspecified, but examples suggest individual psychotherapy primarily	More neophyte therapists tend to be more defensive than senior therapists in addressing reactions to their pregnancies.
Naparstek	1976	32 therapists	Brief questionnaire yielding retrospective data	Individual and group psychotherapies	Patients exhibited fears of abandonment, increased sexuality, identification with the therapist and envy. A therapist's tendency to minimize male patients' reactions was observed.
Fenster	1983	22 therapists	Two interviews (longitudinal design) yielding current* and retrospective data	Primarily individual psychoanalytic with some inclusion of psychotherapy groups	Fenster documented patterns of resistance during the therapist's pregnancy and found that the characteristics of the patients made a difference in degree of resistance.

Table 1.1 (Continued)

Author	Year	Participants	Methodology	Type of Therapy	Salient Finding
Bassen	1988	18 analysts, 61% of whom were in training at the time of their pregnancies	Semi-structured interviews yielding retrospective data	Psychoanalysis and individual psychotherapy with adults	Patient resistance increases during the therapist's pregnancy.
Bashe	1989	15 therapists	Interviews yielding current data	Psychoanalytic/ psychodynamic orientation in individual, group, family and couple therapy with children, adolescents and adults	Therapists retrospectively recognize the need for greater self-care and respite from work during pregnancy.
Katzman	1993	24 bulimic outpatients	Behavioral checklists (completed by therapists and secretarial staff), process notes yielding current data and a 1-year follow-up multiple choice questionnaire sent to patients. Retrospective data.	N/A	Patients exhibited themes of abandonment and loss, envy and jealousy, and sexuality. Borderline patients exhibited more intense reactions and dysfunctional behavior patterns in relation to the pregnancy.
Napoli	1999	6 clients	Examination of client cancellation rates and fee-paying patterns during pregnancy		Appointment patterns changed, with a greater number of missed sessions, but fee-paying patterns did not.
Matozzo	2000	10 psychologists and 10 non-psychiatrist physicians	Semi-structured interview and questionnaire yielding retrospective data	Unspecified	Interdisciplinary differences exist in terms of the challenges of pregnancy in the workplace.

(Continued)

Table 1.1 (Continued)

Author	Year	Participants	Methodology	Type of Therapy	Salient Finding
Byrnes	2000	24 child therapists	Longitudinal design with one interview during the third trimester and another 207 months postpartum	Diverse	Therapists encountered many reactions, but the most common were excitement and anticipation.
Baum	2010	10 married social work trainees	Semi-structured interview with cross-case thematic analysis		Social work trainees revealed that their preoccupations with their first pregnancies interfered with their work to an extent that evoked guilt and feelings of inadequacy.
Vandereycken & DeKerf	2010	60 eating-disordered patients ranging in age from 14 to 43 years	Questionnaire	Unspecified	Patients reported that staff members' pregnancies had a positive effect on patients' views of motherhood.
Toomey	2011	5 trainee therapists drawn across 3 years of training	Semi-structured interview	Unspecified	Trainee-therapists reported a lack of support in dealing with the conjunction of their pregnancies and clinical responsibilities. They identified both challenging and facilitative aspects of their pregnancies for their work with patients.

Table 1.1 (Continued)

Author	Year	Participants	Methodology	Type of Therapy	Salient Finding
Tonin, Romani, & Grossi	2012	8 therapists	Semi-structured interview	Unspecified	Dominant feelings exhibited by patients include fear of abandonment, envy and conflicts related to identifying with a maternal figure.
Zackson	2012	20 therapists	Two semi-structured interviews, once during and once after pregnancy	Diverse—included cognitive, behavioral, psychodynamic and integrative, among others	Having a baby and experiencing primary maternal preoccupation demonstrably affects one's work as a therapist in such important areas as empathy and attunement.
Wolfe	2013	13 psychotherapists from varied disciplines	Semi-structured interview	Diverse	Patients manifested a variety of boundary-crossing behaviors to which therapists reacted with a continuum of responses.
Shaw & Breckenridge	2014	9 therapists	Written semi-structured interview	Diverse and included CBT and psychodynamic, among others	The therapists attested to the reciprocal and often positive influences of being a mother and a clinician.
McCluskey	2016	Clients of pregnant therapists and formerly pregnant therapists	Interview	Psychoanalytic and psychodynamic	This study is one of the very few that captures not only the therapist's perspective but also the patient's. This study reveals that patients feel pressure to suppress particular thoughts and feelings about the pregnancy. Introduces the valuable concept of feeling rules (Hochschild, 1979) in understanding the patient's experience.

Yet, at the time we wrote the first edition of this book, almost all of the scholarly works limited themselves to the pregnant therapist existing within a traditional family. That is, invariably the case material or study focused upon a pregnant therapist, married and building a family within the context of a heterosexual relationship. In the last 15 years, a great deal of literature has emerged in terms of the diverse family structures themselves (Parke, 2013). We know much more than we did on single parenting, same-sex parenting, cohabitation parenting and so on. This knowledge is useful for expectant parents for whom one of these structures is relevant. However, the lack of attention to the implications of these parenting structures for therapists continues with a few notable exceptions, which we will cover in later chapters.

Another limitation in the literature has been the lopsided focus on the mother as the expectant and new parent across parenting structures. For expectant fathers, this transition is momentous just as it is for expectant mothers. Fathers, too, experience great upheaval with the arrival of the child and the expansion of the family. Fathers, too, are presented with challenges involving the juggling of multiple roles. If the father is a therapist, this significant life change has the potential to enter the therapy room. In this text, we capture the emerging work that has been performed vis-à-vis the expectant and new father, and develop its implications for the expectant and new father as therapist. Unfortunately, because far more prior theoretical and empirical work is available upon which to draw, in this text, we continue the trend of giving more emphasis to the mother. However, we have attempted to significantly expand our focus on the father relative to the last edition.

Our Theses and Why We Wrote This Book

Being an expectant or new parent is both an exhilarating and profoundly disruptive event in the life of the therapist. For therapists deeply committed to their work, these same contradictory feelings are paralleled in their feelings about the therapeutic situation. Our aim in this book has been to reduce the isolation of expectant and new parent-therapists and diminish the anxieties attached to questions of how therapists' personal and professional lives will mesh. We offer vignettes with which therapists can identify, and seek to aid therapists in understanding the effects of child expectancy on the therapeutic situation, to augment their appreciation of their own dynamics as they might affect the therapy hour, and to provide practical suggestions based on how others have handled administrative issues and deviations in the traditional frame of psychotherapy.

The expectant or new parent who also happens to be a therapist will find that certain anxieties are inevitable. Often these anxieties are rooted in a concern about disruptions in treatment and variations in the usual frame of therapy. It is true that for the most part, disruptions in treatment—whether due to vacation, illness, moving or the arrival of a child—are less than ideal for the patient. In some cases, even the best therapists are unable to prevent negative effects on the patient's work.

Indeed, the arrival of a child, imminent or actual, like all other major life events, can have a significant negative influence on the therapy process. However, we believe that the process of awaiting and ultimately welcoming a child offers an enriched stimulus for facilitating emotional growth of both the patient and therapist in at least four ways.

First, the special psychological states into which therapists enter highlights particular countertransference reactions:

> Gina, an expectant parent, found herself to be bored during a family therapy session. In her supervision group, she expressed perplexity over this reaction. The group's explorations led her to recognize that she felt she needed to disattune herself, lest she be drained of valuable resources she needed to maintain a state of tranquility that would benefit her developing child. She recognized that she identified with her mother, who when pregnant with her sister, made herself unavailable to the older children. Her boredom, she believed, was both self-protection and a defense against the recognition of this painful childhood memory.

Given the kind of fecund material that can emerge at this time, the self-aware expectant therapist can work through more deeply unresolved conflicts in the service of improving his or her clinical skill.

Second, the experience of building a family can strengthen the therapist's empathy for real-life problems that the client faces, particularly related to family. Therapists would be limited indeed if they needed to have exactly the life experiences of their clients in order to appreciate those experiences. Yet, certain transitions in life are so momentous as to transform the individual passing through them. The birth of a child requires a sustained process of adaptation on the part of the parent (Dyrdal, 2012) and a re-negotiation of roles with one's partner, if there is a partner. In short, having a child requires an individual to undergo a maturation process that can benefit not only the therapist's family, but also those in the therapist's professional life. Therapists who are actively reflective about the transformational process they are undergoing may be better positioned to use their new understandings to benefit their clients.

Third, the therapist's expectant state can be used creatively to aid patients in the successful reworking of their own earlier painful experiences attached to these same developmental milestones. It is our thesis that with each of these treatment "disruptions," for many patients the potential exists for a special growth opportunity—a chance to work with the patient around the perturbations of life. Under ideal circumstances, this break in the usual frame of therapy makes salient an important aspect of the patient's functioning (or dysfunctioning) that might otherwise have remained obscured or neglected. It presents an immediate and often potent stimulus to explore conflicts over sibling rivalry, loss and abandonment, envy and guilt, early mother/father–child relations and sexuality (Dyson & King, 2008). In a survey of therapists, the most widespread regret they had was that they had not made the best use of their pregnancy status for the evocative and powerful stimulus that it was (Naparstek, 1976). This same potential exists for fathers and adoptive parents. Although in neither of these cases does the client see a physical change in the person of the therapist, changes will occur nonetheless. For example, the father-to-be who is also a therapist might need to inform the client that he may need to cancel a session with little notice. If he chooses to disclose that the reason is the arrival of a child, this becomes a stimulus to various reactions. Similarly, for parents who adopt internationally and are also therapists, it might be necessary to take a sabbatical from treating patients due to their need to travel to another country to emigrate the child, and also to be fully present as the child acclimates to his or her new home.

Fourth, the therapist's expectancy status provides opportunities for the therapist to strengthen his or her clinical capabilities. Some of the circumstances surrounding expectancy and the arrival of a child may bring dilemmas into such bold relief that they invite the therapist to grapple with them actively. For example, in our clinical work, we have found a subgroup of patients that denies the therapist's pregnancy, even when it is advanced. This situation is interesting, in that it requires the therapist to make a self-disclosure that has not been requested by the client, and could even be seen as discouraged by him or her. Thinking about what is best to do opens the door to a broad exploration of issues related to self-disclosure. What is its purpose? What are its potential benefits and dangers? The therapist who perhaps never needed an entirely clear policy now has an opportunity to form one, and thereby face other self-disclosure situations with greater consistency and thoughtfulness. Another issue is what can or should be accepted from a client. The therapist who has a hard and fast rule about not accepting presents may be led to visit that policy anew when a 13-year-old patient arrives with a handmade blanket for the therapist's newborn.

Organization of the Text

We begin our text with several chapters about the pregnant therapist. As mentioned earlier, this topic relative to others we explore in the book is the one that has generated the greatest scholarly interest to date. However, in these chapters, we do not assume that the therapist is necessarily in a heterosexual, monogamous relationship. A woman in any relationship context could be a pregnant therapist. Another aspect, however, is that the pregnancy enters the room in a different way than other routes to building a family. Patients, if they allow themselves, can witness the growth of the therapist's abdomen over the course of treatment (Stuart, 1997). The gradual but dramatic change in the therapist's exterior makes pregnancy an extremely evocative stimulus and, as the literature suggests, gives rise to various phenomena. Other expectancy situations— fatherhood, adoption, stepparenting—tend to provide stimuli that are more circumscribed and subtle.

In Chapter 2, we discuss pregnancy as a developmental stage in the life of the therapist. We consider how this developmentally significant event affects her work as a therapist over the trimesters of the pregnancy and her return to work after her maternity leave. In this context and in many others in the book, we will take into account the effects of the therapist's own pattern of relationships, familial and otherwise, on her construal of this momentous transition. Research has shown that such factors as the availability of the pregnant woman's mother to reminisce with her daughter about her own pregnancy, labor and the delivery influence the daughter's confidence and ego strength (Lederman, 1996). We explore how responses of important figures in the therapist's life, such as her spouse, partner, close friends and in-laws shape how she experiences her pregnancy and her work during her pregnancy.

In Chapters 3 and 4, we look at the patient's and therapist's reactions, respectively. The therapist's reactions may be directly responsive to the pregnancy itself (e.g., when a therapist may find it onerous to see a patient because of excessive fatigue from the pregnancy), or may be secondary to the patient's reactions (e.g., the therapist dreads seeing a particular patient because of fear of the patient's envy vis-à-vis the pregnancy). We have used the terms *transference* (patient reactions) and *countertransference* (therapist reactions), a nomenclature consistent with the vast number of dynamic theoretical analyses and case studies in the literature. However, we believe (and have some evidence to suspect) that therapists of all persuasions see in their patients many of the reactions documented by psychodynamic therapists and experience the range of reactions that psychodynamic therapists report. We also believe that therapists of all orientations achieve better clinical decision making through knowledge of the common reactions to this life event. Still, how the therapist in non-psychodynamic therapy uses this information may differ from how the psychodynamic psychotherapist employs it. For this reason, we consider examples of the usefulness of patient–therapist reactions within various orientations throughout this book. We seek to broaden theoretically the discussion of the effects of the therapist's pregnancy on treatment, but we also hope that others are inspired to pursue this effort.

Chapter 5 examines the psychological situation of the therapist who is an expectant father, a topic that Guy, Guy and Liaboe identified in 1986 as neglected, and which continues to be. As in the case of the mother, the father-to-be proceeds through a developmental stage, the outcome of which ideally is of himself as a competent, loving caregiver. An emerging cross-cultural research base (e.g., Boyce, Condon, Barton, & Corkindale, 2007; Finnbogadóttir, Svalenius, & Persson, 2003) suggests that the period of expectancy is often one of upheaval for the expectant father, who experiences a high level of stress at the beginning of the pregnancy and throughout its duration (Condon, Boyce, & Corkindale, 2004). In part, this stress might be rooted in the relative neglect of the expectant fathers' feelings in relation to the profound changes occurring in his life. For example, Friedewald, Fletcher and Fairbairn (2005) point out that childbirth classes almost exclusively focus upon the emotional reactions of the pregnant woman. The prospective father is limned as providing a support role for the mother-to-be, and is typically encouraged to keep any of his own difficult reactions hidden, lest they distress her.

The stress experienced by the expectant father who is also a therapist is likely to enter the therapy room. Shapiro, Brown and Biegel (2007) note that elevated stress produces lower levels of attention and concentration, less effective decision-making skills, and reduced self-esteem, to name a few negative consequences. Additionally, the therapist-father has some tricky decisions to make in handling his partner's pregnancy. Whereas the patient will generally detect a woman's pregnant condition unless some specific resistance is present to recognizing it, for the expectant father, because this disclosure is optional, responses of male therapists are variable (Guinjoan & Ross, 2000). Some male therapists may elect to disclose considerably before the partner's due date, while others may refrain from disclosing altogether. What factors should be considered in forming a decision? Should the decision hold for all patients in their therapist's practice or should it be customized? Therefore, we believe that the range of issues faced by the therapist-father need to be addressed thoroughly, with an identification of those resources that will diminish stress and enhance functioning both at home and at work. We also see as useful the anticipation of decision-making points for the therapist with a view toward the advantages and disadvantages of each alternative.

In Chapter 6, we move on to difficult events that therapists face in their expectant state and how these occurrences influence a therapist's work. During the expectancy period, an array of difficult events can prompt in all prospective parents feelings of sadness, irritability, anxiety, guilt and shame. Examples of such events include miscarriage, infertility, the failure of an adoption to be completed after the assignment of a child, serious medical complications during pregnancy and difficulties with use of assisted reproductive technology. All of these events, while varying in intensity, constitute life crises. Although some of them make the expectancy period extremely difficult, others bring the period to an anguishing close—a close without the arrival of a child. The nature of these events may require that the therapist remove himself or herself from work altogether, as in the case of the pregnant therapist who must be on bed rest. The therapist may have little or no preparatory time to make this transition. In other cases, work will be interrupted by medical visits, for example. All of these events are likely to affect the therapist's patients in some fashion. How to manage the range of painful feelings while still being present for patients, and what to disclose, are issues that inevitably occupy the therapist, and are issues that we will address.

Chapter 7 looks at the family context of child expectancy and new parenting. Here we focus on those structures that depart from the traditional family. For most if not all major events in the course of family life, family structure makes a difference in the particular challenges the family faces and the resources at its disposal. We will home in on three structures in particular: adoption, same-sex parenting and single parenting. We have chosen them because they help us to make the point with special clarity that what you face personally and professionally as an expectant or new parent who is also a therapist depends upon who you are and how your family came into being.

Good clinical decision making must always be predicated upon an understanding of the patient himself or herself. What therapist interventions might be appropriate for a 7-year-old girl with conduct issues may be very different from those for a 31-year-old man with a schizoid disorder or a 70-year-old woman who recently lost grown children. In Chapters 8 and 9, we address how the client's developmental and diagnostic statuses might shape how the client might be affected by the therapist's expectant state, and how the therapist's consideration of these statuses aids in the therapist forming a helpful response.

In addition to the characteristics of the patient, the expectant and new parent-practitioner must be thoughtful about the workings of the modality that the practitioner is employing in working with an individual. In Chapter 10, we focus upon modalities. Much of the literature has centered upon the individual therapy relationship. A cluster of articles exists in the group psychotherapy literature (e.g., Fenster, Phillips, & Rapoport, 1986, chap. 8) on the circumstance of an expectant parent, especially a pregnant woman, leading a group. There are even fewer offerings on couple and family literature. We also want to give some attention to psychological assessment and clinical interviewing because these professional activities can have therapeutic aspects.

Chapter 11 goes beyond the therapist–patient relationship to an examination of the system in which the therapist functions. This chapter explores how other professionals in the therapist's work setting and the expectant therapist respond to one another. We will point to broader societal influences on a work setting's perspective on a professional moving into parenthood, and how the gender of the professional may alter others' perspective.

Our final chapter, Chapter 12, provides an integration of understandings from prior chapters and offers a summary of many of the practice and management issues that expectant therapists confront over time. We identify what factors the therapist should take into account in formulating a decision.

Throughout the book, we primarily talk about the mental health professional qua psychotherapist. Because the literature has concerned itself almost exclusively with this role, we feel that this emphasis is appropriate. However, it is likely that many of the research findings have applicability beyond the psychotherapist role. For example, individuals who are in administrative roles may well find many of the reactions we describe as relevant to their own interactions with the patient. At the same time, we do believe that the role of therapist carries with it uniqueness and specificity. This belief is supported by Matozzo's (1999) study comparing 10 psychologists and 9 physicians, none of whom was a psychiatrist. She found significant differences between therapists (all psychologists) and non-psychiatrist physicians' observations of their work during pregnancy. For example, whereas most therapists felt anxiety over disclosing the pregnancy to patients, none of the physicians did. The therapists commonly reported anger as a patient reaction to the pregnancy, whereas none of the physicians observed overt hostility in their patients' reactions.

This text is intended to help the therapist anticipate many of the challenges of expectant and new parenthood. It is designed to provide, by example, a foundation for the therapist in thinking through solutions to whatever emerges with patients during these life transitions. Undoubtedly, this process will necessitate flexibility on the part of the therapist and a capacity to improvise. What is possible will rest upon the therapist's own proclivities and those of the patient, and their unique circumstances. If a therapist remains open to her own changing demands and those of the patient, that therapist will be better able to evaluate what is needed, acknowledge mistakes and assess anew the meaning of the therapeutic interaction. As Lerner so aptly put it, "Luckily every day of motherhood [or parenthood] gives you the opportunity to revise your revisions from the day before and to rethink your thinking" (1998, p. 71).

Note

1. We use the terms "expectant parenting" and "prospective parent" to talk about any circumstance in which an individual anticipates bringing into the home a child whom he or she can parent. It is inclusive of a variety of situations. For example, as we will discuss, it encompasses pregnancy, adoption in all of its forms and the use of assisted reproductive technology.

CHAPTER 2

The Developmental Journey From Pregnancy to Motherhood: Psychological and Physiological Changes and the Management of Their Impact on Treatment

Framed within a sociocultural context, pregnancy and giving birth, like puberty and menopause, are significant, irreversible psychological and biological land-mark experiences (Benedek, 1959; Bibring, Dwyer, Huntingdon, & Valenstein, 1961; Gross & Pattison, 2007). According to Deutsch (1944, 1945), the desire to achieve the status of motherhood is a powerful and guiding wish. At the same time, it produces significant perturbations in the psychic balance of all women, reactivating early conflicts and ambivalence and precipitating intense self-absorption, time-limited regression and identification with the soon-to-be baby. Although this "maturational crisis" is considered a normal and crucial step in the woman's development from a state of childlessness to motherhood, it is a time of profound psychological upheaval, as hormonal influences compound the general loosening of defenses, resurfacing of childhood conflicts, and unfolding of primitive anxieties (Bibring, 1959; Lester & Notman, 1986). Reactions to the stresses of the biological changes and the naturally occurring developmental process of pregnancy lead to heightened physiological and psychological vulnerabilities that are bound to affect the way the therapist conducts her therapy (Nadelson, Notman, Arons, & Feldman, 1974).

How the therapist responds to this array of stressors depends on her personality, level of adjustment, life circumstances and family supports. Even the types of patients the therapist sees and the dynamics of the setting in which she works will affect the experience of her pregnancy. These vulnerabilities can potentially make the therapist more sensitive to material proffered by her patients, but they also can induce countertransference. The pregnant therapist may experience subtle pressure from the professional community and from general society to deny the impact that these psychological and physiological stresses have on her (Lyndon, 2013). At the same time, she may feel a public surveillance where colleagues, family, patients and even strangers feel entitled to scrutinize and advise her nurturing her fetus (Gross & Pattison, 2007). Neither of these pressures is openly acknowledged, which may leave her feeling isolated, fueled by the perceived lack of acceptability in acknowledging these forces. Thus, understanding the sociocultural, psychological and physiological changes that occur over the course of pregnancy may help place the swirl of emotions that the pregnant therapist is experiencing in an understandable context.

Classical psychoanalytic writings on pregnancy have focused on three critical dimensions of a woman's psychological response to her pregnancy. The first is the resurgence of the woman's feelings and memories about her own mother. Early memories of their relationship are juxtaposed and compared to the pregnant woman's relationship with this growing fetus. The appreciation and reconciliation of these feelings is an important developmental milestone in the separation individuation of a woman from her mother (Ballou, 1978; Deutsch, 1945;Brabender & Fallon, 2013; Pines, 1972, 1982). A related task that parallels the biological process is the metamorphosis of the woman's experiences in terms of her own identity and boundaries with the developing fetus; the initial experience of the fetus as a foreign body metamorphizes to a feeling that these boundaries have dissolved. Ultimately, the mother must relinquish this union and reconcile that the infant and, later, growing child has a separate identity (Ballou, 1978; Trad, 1991). The third very important task discussed in the psychoanalytic literature for the pregnant therapist relates to her own sexuality. It consists of an acknowledgment to the outside world that she is a sexual being and an acceptance of the internal representation of her sexual partner (Pines, 1972). Although all of these tasks involve changes in identity, femininity and the familial relationships, the focus is primarily on the internal transition (Stern, 1998). From a slightly different perspective, feminist writers have identified related tasks that focus more directly on the identity and relationship transformations that occur in accommodating the pregnancy and childcare responsibilities in terms of time and role changes (Deutsch, 2001; Hochschild, 1989, 1997).

The focus of this chapter is on the pregnant therapist and new mother as a person—her changing biological, psychological and role status serving as a backdrop to her reaction to her client and their work together. It fleshes out how the therapist's physiological state, social and professional role changes, and feelings about pregnancy may color her feelings toward patients apart from how the patients themselves may be responding. We provide a broad overview by trimester of the physiological and psychological changes that are likely to be occurring during pregnancy, so that the pregnant therapist is able to appreciate the potentially profound influence that this transformation and its resulting psychic disequilibrium may have on her and her work. We consider how the therapist might address treatment management issues that arise when the therapist is pregnant (e.g., when and how to inform patients of the pregnancy, the issues of gifts, and the framework of time off). We then focus on factors that influence when to return to work and management of new childcare responsibilities that affect and potentially complicate the therapeutic relationship.

First Trimester

The Phenomena of the First Trimester Have Major Repercussions for the Therapist Both as a Person and as a Professional

The Phenomena of the Trimester: Becoming Pregnant

For many therapists, achieving pregnancy is planned to coincide with life events of the couple (e.g., after completion of school). Couples have pursued this desired state with an admixture of science, passion and planful activity. In this pursuit the therapist often experiences a hyperawareness of physiological changes that result in an emotional roller coaster that coincides with the monthly menstrual cycle and hormonal changes. Emotions ranging from elation to despair pull her attention away from her patients, as every little bodily sensation is interpreted in terms of whether or not she has achieved pregnancy status. Technological advances of home pregnancy kits allow us to know without a doctor's visit whether we are pregnant or not, even before a missed period. As the months continue to pass without successful achievement of a pregnancy, the therapist may find herself acutely attuned to pregnancy status of those in her environment, including her patients. She can experience a lack of empathy or sense of envy for patients who become pregnant while in treatment. (See Chapter 5 for a more detailed account of awaiting the pregnancy.)

The achievement of a pregnancy is accompanied by an element of surprise, disbelief and even derealization (Campbell, 1989). One therapist who had been trying to get pregnant put it this way: "Even though we had been trying to get pregnant for several months, when I finally got pregnant, I couldn't shake the notion that perhaps it was the flu." This in part may be because there is initially nothing external to perceive. This reaction may also be in response to the normal ambivalence that women experience on conception: the elation and excitement juxtaposed with the fears and recognition of the psychological and practical losses by this upcoming drastic alteration in lifestyle.

If the pregnancy is unplanned, this normal ambivalence is exacerbated, further impacted by the family's financial situation, the relationship to the male partner, and support from significant others (Campbell, 1989). The task for the pregnant woman is to accept whatever feelings exist on both sides of the emotional ledger. Doing so will not only support an optimal emotional climate for her baby, but will also create a hospitable environment for the patient's exploration of conflicts related to the pregnancy.

In sharp contrast to the lack of external evidence of the pregnancy, a multitude of internal events, both physiological and psychological, are brewing. The early months of pregnancy are often characterized by endocrinological changes producing physiological reactions such as nausea and fatigue.[1] In addition to this interference, the therapist's attention is concentrated on her own bodily sensations (Penn, 1986). These somatic changes create many realistic concerns. The therapist may worry that her nausea will require her to interrupt her sessions precipitously to seek a bathroom facility or she may be apprehensive that her compromised physical state may decrease her attentiveness during the therapy session. Actually, despite the pervasive fear of vomiting, our survey of group therapists revealed that very few were forced to leave the office during a session (see Chapter 4 for a detailed example).

Fatigue is also another symptom commonly reported in the first trimester. In our interviews, many therapists perceived their fatigue to interfere with their session concentration. Although nausea was more prevalent in the morning, fatigue reached its height in the evening for most women. Concomitant with these symptoms, therapists may experience a wide array of heightened emotional states or moods that are not very stable (Balsam, 1974). These may make her feel as if she is losing control; they are particularly unwelcome for therapists who work best when they are able to maintain tight control over their personal and professional lives.

Coinciding with these endocrinological changes are sometimes intense positive and negative emotions. In the first trimester, most pregnant women experience some elation and excitement. Therapists often describe a self-satisfaction or even a certain smugness (Pines, 1972). This increased self-fulfillment and pleasure can have several effects. It may interfere with the therapist's ability to empathize with her patients' suffering (see Lazar, 1990, for an excellent clinical example of how her smugness impacted on therapy with a man who entered analysis with anxiety and depression). The therapist may also experience a certain emotional distance, numbness or sense of derealization from her patients before they are aware and can consciously deal with the pregnancy (Balsam, 1974; Bassen, 1988). Other therapists feel a certain amount of guilt that they carry a secret that, in the not too distant future, will affect their patients. One therapist told us, "I was excited and distracted. I had a feeling I had a secret which was burdensome, but I also felt protective of it."

At the same time that a therapist is struggling to incorporate this potential being into her identity, the pregnant woman may perceive the fetus as a "foreign object" or intruder (Lester & Notman, 1986: Pines, 1972, 1982; Trad, 1991). A pregnant therapist gave us this description.

Vignette 2.1

I knew very early on that I was pregnant. When I would try to visualize the size of the embryo it was, initially, often the visual image of some kind of food perhaps because I was always so nauseated which made me want to put something soothing in my stomach. When I first found out that I was pregnant, I thought of the embryo as a speck of pepper. A few weeks later I was thinking of it as the size of a peppercorn. The peppercorn turned into a coffee bean, and then a grape. Looking at pictures in a book did not change this image. Sometime after my first ultrasound, seeing the shape of the fetus, my baby, as considerably more differentiated with little arms and legs, the food images faded and I began imagining this growing little one as a toddler running through an open field.

Here the therapist first experiences the fetus as a foreign body that transforms with the ultrasound into a more positive, alive, more differentiated fantasy of her infant. The pregnant woman not infrequently also can experience negative feelings toward the unborn infant (Condon & Corkindale, 1998). Deutsch (1945) claimed that all women experienced these to some degree. Ballou (1978), Benedek (1973), Pines (1972) and Raphel-Leff (1980) have also reported pregnant women to have fantasies of the fetus as a devouring force or destroyer (Trad, 1991). Without acceptance of this imagery as a part of her inner life, the therapist may be more focused on themes of aggression in her patients, a projection of her own ambivalence denied (see Vignette 4.2 as an example).

During the first trimester, fantasies of adolescence and puberty are reawakened, partly as a result of the physiological changes of weight gain and breast swelling, mimicking those of adolescence (Lester & Notman, 1986; Pines, 1972; Trad, 1991). Some pregnant women experience a diffuse anxiety that may be related to the reawakening of primitive fear of engulfment by their own mothers (Lester & Notman, 1986). Here is a compelling example of how it threaded its way through the layers of relationships in the supervisor/supervisee and transference/countertransference relationships.

Vignette 2.2

At 12 weeks, when my fears of a miscarriage were held in check by the statistics available to me, I told my supervisor that I was pregnant. After he congratulated me, he pointed out that the dream that one of my acutely sensitive, borderline patients had had several weeks before indicated that she probably had some awareness of my pregnant state. I felt annoyed with him and resisted his suggestion to explore it more in detail with my patient. I reasoned that her material, now, several weeks old would not be seamlessly drudged up. One month later she had another dream. Part of the dream involved her finding out a secret about someone at work. Her associations involved her feeling that her mother and two older sisters were always keeping secrets from her. Again my supervisor thought that I should have brought it up to my patient. I recognized that I should have brought it up, but I had not rehearsed how to say it. I feared that the patient would attack me and that I was not ready for the attack. At the same time, I felt annoyed with him and everyone else around me, but was unable to point to a rational source for this irritation because he had been supportive of becoming pregnant and non-judgmental in my not pursuing the patient's associations. Later, I realized that I felt that I was being told what to do and resented this intrusion into my autonomy. I put this together the following week when I reacted with irritation to a telephone conversation with my mother. In a loving gesture, she had purchased and sent me a book on exercising during pregnancy as well as some vitamins. I felt that she had been trying to tell me what to do about diet and exercise while I was pregnant. I had been living on my own for more than a dozen years, comfortable in my relationship with her. She had learned to respect my vegetarian lifestyle. Now that I was pregnant I felt annoyed at her gifts, for they represented the same struggles of control over my body that had characterized my adolescence.

In this complicated case, the therapist has shared her news with her mother and supervisor, but does not yet feel ready to do so with her patient. The patient's uncanny dream may have been an indication of an unconscious recognition of her pregnancy. This dream, the supervisor's exploration of the patient material around her pregnancy and urging to explore her pregnancy with the patient, and her mother's gifts of vitamins and exercising books are seen by the therapist as an intrusion into her space with her baby, threats to her autonomy and identity, and perhaps even fears of engulfment. She resists this intrusion into her private space by not exploring the patient's material and not utilizing the advice of the supervisor. The therapist's pregnancy has probably created disequilibrium in her previously found resolution with her mother. With the pregnancy, the therapist felt that her mother was challenging identity as a vegetarian (the vitamins) and hard-won sense of autonomy (exercise book). This was replicated in her transference to her supervisor with whom she felt a parallel intrusion, as he asked her to explore her patient's fantasies about the dream (i.e., the pregnancy). She perceived the supervisor's suggestions of pursuing her patient's associations as similar to her mother's vitamins and exercise books. The therapist in a parallel process to her patient had reacted to the patient's dawning awareness of her pregnancy as a threat to her autonomy and identity. In addition to the therapist's unconscious reactions to her supervisor, patient and mother, the supervisor did not appear to recognize the parallel process between the patient and the therapist and the therapist and him. In reality, he, like the therapist's mother, may have been intrusive in the same way her mother had been. We believe that the therapist may have been aided by the supervisor's acknowledgment and exploration of his disattunement to her timing needs.[2]

During the first trimester, the pregnant therapist may have tremendous anxieties associated with the viability of the pregnancy and the health of the growing fetus (Hart & McMahon, 2006). Fear of miscarriage and deformity are common and may be realistic (Leifer, 1977).[3] Most women worry about the outcome of their pregnancy (Gross & Pattison, 2007). However, depending on age and other risk factors, the possibility of miscarriage in the first trimester ranges from 30% to well over 50%. If a woman has had a previous perinatal loss, this fear can be especially intense. She is likely to suffer with considerably more anxiety concerning the integrity of her pregnancy than a woman without such an experience (Franche & Mikail, 1999). See Chapter 5 for a more detailed discussion.

Through most of the twentieth century, pregnancy has been established mainly through a woman's symptoms of missed periods, nausea and later physical changes in the body. Medical research has created a more in-depth understanding of the physical processes, and lowered the risk for morbidity for both mother and baby, by identifying possible hazards. With this has come a perception of the woman's agency involved in having a successful pregnancy (Gross & Pattison, 2007). Quantifying these risks is mainly through extrapolation of epidemiological data. Concomitant with identifying these risks have been the development of many screening and diagnostic tests that allow couples to not only visualize what had previously been a psychologically embodied experience of the woman, but also aid in the identification of problems. However, some of these test findings are challenging even for professionals to interpret (Gross & Pattison, 2007), with high levels of false negative and false positive results, concepts that most couples do not understand. Yet, a consumer society encourages couples to act accordingly and responsibly.

Much information is also available through social media; even though the risks are often probabilistically very small, its presentation at all alters the perception of its likelihood and encourages a perceived amplification of the hazard. Technology and research have created the illusion that pregnancy and healthy babies are within the woman's locus of control. Such perceptions can promote anxious surveillance of the environment and one's behavior and self-blame if things go awry (Gross & Pattison, 2007).

Endocrinological changes, intense anxieties and other emotional reactions can lead the therapist to experience a great deal of emotional vulnerability. This may translate into a desire to be alone so that she can replenish herself physically and emotionally (Leifer, 1977). This time period has been described as a phase of introspection or "investment in the self" (Campbell, 1989). The therapist's reactions to these changes vary depending on her own psychology. Some harbor a belief that pregnancy is a private event (Gavin, 1994). One therapist expressed it this way: "initially I saw my pregnancy as a personal matter that had no business interfering with my patient's therapy session in the same way that a headache or getting married was part of my private life that should not impact on her (the patient's) session." Other therapists, aware of their desire to be alone, may feel guilt for being self-indulgent and for cheating their patients because of their self-absorption (Balsam, 1974; Bassen, 1988; Goz, 1973). One of the authors remembers being excessively active in some patients' sessions as a compensation for her desire to absent herself totally.

Technical Considerations and Implications for Intervention

Introducing the Pregnancy

For many therapists, this may be the first time personal material (beyond the ordinary vacations and illnesses) has entered into the therapeutic area. A therapist may need to attend to two major areas in the first trimester: her altered physical and emotional state, and her patients' potential awareness and questions concerning her pregnancy status.

At times, the fatigue, nausea and emotional lability may feel unbearable and never-ending when it continues day after day. As a practical matter, consideration of the time and placement of sessions may improve attention and well-being. Decreasing early morning hours may minimize the nausea experience. Cutting down on evening hours and allowing for some "downtime" after meals for relaxation and even a brief nap may help with fatigue and improve concentration. If it is difficult to rearrange one's schedule, it is important to remember that for most pregnant women, the nausea and fatigue usually dissipate by the fourth or fifth month.

Many therapists complain of decreased perspicacity in this trimester (Zackson, 2012). The evidence is mixed as to whether this is primarily due to endocrinological changes or a "cognitive overload" from attempting to learn and integrate a wealth of new information about the pregnancy and parenting (Gross & Pattison, 2007). Also, decreased caffeine intake may also contribute to this cognitive change (Kuhman, Joyner, & Bloomer, 2015).

What are often more difficult to recognize and manage are the psychological perturbations occurring within the pregnant therapist. Recognition and understanding of these potential emotional eruptions and disruptions can significantly aid in recognizing the limits of one's emotional availability and in minimizing their impact on the patient's therapy. They are more likely to be problematic if the therapist denies or is overwhelmed with any of these feelings; her response to her patients will likely involve her usual psychological armamentarium. For example, some therapists may be more likely to read a similar feeling in their patients as they themselves are feeling (Balsam, 1974). Paluszny and Posnanski (1971) noted that their own reactions toward their patients were often complementary to the patient's reactions, with their daydreams revolving around their heightened sensitivity of their own physiological changes and their thoughts and dreams of their unborn infants. It was their experience that this hyperawareness of their pregnancy status unconsciously stimulated more discussions about children from their patients.

In our survey, most of the pregnant group therapists felt that their physical or emotional state impacted the way that they attended to the session material; they felt elated, distracted, tired and inundated with worries. Yet, most felt that despite these feelings, it did not in major ways affect the manner in which they conducted their sessions. Those who felt that their behavior was altered in the session acknowledged that they may have been less active and less confronting in the session. This adaptation does not necessarily yield negative consequences, as long as there is some awareness of this change and some willingness to explore and find meaning in it if the patient notices and is able.

This exploration is often not undertaken for fear that it will lead to the pregnant therapist's second anxiety: that this excursion will force the therapist into acknowledging her pregnant state before she is ready. With the technological advances that medicine has accomplished, it is possible to know of one's pregnant state much earlier than in prior decades, even before a missed period. It is true that more sensitive patients often perceive physiological changes in the

therapist, in combination with her awareness of her altered state. Many therapists, knowing of their newfound status, decide not to reveal the news to patients, colleagues and even families. There are good reasons for not announcing the news in the first trimester. The pregnancy has less durability in this trimester. Depending on one's health and age and previous obstetrical history, the possibility of miscarriage may be high, which decreases as the first trimester progresses.

Therapists may also wish to wait for disclosure until they have some assurances of low risk of fetal abnormalities because they intend to terminate the pregnancy if the test detects certain abnormalities in the fetus. New screening and diagnostic procedures are available as early as 10 to 13 weeks, but the most definitive—amniocentesis—cannot be done until 16 weeks.[4] Many do not want to share the vicissitudes of the early pregnancy miscarriage roller coaster with either patients or colleagues. Also, many therapists feel they would like to be better prepared for questions related to future professional plans and goals. Another very important reason for waiting has to do with coming to terms with her new identity. Particularly with the first pregnancy, the therapist may feel that she has not worked through enough of her own questions about her state to handle the patients' concerns with equanimity. The therapist may also simply wish to have more control over what is known about her.

Inquiries of patients suggest that more than half suspected their therapist's pregnancy before it was disclosed (McCluskey, 2016). For patients, knowing and recognizing the pregnancy take place on many levels. Many therapists with whom we spoke thought that patients, for the most part, seem to respect our unspoken wishes and rarely raised the issue in the first trimester. When asked directly, all stated that they did not want to pry (McCluskey, 2016). Some have suggested that patients follow implicit cultural guidelines in their decision making about broaching the topic of the pregnancy: one does not spontaneously speak about it until it is announced (McCoyd, 2009; Tinsley & Mellman, 2003).

Nevertheless, many therapists live in fear of the audacious, astute (usually female) patient who confronts the therapist with "Are you pregnant or are you just getting fat?" Although how to respond to inquiries and introduce the pregnancy is discussed in the next section, here we wish to consider the approach when patients have correctly anticipated the pregnant state, but the therapist does not feel ready to address it with this patient. This is a complex issue for several reasons. In other circumstances, an answer to such a patient would reflect the therapist's style, the kind of therapy being attempted, and the extent of the patient's psychopathology (i.e., some may choose to answer personal questions that are deemed "harmless," whereas others almost always explore what lies beneath the superficial question).

For more psychoanalytically inclined therapists, the patient's associations clearly provide the context in which to explore the multiple layers of meaning to these questions. Therapists who often share parts of their personal lives are likely to find such a question more difficult. When the patient does not directly question the therapist, but rather presents derivative material that indicates some awareness of the therapist's state, we suggest looking at other levels on which to respond to the material. For example, if a patient remarks that the therapist appears tired and pale, one might explore what it feels like trying to talk with the therapist about important matters when she appears tired or not giving her full attention. If the patient is aware, additional derivative material (e.g., growing up in a household with a mother who was so worn out from taking care of younger siblings) might appear. This derivative material can be explored without relating it directly to the pregnancy. This moves the material away from the pregnancy, but still permits valuable transferential aspects related to the consequences of pregnancy to be examined. If there are any negative consequences from the direction of this discussion, they may not be manifested until some time after the pregnancy has been openly acknowledged. At that time, it is possible to return to this discussion, a direction that might be particularly important to pursue if the therapist, in retrospect, is aware that the patient has been confused or hurt by the earlier discussion.[5]

If a patient does directly question (perhaps a psychotic or personality disordered patient), one can simply refuse to answer. After all, even the most revealing of therapists does not tell her patients everything. However the material is handled, we would strongly discourage answers that directly deny or discount the patient's perceptions.

On a final note, as one begins this auspicious metamorphosing journey, the most important thing to remember about managing the therapeutic interaction is the inevitability that the pregnancy will impact all relationships, including the therapeutic one. The extent of its "intrusion" will be dependent on the particular patient and the interplay between therapist and patient. Whether the pregnancy will go smoothly and its effects on one's patients cannot be predicted with certainty. As Lerner (1998) so aptly stated, "pregnancy is still a lesson in surrender and vulnerability. . . . No matter how well you prepare yourself, you are not going to be able to run the show" (p. 9). One cannot prepare for all contingencies, no matter how intelligent, well-read or well organized one is. It is likely that in both one's personal life and with one's patients, the many anxieties worried about the most will be managed surprisingly well, whereas other unattended surprises may create significant challenges.

Second Trimester

The Phenomena of the Second Trimester Are Often Less Dramatic but No Less Important

Phenomena of the Pregnancy: A Time of Relative Quiescence and Growing Visibility

As the pregnancy progresses into the second trimester, the body seems almost to have made its peace with this new physiological state as the intense nausea and fatigue begin to subside. In contrast to the first trimester, many therapists report feeling exhilarated and full of energy for their families and patients. This shift in combination with a therapist's guilt over her pregnancy and/or fear of having her personal and professional life encumbered by the new baby may lead her to a denial of its impact and an over-commitment professionally and personally.

Physiological Phenomena

At the commencement of the trimester, the miscarriage rate plummets as the mother's relief at having reached this benchmark soars. However, a cardinal event for many pregnant therapists— particularly those who are well into their thirties—is the amniocentesis. The beginning of the second trimester is fraught with anxieties centering around fetus normality and being "found out" by colleagues and patients before the amniocentesis results are available. Many are hypersensitive to their appearance and the way they carry themselves in order to try to hide their enlarged breasts and expanding waistlines.[6] One colleague told us:

> I remember hiding in my office during my free time, avoiding places like the cafeteria. On the weekends, I would shop for clothes that were loose fitting which would hide my waist and bust and make me look thin. I wanted to wear regular clothes as long as possible.

Most women are able to adjust their body image ideal over the course of the pregnancy (Skouteris, Carr, Wetheim, Paxton, & Duncombe, 2005).

When the results of the amniocentesis reveal the lack of any genetic abnormalities,[7] therapists experience an immense relief; emotionally they feel a sense of calmness or self-satisfaction. Some therapists become even more rapt with their inner lives than they felt in the first trimester (Turkel, 1993). For a primiparous woman, this withdrawal and preoccupation is more pronounced than it is for the multiparous women (Campbell, 1989). It is, however, at this point that many therapists feel a decrease in uneasiness about others, including patients learning of their pregnancies. Most therapists seem to have some ambivalence about the discovery of their pregnancy, with a desire to withhold their status from their patients as long as possible, and a concomitant wish to brandish their newfound state to family and friends (Imber, 1990). Whereas the majority of pregnant therapists we interviewed felt that their physical and emotional state did not impact the way therapy proceeded in this trimester, anxieties about when and how to announce the pregnancy, what to reveal, and how to integrate professional and personal needs begin to take center stage in their professional thoughts. These are discussed in the intervention section.

During this trimester, the pregnant state activates a feeling of the fluidity of body boundaries as the woman begins to share her body with this burgeoning life within her. The boundaries between the mother and her unborn infant become blurred as psychological and physical identities merge (Blos, 1980; Lester & Notman, 1986; Trad, 1991). For those therapists not undergoing ultrasonography, "quickening" or fetal movement is the first harbinger that there is a living entity that is separate from themselves. The fetus—growing, moving and kicking—felt exclusively by the pregnant woman, has been considered for many women the turning point in acknowledging the realities of their pregnancy (Lester & Notman, 1986). As the baby becomes active and the presence of a viable life is felt, many women experience more self-absorption and withdrawal (Bassen, 1988; Paluszny & Posnanski, 1971). This experience separates the pregnant therapist from the world and at the same time ensconces her and her fetus in a special space that can potentiate her gradual disengagement from social and work-related activities. This fetus activity also may be a distraction to the therapist (Ashway, 1984; Nadelson et al., 1974). The patient's experience of rejection can be fueled by this withdrawal of energy from therapy. Whether distracted by the fetus's movements or absorbed by the special developing bond, the therapist may experience anxiety and guilt as she begins to experience the divergent demands of her roles (Baum & Itzhaky, 2006; Lyndon, 2013).

Experiences With Patients

Although the experience of fetal movement signals a oneness with her infant, it also alerts the pregnant woman that it will soon become a separate being. In doing so, pregnant therapists may recognize in their patients their own personal issues regarding symbiotic desires, an awareness that potentially enables pregnant therapists to feel greater empathy for patients' wishes for merger, or it may frighten them leading to their engagement in psychological maneuvers that will defensively distance this material and patients (Penn, 1986).

Vignette 2.3

A therapist had been seeing a schizophrenic woman for a number of years. Routinely, the patient brought a soda to her sessions. The therapist had never challenged this partaking because she felt it enhanced the patient's sense of safety within therapy. However, at the end of a therapy session one day she was having thoughts that she should encourage this patient to give up the beverage and thereby possibly have access to new elements of her experience. She discussed the matter in a supervision group. One participant said it was strange that she would take this stance so soon before her maternity break. On reflection, the therapist recognized that she had begun to experience sessions as a tea party. It was pleasurable to think of herself as having a special connection with this patient. In urging the patient's abstinence, she was banishing a wish that she saw as forbidden.

Concurrent with self-absorption is a heightened physiological and emotional vulnerability (Coleman, 1969; Nadelson et al., 1974; Penn, 1986). Harriet Lerner, a psychologist author of *The Mother Dance*, put it poignantly,

> Containing my anxiety was not easy. . . . Having a baby was now almost all I cared about. I wanted this baby with a fierceness I had not known was possible, and I would burst into tears if I found myself in line at a super market with a mother and her infant. I'm not sentimental about fetuses, so there was no way I could have anticipated the searing intensity of this bond. . . . having children, even in so called ordinary circumstances, is a lifelong lesson in feeling out of control.
>
> (1998, pp. 5–6)

In an effort to manage the out-of-control experience, many mothers-to-be begin to read about child development, whereas others shy away from becoming knowledge experts, each group attempting to cope in its characteristic manner with this developmental transformation (Leifer, 1977; Lerner, 1998). Regardless of their style of contending, most find themselves more interested and attuned to other young children and infants around them (Leifer, 1977).

At the same time that self-absorption may be prominent, pregnant women are also reporting a sharpened receptiveness and intuition associated with pregnancy, which functions biologically and psychologically to prepare them for their relationships with their newborns (Dagan, Lapidot, & Eisenstein, 2001; Tudiver & Tudiver, 1982).[8] Although potentially regressive, when carefully monitored, therapists' observations, intuitions and other reactions can provide a conduit to unconscious processes and conflicts that often stay outside our awareness. For many therapists, this relatively heightened access to the unconscious results in greater intuitive powers and enhanced alertness that may be employed to become more aware of the subtle changes in their patients' presentation; this potentially translates into a more empathic sensitivity to their patients and their issues (Barbanel, 1980; Fenster, Phillips, & Rappaport, 1986; Pielack, 1989; Rogers, 1994). Therapists describe themselves as more affectively available and experience a greater openness to the conflicts that their patients present (Penn, 1986). Balsam (1974) suggested that this greater openness and availability may aid the pregnant therapist "to withstand the many ungratifying passages in therapy, and . . . allow the patient more leeway to express his or her painful emotions without requiring evidence of improvement to give the seal of approval to her work" (p. 268). The same therapist presented earlier in the chapter, who had resented the intrusion of her mother, her supervisor and her patient into her pregnancy, felt differently during her second trimester as she had developed a new sense of mastery.

Vignette 2.4

Armed with my newfound understanding of my mother's continuing impact on my therapeutic work, I felt quite differently about this patient and my supervision in the second trimester. I did not feel as if the patient was intruding into my space. I felt ready for her to know of my status and sturdy enough to weather her attacks. I felt I could be a part of her world, aware of her pain and conflicts and able to contain her rage, yet separate from her. Her struggles for intimacy and independence were hers, not mine, just as my baby was part of me, but doing his own thing as he chose to kick me whenever he felt like it—during sessions and at night.

Here, the therapist has developed a sharpened perspective both with regard to the dualism of fusion and separateness in relation to the developing fetus within her and the layers of her relationships that are affected by her developmental status. We see the potential of the mother's relationship to the child as having "distinctive characteristics of freely changeable fusion . . . they will always remain part of herself, and at the same time will always have to remain an object that is part of the outside world and part of her sexual mate" (Bibring et al., 1961, p. 16). At the same time, she appears not to feel invaded or challenged by her supervisor's comments or her patient's verbal attacks.

We also suspect that a maturational resolution in this therapist's relationship with her mother enabled her to enter a new phase of identification. This reconciliation is often mutual. From the pregnant woman's perspective, she experiences a more positive sentiment toward her mother's gestures, a greater acceptance of her own dependency needs, a reallocation of her mother's role in her life as more benign, and the development of a more adult sense of self (Ballou, 1978; Leon, 2009). This process may occur in concert with her mother's greater acceptance of her daughter as an equal adult. Being a biologically mature woman with the power to create life within her, along with this reconciliation, then, allows her to move psychologically toward her new role as a mother herself. Interestingly, as a more positive relationship with her mother evolves, an often increasing underlying tension is experienced with her mother-in-law. Pregnant women also report their relationships with their mothers-in-law (and other maternal representations) to be increasingly problematic; they perceived them as being more critical and attributed this shift to envy (Leon, 2009; Zheng, 2014). Ballou (1978) suggested that this intensification of negativity occurs in order to protect their newly attained positive relationships with their own mothers by way of displacing any competitive feelings from their mothers to their mothers-in-law. Also, the mother-in-law might convey more envy and competition whose identification with the pregnant woman may be less and who may be more explicitly excluded.

Some therapists can experience a magnified interest in exploring their patients' conflicts and issues particularly related to their pregnancies; it is important that their personal zest does not result in them overzealously attempting to interpret all their patients' responses as symbolically related to the pregnancy (Bassen, 1988). Some make premature interpretations, worried that therapy will end early due to patient dissatisfaction, fear of abandonment or the premature arrival of the baby. This may occur for any number of possible reasons: (a) as a counter-phobic response to talking about the pregnancy; (b) because the intensity of needs and emotions of the pregnant therapist (or any preoccupation) naturally leads to their use as a selective filter; and (c) to the extent that the patient's negative experiences are attributed to the pregnancy, it constitutes a self-flagellation, penance for guilt over the misdeed of getting pregnant and inconveniencing the patient. An awareness of the material, presented in the context of the patient's constellation of personality dynamics and current problems, may shield the therapist from automatically viewing this highly consequential event as disproportionately meaningful for the patient.

In contrast, some therapists feeling guilt or anxiety over the pregnancy belabor the real aspects of the intrusion of the pregnancy on the therapeutic situation; they, unlike the previously mentioned therapists, miss the opportunity to explore the transferential aspects of the patients' reactions (Baum & Itzhaky, 2006; Lyndon, 2013; Penn, 1986). Guilt or other strong preoccupations erode an intellectually accepted perspective that pregnancy can be an opportunity to stimulate existing conflicts and to explore creatively its impact on the patient. For example, Hannett (1949) found that even with her miscarriage, each of her patients reacted consistent with their own psychopathology.

As the pregnancy progresses, many women experience both a desire to nurture and be nurtured. They report a more intense need for succorance from their significant other, extended family and friends, particularly when experiencing physical discomfort or anxiety about the fetus. Many display an exacerbated sensitivity to perceived rejections or insults with increased emotional manifestations of anger and hurt over minor incidents (Leifer, 1977). Although this sensitivity may increase the therapist's attunement to the patient's vulnerabilities and need for caring, the therapist may allow her own needs to permeate the therapy session (Naparstek, 1976).

At the same time, many pregnant women increase their own nurturing role with those around them, perhaps in an attempt to psychologically rehearse the maternal role.[9] Pregnant therapists can find themselves beginning to enact this role with their patients. The therapist should pay particular attention to her own insecurities concerning her mothering so that she does not burden her patients by cultivating their view of her as an idealized mother. (This point will be considered in greater detail in the section on the last trimester.)

As the second trimester progresses, the concrete visual evidence of the fetus is undeniable. Some women feel a sense of pride in their appearance and are temporarily freed from the cultural expectations to be slim and fit (Clark & Ogden, 1999; Loth, Bauer, Wall Berge & Neumark-Sztainer, 2011). For many, the changes in bodily shape, particularly the enlargement of the abdomen, evoke negative feelings and they describe themselves as "feeling fat" (Chang, Chao, & Kenney, 2006; Clark, Skouteris, Wetheim, Paxton, & Milgrom, 2009; Lester & Notman, 1986). Women who have previously experienced shame over weight-related issues often have difficulty in adjusting to the increase in weight and change in shape from a slender or curvy shape to a more matronly one (Pines, 1972). The body image dissatisfaction often increases as the pregnancy progresses, culminating in the postpartum phase (Earle, 2003). The pregnant therapist may find herself feeling envious and jealous of those female and even male patients and friends who maintain a svelte figure. One therapist said, "I felt like a beached whale. It was summertime, these adolescent girls would come to my office with these cute little short sets with their flat midriffs exposed. I could hardly stand it." In response to these internal and external challenges, many therapists struggle to hide their physical appearance and discomfort (Lax, 1969). If the therapist is treating a population that shares body image difficulties, her discomfort may intensify further.

One of the group therapists interviewed reported how difficult it was for her treating a group of eating disordered women who intensely focused on her progressive changes in body shape. Some patients will sense the therapist's vulnerability on this issue and astutely exploit this vulnerability, using it as an outlet for hostility. One therapist running a cognitive behavioral group told of how a patient began remarking that the therapist was fat in the second trimester. This and other insults continued throughout the pregnancy. If a therapist finds herself struggling unduly with this body image change, some self-reflection may be helpful; the therapist's discomfort with her changing body image also may metaphorically represent the desire for the unencumbered lifestyle. At the same time, a therapist who has never grappled with weight issues may cultivate, as a result of her experience with the pregnancy, a new appreciation for the psychological problems correlated with body image and the weight gain/loss cycle (Allison & Sarwer, 2016; Perlman, 1986).

Although some therapists operate in solo practice, many are functioning within group or organization settings. Many therapists report that female colleagues often take more of an interest in the pregnancy than male ones do. Gross and Pattison (2007) suggest that male colleagues often resent maternity benefits, although laws now require that equal leave be available to both parents. More disturbing are the many studies that report that pregnant women perceive both disadvantage and discrimination in the workplace (see Chapter 11 for further discussion of workplace dynamics). Women who feel supported at home and on the job are more likely to return to their work after childbirth (Killien, 2005); those that perceive maltreatment are less likely to return to their positions post-pregnancy (Lyness, Thompson, Francesco, & Judiesch, 1999).

Technical Considerations and Implications for Intervention: Introducing the Pregnancy

Broad agreement exists that announcements and information involving any interruption of treatment—whether the result of serious illness (Abend, 1982), relocation (Martinez, 1989) or pregnancy (Uyehara, Austrian, Upton, Warner, & Williamson, 1995)—must be tailored to the therapist's style, the environment in which she practices, the nature of the therapist–patient relationship, its anticipated impact on the patient, and whether the therapist intends to return after pregnancy. The amount of notice given until the therapist departs (at least temporarily) varies widely. The general rules for therapist revelation in ordinary therapeutic discourse suggest that in order to avoid unnecessarily introducing a therapist's agenda or her personal life into the treatment, a therapist waits until the patient "notices," questions or comments on it. In the case of pregnancy, the revelation ideally would occur only after the patients' comments manifest a conscious or unconscious acknowledgment of her state.

Awareness by the patient can be indicated by manifest articulation ("Are you pregnant?"), or it can be displayed derivatively in the form of dreams (e.g., dreams of babies and mothers), metaphorical associations (e.g., feeling the therapist is taking better care of someone else, suddenly thinking about getting pregnant) and/or acting out (e.g., missed sessions, unprotected sex). To allow patients the flexibility to acknowledge the pregnancy in their own way and time has the advantage of allowing them some degree of control over their "psychological readiness" to deal with the therapist's pregnancy (Fenster et al., 1986). Generally patients' responses to the discovery and ongoing interest and concern about the pregnancy is characteristic of their other interactions (Bassen, 1988). Such advice is offset by the need to allow adequate time for patients to work through whatever their responses may be. In addition, therapists must prepare for the possibility that premature labor or pregnancy complications may attenuate therapeutic time together before the baby is born. Time also may be curtailed if the therapist desires to temporarily discontinue prior to her due date. McCluskey's study (2016) revealed that almost 40% of the therapists had their babies before they were due or required premature bed rest.

If a therapist has the urge to inform patients of the pregnancy before there are any overt intrusions (obvious morning sickness, changing appointments) or before they are "showing" (either literally or metaphorically), careful thought ought to be given to the rationale for doing so in order to ensure that the therapist's countertransference is not driving the announcement. Technically, informing patients of the pregnancy too early may focus the patient on the realities of the pregnancy, but also may eclipse their awareness of feelings of exclusion or other more transference-based reactions (Goldberger, 1991). Disclosures before patients are aware of them also may be motivated by the therapist's own anxiety, fears and ambivalence; in anticipation of their patients' responses to their discovery, most therapists report feeling apprehensive, eager and nervous (Bashe, 1989). One of McCluskey's (2016) therapists, who was tempted to reveal her pregnancy, said, "There was something secretive about waiting until someone brought it up. . . . I'm glad I didn't just jump to tell straight away because I don't know that some of the material would have emerged if I had disclosed prematurely" (p. 2). A trusted colleague, supervisor or therapist can aid in teasing apart the pregnant therapist's needs from those of her patients.

Most patients, either directly or derivatively, give some indication of their awareness during the second trimester or even earlier (Bashe, 1989; Bassen, 1988). It is generally accepted that under ordinary circumstances, the therapist can wait for this spontaneous discovery no later than the end of the second trimester in order for sufficient processing time prior to the therapeutic hiatus (Fenster et al., 1986; McCluskey, 2016; Uyehara et al., 1995).

Exceptions occur. In those settings in which many patients have access simultaneously to many staff members in multiple roles (e.g., residential and inpatient facilities, day hospital programs), it may be better for the pregnant therapist to announce to both staff and patients at the same time, as dissemination of this knowledge spreads quickly and in a less controlled fashion if such an announcement is not made (Benedek, 1973). In our interviews, a few therapists felt it necessary to discuss/announce their pregnancy early because news spread on their units or patients overheard staff discussing it. Particularly among our group therapists, the need to announce it earlier (8 to 16 weeks) than they might otherwise occurred because one of the group members might confront the therapist in an individual session. Were he or she to be successful, potential negative ramifications would occur for the group as a whole. When dealing with two or more people as a unit (group, family, children and their parents), where possible, the individuals should be given information in the same session. For example, when a patient in an individual session questioned a group therapist about her pregnancy, the therapist requested that the patient bring it up in the group where she confirmed the patient's inquiry. Other group therapists we interviewed reported that the disclosure frequently occurred in response to a question in an individual session, and that individual then announced it to the group either before or in the group session. In this latter instance, the unfolding of the information might occur in variable ways because it is filtered through the dynamics of the informant. For example, the individual may withhold the information from the group or use it to display her special relationship to the therapist.

When the therapist is not planning to return to her practice after childbirth, the therapist is forcing a termination or transfer. More notice may be required in order to work through this forced termination. The longer the tenure and more intense the therapeutic relationship has been, the earlier a notice is required. In the psychoanalytic relocation literature, 5 to 6 months' notice is suggested (Martinez, 1989; Uyehara et al., 1995). We concur that if a therapist is involved with long-term patients (more than one year), intensive therapy (two or more times per week), or an individual with serious abandonment or dependency issues, and the therapist intends not to continue after childbirth, we recommend introducing the topic shortly after a normal pregnancy has been confirmed (20 weeks). A definite date for termination should be set in order to avoid patients' not being able to say goodbye to their therapist. In any other circumstance this is standard technique, yet not uncommonly in agencies and clinics, pregnant therapists one day disappear and patients only "hear" that their therapist had her baby. If the therapist expects to return, and has no history of obstetrical complications, she has greater leeway as to when her pregnancy can be introduced.

In general, then, informing patients should be considered on a case-by-case basis: there is, however, some agreement that in the early months (first trimester and the early part of the second trimester), the therapist can wait until the patient indicates awareness of the pregnancy directly or indirectly. It seems prudent that therapists prepare for questions and discussion about it. Patients have reported that if they were not informed until late in the pregnancy, they felt that they were not prepared; when they were told "early enough," they expressed a greater trust in the therapist (McCluskey, 2016).

If a patient asks directly, the therapist may simply confirm the patient's observations with time and space to explore the patient's thoughts and reactions, or fantasies can be explored first before therapist confirmation. The order should follow the therapist's customary stance, as it provides one of the first indications that the therapist's enthusiasm and interest in her baby has not overshadowed her ability to concentrate on the patient. Such a reassurance is likely to be important regardless of the therapist's theoretical orientation. At the point of discovery, the patient may offer a congratulatory comment. Here the therapist's responses may need to balance a reflective stance with the more "human" response. A genuine, gracious, but not overly ebullient thank you or acknowledgment of the patient's comment is in order. To offer only silence and treat the comment as an emotionally charged, highly loaded comment (which it may be), at least initially, may be perceived as being rejecting. The therapist can answer directly or show some delight without ruining even the more analytically based therapies (Naparstek, 1976). There are likely to be many opportunities throughout the pregnancy to explore the patient's reactions, including surprise at the therapist's warm response. At the same time, to use it as an opportunity to disclose further about the pregnancy may satisfy the therapist's own needs and curtail the patient's transferential responses.

What is more difficult to discern in the early months is whether there is metaphorical or derivative material that suggests a patient is aware of and ready to deal with the pregnancy. There are many common themes that give the therapist a clue that patients are reaching some level of awareness. Some of these are themes of changes in physical appearance, birth control, abortions, pregnant friends, gardening, desiring children, being taken care of, memories of childhood, and being excluded (Naparstek, 1976).

Where the patient makes only indirect references to the pregnancy, the therapist may not be able to discern whether her own enthusiasm and self-involvement is transcending her patient's interest in her pregnancy, or in contrast, whether her own discomfort about disclosing is minimizing its centrality in the session. The salience of this psychological event for the therapist reawakens old conflicts and intensifies the self-perspective that will affect the timing of the disclosure (see Chapter 4 on countertransference). For therapists desiring to spread the good news, patients' verbalizations can almost always be interpreted as derivatively relating to the pregnancy (Baum & Herring, 1975). For those therapists who wish to hide their status as long as possible, they miss material that is there. Anxiety and guilt may preclude them from even hearing patients' comments related to the pregnancy.

Some therapists report that their patients are not aware because they are not "showing." It is our experience, however, that subtle changes are apparent for our more astute patients even if an enlarged abdomen is not. If a pregnancy has not been acknowledged by someone authorized to provide the information (McCluskey, 2016), a cultural taboo prohibits mentioning it. The initial lack of dramatic changes often colludes with the therapist's wish to hide her pregnancy from her patients as long as she is able. She, then, is likely to miss important subtle initiations by her patients into this domain (Imber, 1990). The traditional wisdom to allow patients the freedom to determine their own psychological readiness does not correct for the therapist's desire to delay the announcement. Some therapists report that they were aware in retrospect of patients' material related to the pregnancy, but they nevertheless remained reluctant to clarify. This bias to delay seems more prevalent among primiparous therapists (Naparstek, 1976; Van Niel, 1993).

A guiding principle is that as time passes, the therapist needs to increase her level of activity in exploring derivative material. In the early months, patients' reactions ought to be more overtly or directly expressed for the therapist to pursue this line. As the pregnancy moves well along toward the end of the second trimester, the therapist should be more active in monitoring derivative material in order to introduce the pregnancy into the conscious realm. Bashe (1989) reported that although many patients do not express an awareness of the pregnancy, when told, they revealed that they had thought about it, but felt reticent to ask.

Sometimes, in spite of the clinician's best efforts to hear and work with the material, a few patients seemingly give no evidence of having "noticed" the therapist's pregnancy, even by the end of the second trimester. This requires the therapist to announce her pregnancy rather than explore and clarify her patient's curiosities and concerns. *We know of no instance in which not informing patients of the pregnancy is therapeutic.* Such behavior on the part of the therapist most often involves acting out (Fenster et al., 1986).

Therapists are often in a quandary about how to introduce it. The announcement ideally is made in the first half of the session so that the patient has the opportunity to process at least some of this disclosure. Depending on the patient, the therapist can simply say, "I have something I want to let you know." If the therapist wishes to address the denial or defensive aspects of the lack of awareness, she can comment, "I think that you are hiding the knowledge from yourself that I am pregnant."

With these discussions, whether the patient spontaneously asks or the therapist must point out her status, many therapists wonder what other information should be revealed. This answer depends on the type of treatment, the therapist's style and the patient's difficulties. We suggest that each therapist wait to hear their patients' interests and concerns before offering other information. Some therapists wait to announce their pregnancy even after derivative material is present, with the rationale that they wish to finalize their maternity leave plans before announcing the pregnancy so as to give all the "bad" news together. However, some suggest that it may not be advisable to spontaneously offer maternity leave plans at the time of the pregnancy announcement or confirmation (Imber, 1990; Uyehara et al., 1995). Focusing the patient's attention on the separation aspect potentially colludes with the patient in avoiding other meanings of the pregnancy.

Patients are entitled to receive answers to those questions that have practical significance for them, such as the scheduling of their sessions. Questions such as the baby's due date are directly relevant to the timing of the therapeutic hiatus. Other questions regarding the sex of the baby, preferences of the therapist, marital status, number of children and physical health should be considered on an individual basis, evaluating the potential benefits in sharing this information against the negative impact of intensifying the real relationship or burdening the patient. Although Bashe (1989) and Fenster (1983) found that therapists were generally more revealing about the pregnancy than they were in other circumstances, therapists vary on how much they disclose to their patients. Not all are self-disclosing. Other therapists working in less interpretive psychotherapies may engage in self-disclosure on a routine basis, and the disclosure of the pregnancy may be consistent with the therapist's stance. Furthermore, each therapist may be comfortable with varying their level of disclosures among patients, based on clinical decisions. Most acknowledge that they often struggled with finding the right balance between the patient's interest in the therapist and baby as a transference phenomenon and being appreciative of their patients' sincere concerns (Bassen, 1988; Turkel, 1993). Self-disclosure should neither be for self-gratification nor used as a method to deflect anger or elicit sympathy; however, it may serve a valuable function in creating a trusting, safe atmosphere for the patient (Uyehara et al., 1995).

Personal disclosures do not necessarily ruin a reflective stance, and they can sometimes enhance neutrality (Greenberg, 1986). Some of the therapists who were more revealing of personal information felt it was common courtesy, yet in hindsight they felt that such information did not serve as a role model or further the therapy process, and they often regretted divulging certain information (Bassen, 1988). However, most of these regrettable revelations can be grist for the therapeutic mill. After deciding how much information to reveal, the challenge is to remain neutral and to hear all the patients' expressions of emotion (Counselman & Alonso, 1993). Therapists who are pregnant for the second time report that the second time around they are more relaxed and prepared for the disclosure (Bashe, 1989; Van Niel, 1993). We offer a cautionary note on disclosures. Therapists may be surprised when patients get upset about a therapist's refusal to answer a particular question if she had previously been forthcoming, as in the following example shared with us.

Vignette 2.5

I had been seeing this mother and her young adult son who was cognitively disabled and schizophrenic with episodes of aggressive behavior. We had effectively reduced positive symptoms of schizophrenia and his aggressiveness. The mother and I seemed to have a good relationship when I became pregnant. All the way through the pregnancy, she was quite solicitous of my state and comfort, empathizing with me as I waddled through my ninth month. After I returned from my leave, she had asked a number of questions about the baby (sex, how big, features, normality), but when it came to his name, I became protective and told her that my husband and I discussed that I would not reveal the name when I went back to work. The patient became angry and pushed insisting to know why my husband should get to decide this. She ended up walking out of the session prematurely and was very distant in the sessions that followed wanting to quickly get the meds for her son and leave. In supervision I remembered that she said, "I bet he (baby) is so smart" and we discussed that she may have been experiencing some envy or jealousy because her child was cognitively impaired, requiring that she would need to care for him the rest of her life.

This example has a number of interesting elements. The patient's mother and therapist seemed to function more like peers before the pregnancy, a pattern that continued until the therapist returned from leave. Upon her return, the therapist perceived the woman as intrusive rather than simply interested and compassionate. In response, the therapist set a boundary that re-established a more traditional frame of therapy. The patient experienced this posture as a rejection of their previous level of intimacy and withdrew angrily, ending the "buddy" nature of the relationship. The therapist also became protective of patients knowing her baby's name, and it would have been interesting for the therapist to explore what was behind this sensitivity, as many therapists would reveal this fact if they had revealed other similar facts. In retrospect, the therapist may have been getting some emotional reassurance and support from this patient by her disclosures prior to the birth. The solicitations of the patient masked the envy and jealousy that the mother was feeling, which became more obvious after the birth. The last point worth noting is that the therapist bolsters her reasoning by including her husband in her refusal to disclose her baby's name. In doing so, the patient is reminded of her exclusion from the intimacy of the therapist's family, and that someone not part of the therapeutic triad had a say in the therapist's decisions.

Pregnant therapists often have mixed feelings about accepting new referrals. On the one hand, they fear the dissolution of their practice and financial ruin with the coming of motherhood. On the other hand, because of physical limitations and emotional energies going elsewhere, they would be happy to have patients see a colleague. We advise informing all prospective patients and new referrals of the pregnancy and the upcoming interruption in treatment from the outset (Fenster et al., 1986). Not revealing the pregnancy at the commencement or as soon as the therapist knows can be very disruptive in treatment and can likely result in treatment dropout (Bassen, 1988; Fenster et al., 1986). Perhaps it is the inability of new patients to process the announcement and its associated feelings in the context of a prior healthy therapeutic alliance that shades their initial experience of the therapist as one of deprivation. This then exaggerates the patient's sense of betrayal. Likewise the therapist is cautioned to think carefully about taking on "difficult patients," as most therapists find it hard to tolerate the intense demands and the often primitive expressions of rage, jealousy and envy that these patients so readily verbalize. Some therapists expressed regret at having committed themselves to individuals who required intense vigilance; therapists may find themselves subtly encouraging the discontinuation of difficult individuals.

Some thought should be devoted to preparing for the disclosure with an emphasis on what will be disclosed with each patient. Gerson (1996) suggested scrutinizing personal needs, countertransferential tendencies and transferential aspects before making or withholding a disclosure. Self-disclosure should be connected with a specific patient's need. Finding the balance between the patient's genuine curiosity and expression of appreciation and caring, and recognizing and dealing with their interest in terms of its meaning in their lives, is most difficult. Gerson (1996) offered a few specifics, suggesting that she would not disclose when the question violated her privacy, had a hostile intent, or appeared to function as a resistance. In retrospect, many therapists felt that what was disclosed was secondary to the exploration of the patient's reactions around the disclosure. It was often the therapist's anxiety or countertransference that did not permit full exploration of the meaning of the disclosure to the patient (Dewald, 1994). How it is explored is more important than what is disclosed, and this often continues well after the therapist has returned from leave (Gerson, 1996). As Gerson (1996) aptly stated, "the patients' 'real' experiences with me during this time brought to the foreground core transference-countertransference issues. In struggling with unavoidable realities the nature of our relationships emerged with clarity" (p. 61).

Third Trimester

As the Therapist Anticipates a Revolution in Her Life, a Whole New Set of Phenomena—Physical, Emotional and Interpersonal—Is Ushered into Her Psychological World

Phenomena of the Pregnancy: Preparing for Separation and Motherhood

By the third trimester, most pregnant women experience a disequilibrium in their emotional life (Fatoye, Adeyemi, & Oladimeji, 2004; Hart & McMahon,

2006). Tension and irritability increase, and the ability to cope with stressful events decreases. As patients present their curiosities, tenderness, envy and rage, the "graphic visibility" of the therapist becomes undeniable. The therapist must come to terms with the way in which her emotional vulnerability limits her capacity to see patients and relate to colleagues and supervisors (Balsam, 1974). This emotional vulnerability seems most prominent among primiparous therapists, who report feeling unprepared for both parenting and managing their patients' questions (Bashe, 1989).

It is during this trimester that there is preparation for labor and delivery. This process is tripartite, characterized by engaging in practical steps to collect information (e.g., talking to other women, reading books, watching films, taking prenatal classes), active imagery or fantasizing about labor and delivery (thinking about contractions, breathing, transition, pushing and maintaining control) and dreams about labor (Lederman, 1996). This intrapsychic work is particularly important because there is evidence that congruence between a woman's fantasies about labor and delivery and the actual experience of it enable her to better handle the experience (Lederman, 1996). However, a realistic perspective on labor involves acknowledgment of work, pain, risks and the unknown, which in turn precipitates doubts and fears about the loss of control over the body and emotions. To the multiparous therapist, labor and delivery fears and anxieties are based less on book knowledge and hearsay from friends and family than on their own memories of previous labor and delivery experiences (Lederman, 1996).

It is during this trimester that many women change their focus from concern about the baby to fears about labor (Furber, Garrod, Maloney, Lovell, & McGowan, 2009; Maloney, 1985). Some therapists experience fears and fantasies of harm to themselves and their babies, which are more intense during first pregnancies (Fenster et al., 1986; Ryding et al., 2015). Fear of death and loss of a spouse are not uncommon (Dagan et al., 2001; Deutsch, 1945; Leifer, 1977). Patients often express similar fears of harm and death of their therapist and her baby. When the therapist has not contained her own fears, it is difficult to explore patient concerns. She may fail to become aware of her patients' concerns and concomitant hostility or be too quick to reassure them. This concern about loss often affects therapists' relationships with their patients, to the extent that therapists may experience patients as being able to harm their baby. Distressing and intruding fantasies of mutilation, the rupture in the membranes, or other harbingers of the onset of labor may encroach with more frequency in therapy as well (Lester & Notman, 1986; Nadelson et al., 1974). Many patients experience a tremendous sense of abandonment at this time. A therapist's fears of loss of the baby, their spouse, or even their own lives may be in part an identification with their patients who are fearing a loss of them.

Anticipatory anxieties about competency to care for the newborn are present. Coleman (1969) described many women in his group as having dreams of feeling excluded from caring for their newborn or relinquishing this task to others. Preparation and acceptance of the mothering role is influenced by her relationships with her spouse, mother and mother-in-law. Anxieties are also influenced by her experience with previous pregnancies and her experience with her other children. When experiences with other children have been positive, the pregnant woman is more likely to anticipate the new baby more positively. In the face of the therapist's anxieties, fears and increasing lack of control, a reversal of roles may unwittingly occur. Patients offer to pick up dropped objects, move furniture and bring food and drink in order to cater to their pregnant therapist. Therapists may be uncomfortable with patients' increasingly solicitous behavior. One therapist told us that a male schizophrenic whom she saw at the end of the day offered to walk her to her car, "saying the neighborhood wasn't safe." The therapist, not previously focused on this issue, became fearful of being attacked. She declined the patient's offer, but wished she had acknowledged and explored it further as she felt that this offer signaled an increased appreciation for others' needs.

"Primary maternal preoccupation" (PMP; Winnicott, 1956), that state of heightened sensitivity and focusing inward during the pregnancy and lasting through several postpartum weeks, becomes more apparent. The therapist may have less energy and interest in her work. For the mother–child dyad, it is essential—enabling the mother to sensitively identify with her infant and his or her needs and aids in the bonding process. Zackson (2012) wrote of her own experience that the patient

> denied any negative impact of the pregnancy, I believe I was contributing to her inability to consciously express her feelings about my pregnancy, perhaps I felt too vulnerable. . . . I found myself in session fantasizing about my infant and at times I was preoccupied and distracted. I sometimes day dreamed about my infant and felt detached.
>
> (pp. 2–3)

"Nesting" behavior is common during this trimester (Anderson & Rutherford, 2013). Toward the end of the trimester, the woman frequently experiences a surge of energy as she prepares the "nest" for her newborn. Nesting commonly occurs in behavior ranging from straightening drawers to heavy cleaning. One of Bashe's participants described this phenomenon as "I just want to stay home and think about what color to paint the baby's room" (1989, p. 109). A parallel process may occur in therapy, with the pregnant therapist desirous of tidying things up before she leaves. One colleague of ours described it as wanting to make certain that each of her patients was "tucked away" before she departed. At the same time, therapists also may feel a growing helplessness, anxiety and guilt both over their waning interest in patient welfare and over "abandoning" their patients. They may worry that the arrangements they made for their absence will go awry and require additional energy. The therapist's changing status and temporary hiatus (or permanent departure) unmask the ever-present delicate balance between personal and professional life and requires the therapist to rethink her commitments. If the guilt is too overpowering, therapists may be unclear with patients and covering professionals about their sabbatical or their continued involvement during their hiatus. Several of our group therapists lamented that they had agreed to a shorter maternity leave and/or continued involvement with patients that they later regretted.

Many of the group therapists we interviewed remarked on the re-emergence of physical symptoms after a relatively intervening quiescent trimester; they felt physically uncomfortable moving more slowly, finding it necessary to elevate their feet, requiring bathroom breaks midway through their groups, and experiencing various other symptoms such as heartburn, shortness of breath, backaches and hot flashes. The extent of the preoccupation with one's physical state may equal or exceed that of the first trimester (Bashe, 1989; Fenster et al., 1986). Therapists struggle with being preoccupied and their lack of control over events happening to them.

Many have remarked on decreased attention, concentration and mental acuity (Henry & Rendell, 2007). This is consistent with pregnant therapists who report that they are less able to conceptualize or synthesize material than previously, despite efforts to increase attention and concentration (Lazar, 1990). Although increasing levels of progesterone and estrogen may contribute, psychological aspects may be equally important as the prospective mother prepares to welcome her newborn into her world. Paluszny and Posnanski (1971) noted that in their final stages of pregnancy, residents' interests in learning new theoretical concepts and case conceptualization waned: "The inner world beckoned too strongly" (p. 274). Our interviewees noticed they were less active, less aggressive about confronting, and went "less deep" because they did not have the energy. Some became weary of the incessant focus on their pregnancies in the work environment. Others wished that it were possible not to have to work at all (Bashe, 1989).

Although many therapists look forward to the end of the pregnancy because of physical limitations and hormonal havoc, concurrent mourning processes take place as the pregnant woman prepares for physical separation from the fetus. Her task is to accept the physical separation and at the same time experience strong bonds of attachment. A parallel process of both mourning and relief may emerge in therapy, as most therapists make final preparations for separation from their patients. Mothers pregnant with their second child may experience a mourning over the loss of an exclusive relationship with their child. Primiparous mothers may mourn the loss of a more carefree relationship with their spouses or partners.

Technical Considerations and Implications for Intervention

This Period is Rife With Decision-Making Moments for the Therapist

Responding to Gifts

We have found that pregnancy, more than any holiday event, is likely to elicit a presentation of gifts to the therapist. The handling of this gesture in pregnancy needs to be explored in the context of what ordinarily occurs. The therapeutic protocol for the acceptance of gifts also depends on the orientation of the therapist. For analytically oriented therapists, both conscious and unconscious motives for gift-giving should be considered. Although societal norms and expressions of care and concern are certainly part of the effort behind the giving of a gift, motives can be multifaceted. These are varied, ranging from bids for special attention, a sense of indebtedness, a compensation for angry feelings, or the expectation that it is required. If explored, these motives, whether conscious or unconscious, become evident in the material the patient presents. The acceptance or refusal of the gift is often considered secondary to understanding the motivation for such an act. Although many psychoanalytically oriented therapists under ordinary circumstances are inclined to explore the motives behind the gesture and refuse the gift, acceptance of the gift (a relatively inexpensive one) almost always occurs when the returning of it would damage the patient, the therapeutic relationship, or both. Acceptance also occurs when the gesture primarily represents an increase in the patient's awareness of socially appropriate behavior. For bought (more impersonal), inexpensive gifts, therapists can accept or refuse them. However, for handmade gifts, acceptance becomes more important; any explanation of refusal is likely to be devastating for the patient, particularly when it occurs shortly before the termination, a therapeutic hiatus or on the therapist's return (Hollander & Ford, 1990). Consideration of a refusal needs to occur in the context of consideration as to what the therapist would be communicating to her patient by refusing a gift over which he or she had "labored." Although therapists in private practice usually receive few gifts, a clinic situation is considered different, perhaps because patients receiving lower fees are realistically more likely to feel indebted to their therapist and express this gratitude with token gifts. It is also possible that clinic populations have diverse backgrounds and perhaps have different rules, norms and expectations around how to treat the expectant mother. Private practice therapists who are showered with gifts ought to carefully scrutinize their therapeutic interactions; acceptance of these gifts in the clinic situation is considered to be common and in part based on the circumstances (Langs, 1971, 1975). There is general agreement that expensive gifts need to be returned.

The analytic pregnant therapists interviewed by Fenster (1983) and Bashe (1989) reported that they ordinarily did not receive or accept gifts. Yet, almost all accepted or planned to accept the gifts offered them during their pregnancy and after the birth of the baby. Although many attempted to explore the gesture, a significant proportion (one-third) did not or did not intend to explore it (Bashe, 1989; Fenster, 1983). In our sample, in which only half were analytically oriented, almost all accepted the gifts and very few processed the gesture. For Fenster's (1983) and Bashe's (1989) samples, this behavior was in marked contrast to their customary behavior, which left many of the therapists experiencing some anxiety about the appropriateness of their behavior. It is with this backdrop of conflict and anxiety that therapists can exhibit a lack of grace and ineptitude when it comes to accepting gifts during pregnancy, as manifested in this next vignette.

Vignette 2.6

An insightful psychodynamic patient brought me a bouquet of flowers upon our first meeting after the baby was born. I took them, thanked her, perhaps in a perfunctory manner, slid them under my chair, and asked her to explore her bringing me the flowers with a question such as "What lead to your bringing me these flowers?" She dutifully explored it initially at a superficial level talking about how she wanted to get something for me and not for my baby. She did not have children, by design. I remember feeling uncomfortable with her gift, for several reasons. First, I come from the tradition that consider gifts as an indication that things are being acted out rather than talked about. I was anxious to deal with this as any other acting out, rather than the result of a separation imposed by me. Second, I could have accepted a baby gift more easily than a gift for me. Third, I felt that she was angry at me for abandoning her for 7 weeks. She struggled with my absences throughout therapy. She often had difficulty expressing anger and if I made too much of the gift she would find it more difficult than otherwise to express her anger. She did get angry, but also hurt and rejected. This incident was added to the list of incidents that demonstrated my "cold, unfeeling" therapeutic stance toward her and we revisited it many times over the next few years of therapy. Years later, I think that I was too "mechanical" and theory-driven in my approach to her gift. Yes, she was angry and worried that I could abandon her, but she would have gotten to these emotions regardless of whether I had been more genuinely appreciative of her socially appropriate efforts.

In this example, the therapist appears uncomfortable and conflicted about accepting the gift, but does accept it. She then rather immediately attempts to explore the meaning of it. This could be interpreted as a push to return to the dyadic relationship as quickly as possible (Bashe, 1989). Although it was obviously a judgment call, the therapist acknowledges in retrospect that the patient may also have been responding in a socially appropriate way to an event that was foisted on her. She might also have been responding within the real relationship with genuine excitement for the therapist. It may be that the acceptance of gifts around pregnancy may require a response different from our customary ones because patients have no control over the baby becoming a major part of the therapeutic interaction. Acceptance of a gift is reparative for the patient and may be a way of working through an impending loss. In this case, a gift postpregnancy seemed to help the therapist rethink her therapeutic "rules" and develop a better more flexible technique. This is a good example of how pregnancy can be an opportunity to reconsider and renegotiate difficulties in one's prior technique and make one a better therapist.

One inpatient group therapist told us that the occupational therapy department encouraged the patients to make toys and other objects for the baby as a vehicle for talking about the impending separation. Refusal to accept such a token gift would be an insensitive deprivation. Such immediate scrutiny may be more damaging to the therapeutic relationship than no exploration at all. Rather, a genuine and appreciative thank you still allows for the possibility that exploration may occur later in the treatment, perhaps in the context of the patient's reaction to the maternity leave and ongoing concerns of being cared for now that the therapist has an additional one for whom to care.

Within our social world, giving a baby gift is almost a required social behavior. In our interviews, many therapists reported patients discussed giving gifts, but their thoughts did not reach fruition—perhaps because they felt pressure from societal obligations and the lack of an enthusiastic response or implicit prohibition from the therapist freed them from the "obligation." In our sample of group therapists, most received gifts before delivery or at termination. A few came to the clinic while on maternity leave and a few on resuming treatment. Acceptance usually included an appreciative statement. Some who received them before or while on maternity leave wrote thank you notes during the treatment break.

Some therapists who did not get gifts felt disappointed. This reaction, then, becomes another force in the treatment with therapists needing to manage their disappointment at a vulnerable time. This is likely to be more true for private practitioners who may not get showers or gifts from colleagues.

Establishing a Leave: Setting a Date to Leave, Determining the Length of the Leave and Deciding When to Return

The determination of when to stop working, how long to take leave and when to return to work are intertwining decisions and are dependent on a multitude of factors, only some of which are in the therapist's control and can be known ahead of time. The decision can be difficult. For those working in agencies, it sometimes feels like the agency, colleagues and supervisors are not supportive in helping the therapist find a good solution (Chariamont, 1986). The leave date is dependent on the time required for personal needs prior to the arrival of the baby, the length of time desired to be away from work and how much time is desired after the arrival. Some therapists find it preferable to work until delivery, feeling they are more helpful to patients if they allow them to continue until the last possible minute (Bassen, 1988; Naparstek, 1976). Others want more postdelivery time or do it because of their own desire to work, feeling that there may be nothing to do at home (Bashe, 1989). Bassen (1988) reported that one therapist gave patients the option to stop or work until delivery; all chose to continue until it was no longer possible. In retrospect, all those interviewed who took this route regretted their decision and advised predetermining a date to interrupt treatment (Bashe, 1989; Bassen, 1988; Naparstek, 1976).

Setting a date is preferable in almost all instances. Not setting a date may collude with the patient's denial that the therapist is pregnant and fosters the misperception that there will be no baby or break in treatment (Fenster et al., 1986). It places an undue burden of anxiety on patients who are uncertain when they might arrive and find their therapist gone (Naparstek, 1976). It also precludes the working through of separation, dependency and abandonment issues in a defined manner and with closure (Fenster et al., 1986). In addition, there is some evidence that patients found it gratifying when therapists continued until delivery or took short leaves; they expressed less anger at the time, although the effect may have been postponed because it seemed to surface later around other postpartum limits (Bassen, 1988). Setting a leave date that is the week of the due date also can have negative ramifications given that babies not infrequently arrive before their due date. Therapists who set dates close to their due date report in retrospect that they wished that they had discontinued earlier (Naparstek, 1976).

Serious consideration should be given to discontinuing therapy in the late pregnancy because of increasing internal anxiety and preoccupation with the baby, bodily changes, anxieties about mothering and the changes in the marital relationship (Balsam, 1974). Such internal preoccupation may overwhelm the therapist and make it difficult to be responsive to her patients. Often, disturbed patients whose therapists go into labor prematurely typically experience great difficulties (Uyehara et al., 1995). A premature departure due to pregnancy complications can shatter a patient's sense of the therapist's omnipotence. If the therapist is struggling with her own feelings of being unable to control events, she may be even less able to respond to patient's negative reactions. The earlier the leave date, the greater the control over abrupt terminations and the more likely for closure to occur (Fenster et al., 1986).

Setting a realistic leave date will also attenuate the anxiety and fantasies of both the therapist and patient that labor will begin prior to the break in treatment. The ideal leave date allows for the finishing out of obligations and treatment sessions with enough energy left to have some conflict-free time to care for oneself and prepare for the baby. However, many therapists understandably worry about the financial implications and want to maximize the time with their newborns. In one study, three-fourths of the therapists ended 5 or more days prior to the due date (Bashe, 1989). A compromise to discontinuing early might be to cut down on the weekly load if discontinuing completely at such an early date presents a hardship. Of course, if only a set amount of leave is available (as is often the case with therapists in clinical and hospital settings), then the longer the predelivery time away, the less postdelivery time will be available.

Part of setting a leave date requires the therapist to consider the total time she desires to be away from her practice. These decisions need to be made well before the primiparous therapist has knowledge of how she will feel after the birth of the baby. Decisions about length of time needed to balance what the new mother desires in terms of time with her baby against the therapist's financial situation, her desire to maintain her professional identity and the length of time that her patients can tolerate her absence. In Bashe's study (1989) analytic therapists (most primiparous) averaged 10 weeks of leave with a range of 4 to 24 weeks. Our study had similar findings; for those returning to practice, 11 weeks was the average leave with a range of 3 to 26 weeks. Those who took the longer leaves worked in a hospital or clinic setting. The therapists in Bassen's study (1988) and in Fenster's study (Fenster et al., 1986) averaged less time away, with the majority of therapists having leaves of 4 to 8 weeks. Naparstek's (1976) therapists placed between Bashe's and Fenster's study averaging 12 weeks with a median of 8 weeks. Those returning at the earlier dates often regret their decisions; they report that they had not appreciated how much they felt attached to their newborns and how reluctant they felt about returning to their professional lives (Fenster et al., 1986). Guilt over having the baby as a competitor may lead the therapist to accommodate to the detriment of her own needs. It seems that negotiating and learning from mistakes about discounting one's needs during pregnancy better equips therapists subsequently to deal with other issues involving negotiation of one's needs (e.g., scheduling patients, patients' accessibility to therapists). This type of error seems to correct itself with subsequent pregnancies, as experienced therapists report stopping work earlier and taking longer leave (Bashe, 1989; Fenster et al., 1986; McGarty, 1988).

The length of maternity leave also must be balanced with patients' capabilities of managing the separation and the extent to which they can readily reconnect when the therapist returns. Most patients, no matter how disturbed, can manage a 4-week separation if interim coverage is provided adequately. Evidence suggests that therapists who take between two and three months can retain the majority of their practice, although additional crises and precipitous terminations are more likely (Fallon, Brabender, Anderson & Maier, 1995; Fenster et al., 1986). However, when the therapist desires to take a leave longer than three months, the dropout rate increases precipitously. When a longer leave is planned, it may behoove the therapist to weigh for each patient the ill effects that this lengthy separation may have against the effects of termination or transfer. Fenster et al. (1986) reported that lengthy leaves can result in patients feeling bound to the therapist, often unable to take appropriate action for help when they needed it. In addition, many who remain through the hiatus drop out on the therapist's return and have a great deal of difficulty returning to psychotherapy with a new therapist. Some of the difficulties with the separation may be mitigated with some contact and periodic sessions through the latter part of the maternity leave. This is discussed further in the next section.

Difficulties in determining and setting an adequate time for the therapist's leave can result from unresolved therapist and/or patient separation/individuation struggles. In the event that the therapist leaves precipitously, we recommend that she inform patients herself. If this is not possible, Abend (1982) and Dewald (1982) emphasized the importance of knowing what information patients have been given and by whom, as well as the context in which it occurred, so that the patient's responses may be anticipated and later understood in this context. Many of the difficulties arising around these issues could be circumvented with some careful thought about this matter earlier in the pregnancy. Patient confidentiality is always of concern when communication paths are disrupted. We recommend that patients be informed beforehand what professional could potentially call and cover the therapist in the event of a precipitous termination. Having husbands, partners, or other relatives perform this service would be less than optimal. Relying on relatives opens a quagmire of problems around confidentiality and may be too stimulating for many patients.

The professional–personal identity crisis threads through return-to-work decisions and the extent to which the therapist continues her other professional commitments. This conflict and decision is most troublesome for therapists during their first pregnancy. It is difficult to imagine what one's response to becoming a mother will be, and how the symbiotic ties of this newborn will tug on and tilt the integration of professional–personal identity. Psychologically, the new mother/therapist will never have quite the same existence again. For every new mother, there is likely to be an ideal time to return to seeing clients based on one's comfort with mothering and identification of being left and a feeling of readiness to re-establish one's professional identity and connection to the outside world. (Balsam, 1974). But it is not possible to say with certainty how much one will be comfortable being away from the baby and the extent and point at which she will desire gratification from her professional identity.

Factors influencing return are more than just the integration of professional and personal identity. Often, practical considerations such as money and the availability of acceptable childcare arrangements influence the pregnant therapist's decision to return to work. Patients and colleagues and the pregnant therapist's own internal requirements for formulating concrete arrangements postpregnancy push pregnant therapists into making plans long before the birth of the baby. Sometimes this occurs before she has realistically considered what life may be like after the baby is born. (See Chapter 4 for a more detailed discussion of this topic.) A therapist's struggle over letting go of professional activities concomitant with her guilt over abandoning her patients conspire to push a new mother into returning to work too early. Conversely, these anxieties and doubts about her ability to successfully integrate these parts of her life may collude with her patients' fears that she may abandon them in favor of her new child and not return to practice at all (Penn, 1986). Along these lines, the most intense pull for remaining at home may be the symbiotic ties to the infant. The looming presence of an impending return to therapeutic work may be felt as an unwanted intrusion, threatening to put a wedge into the mother–child symbiotic dyad (Balsam, 1974).

Under the most ideal circumstances, the therapist's awareness of her infant's needs would be balanced with her patients' ability to tolerate her absence. However, the therapist may not correctly anticipate her feelings after delivery. For this reason, the pregnant therapist should build in some flexibility as to when she may return to work after the birth of the child (Balsam, 1974). This involves establishment of an approximate date (e.g., 2 months, the beginning of the new year) with instructions for patients to expect a letter providing more specific details of her return 1 month prior to it occurring (Fenster et al., 1986). This communication then serves as a transitional attachment to their therapy. In subsequent pregnancies, the therapist has better knowledge of her response to being a mother and how it interferes with patients' needs and her own professional gratification. She can then make a more realistic decision prior to the birth of the child and in time for patients to work through the impact of her decision on them and on the therapeutic process.

If the therapist's capacity for emotional availability is significantly diminished by her desire to remain with her infant, the ideal solution would be for the new mother-therapist to reassess her return timetable. At a practical level, this is much more difficult to do, although it is almost always possible to change one's mind. One therapist in the Naparstek study (1976) called her patients and extended her leave by 6 weeks, explaining that she had misjudged the way she would feel. McWilliams (1980) made the point that this is the first time some female therapists learn how to set limits. This learning is helpful to them for the rest of their professional lives. In coming to a decision about a maternity leave, it might be helpful to know that a number of those writing in this area report that therapists tend to think they will want to return to work earlier than they actually do (Balsam, 1974; Fenster et al., 1986).

Another alternative to the complete return to practice is to transition into practice from full-time motherhood by initially seeing patients at less than the frequency they had prior to the pregnancy leave (e.g., begin by seeing twice-weekly patients once a week for a specified number of weeks). Another possibility is to have a graduated return by beginning to see those that are more disturbed or have the greatest difficulties with separation first (Naparstek, 1976). Either of these alternatives may be able to increase a part-time leave for several weeks.

Technological advances have enabled therapists to conduct therapy using visual and auditory internet platforms. It may be possible to utilize these as a transition between her leave and return to the office. This would require a HIPAA-compliant platform.[10] If these are considered, the therapist may want to introduce the possibility prior to her leave. Technology is not perfect, so that glitches might be anticipated in the authenticity of the connection. Preparation prior to leave might include a trial run with a few sessions to process the experience (such as loss of connection, asynchrony of audio and video). The therapist should have a suitable space that does not include baby paraphernalia and is largely free from background noises of the baby and home. Given the vicissitudes (variability) of the infant's schedule, it is not always possible to arrange the session during "nap time." The therapist should consider having another (spouse, partner, relative, babysitter) available in case the baby requires attention during these calls. The patients' fears of the therapist's distractibility and commitment are well-founded if the therapist is interrupting the contact to attend to a crying or fussy infant.

Some therapists toy with the idea of not returning to practice or their job, perhaps because they anticipate endless blissful interactions with their new infant or because they find their current position unpleasant or stressful, anticipating this to worsen on their return. They may also feel that multiple roles will be too stressful for them. Women who experience a job as unpleasant, unsupportive and inflexible in terms of time are less likely to return after the birth of a child (Botsford Morgan & King, 2012; Killien, 2005; Meglich, Katja Mihelič, & Zupan, 2016). Factors such as lack of spouse or partner support for working and lack of childcare availability also impact on the decision not to return to work (Kaplan & Granrose, 1993). Zackson's (2012) study suggests that those women who continue to experience high levels of maternal preoccupation had more difficulty returning to full-time organizational positions, whereas those with lower levels were more successful in returning to that work environment. On the other hand, she also found that those with high maternal preoccupation were able to be authentic with patients and respond more empathically than those low on this variable.

A few positive findings from national studies on pregnancy, employment and mental health may comfort the therapist in the decision to return to work or practice. It is true that multiple roles for women increase stress. However, employment per se is not associated with mental health problems among women (Sumra & Schillaci, 2015). Nor is there any evidence that an increasing number of children an employed woman has will increase her risk for mental health difficulties. In fact, there appears to be no overall difference in the mental health of mothers with children under the age of 1 whether they are employed full-time or part-time or remain as a homemaker. However, in a review of European epidemiological data, the longer the leave (over 25 weeks), the better the physical and psychological health of both mother and baby (Staehelin, Bertea, & Stutz, 2007). In contrast, American women who are very involved with their work prior to pregnancy, but do not go back to work by the end of the first year, exhibit low self-esteem and have high levels of depression and irritability (Klein, Hyde, Essex, & Clark, 1998; Wiese & Ritter, 2012). Those who desire a different employment arrangement (e.g., want to work part-time instead of full-time) have significantly more anger, anxiety and depression than those whose preferences match their current situation. Where employment most seems to affect mental health is in the area of job overload and job quality. If a new mother feels overloaded at her job, is not supported and is not enjoying the kind of work she is doing, there is a greater likelihood of her experiencing anxiety, depression, low self-esteem and anger (Klein et al., 1998; Wiese & Ritter, 2012).

Coverage Arrangements and Interim Contact

One decision a pregnant therapist must make prior to her leave is whether she will manage her own coverage or have someone else provide emergency backup. This in part is dependent on the ability of the majority of patients to continue functioning independently without serious repercussions, the number of patients to be covered and the therapist's inclination (Chiaramont, 1986). Therapists have found many variations acceptable. Some provide their own coverage. Others cover their practice, but have emergency coverage if more than a phone call is necessary. Others have found the use of a substitute therapist important for both emergency coverage and for ongoing problem solving. Still others have outside coverage for an initial period and then handle their own telephone contact in the latter part of the leave. The advantage of having someone else cover the practice is that emergencies (often when one is least able to manage them) will be handled by someone whose investment in her practice is not temporarily diminished with the advent of this new little one in her life. As stated earlier, many of the therapists do not realize how involved they will be with their babies. First-time mothers systematically and seriously underestimate how little time there is to handle anything other than taking care of the baby during their time off. The advantage of having additional substitute coverage is that a therapist may feel that she is able to buy additional leave time. However, it still remains a hardship for many seriously disturbed patients. The disadvantage of having substitute coverage is that the permanent therapist is usually in the better position to handle particular crises as they unfold. With arrangements of leave and coverage, it is important that patients and those providing backup have a good understanding of how the pregnant therapist intends to handle her leave and coverage. Being available as a consultant to the individual covering or substitute therapist can spare difficult moments later. If the therapist is open to a variety of alternatives, patients can be included not only in the exploration but also the choice of what transpires for them during leave. As one of McCluskey's (2016) therapists indicated, "Patients seem quite appreciative of my giving them the choice to stop, cutback or continue, as well as the knowledge that things could shift quickly" (p. 7).

Regardless of whether someone is covering for the practice or whether it is self-coverage, the therapist may desire or feel the necessity to have some kind of contact with her patients during her leave. Most therapists in the Fenster (1983) sample had some contact with their patients. Communication can be written or verbal. Many therapists send patients birth announcements, giving some details on the baby and informing or reminding patients of the next appointment (Naparstek, 1976). Patients like this opportunity; it includes the patient in the resolution of a 9-month event that often seriously has impacted on the treatment. It also functions to reassure patients that both therapist and baby survived and that therapy would remain viable. Another variation is to send a letter or birth announcement in an envelope previously self-addressed by the patient that has been specifically designed for patients. Computer technology permits this to be planned prior to the birth and requires only a few keywords to be entered after the birth. They are then reproduced with the click of a mouse! (See Chapter 4 for a cautionary note on sending such communication to all patients.)

Other therapists prefer to telephone. Although the phone provides a more spontaneous interaction that potentially seems quicker and easier, there are potential surprises and dilemmas in handling patients' questions. Therapists experience more pressure to answer questions, particularly when patients have been deprived of therapy sessions and contact for weeks. Most therapists in their phone contacts decide to volunteer, "all is well." There are important differences in the handling and revealing of other information. For instance, some therapists volunteered the name and sex of the baby, whereas others did not.[11] The former group often feels that not answering seemingly innocuous questions is too depriving. The latter group feels that it is important to explore the patient's issues around these questions and not automatically or reflexively answer the questions (Bassen, 1988). In most cases the revealing of some personal information did not preclude being able to explore the meaning of the event and disclosed information with the patient. Other therapists feel intruded upon by questions and find the written note an easier medium to convey information and a sense of ongoing connection. Another alternative is to place a message of the birth announcement and other pertinent information on one's voice mail. This permits a sense of ongoing connection with the therapist albeit a less personal one, allays fears of the therapist's well-being, is less time-consuming than correspondence and is less intrusive than telephone contact.

If the therapist does schedule phone or internet appointments with patients during her leave, as previously mentioned, it is ideal that she be free of infant distraction when conversing with patients. Given the vicissitudes (variability) of the infant's schedule, it is not always possible to arrange these calls during "nap time." The therapist should consider having another (spouse, partner, relative, babysitter) available in case the baby requires attention during these calls. The patients' fears of the therapist's distractibility and commitment are well-founded if the therapist is interrupting the call to attend to a crying or fussy infant. Regardless of whether this contact takes place, it is a good idea to have backup coverage for the handling of emergencies.

Some of the preceding recommendations attempt to help the therapist anticipate areas in which she has no experience. How maternity leave is planned is critical to the preservation of the therapeutic relationship and the psychological development of the patient after the therapist returns (McCluskey, 2016).

Maternity Leave

The Baby's Arrival and Postpartum Phenomenon: Becoming a Mother

Childbirth is an intense event that is unparalleled to any other in terms of passionate emotion. Rubenstein wrote (1998):

> children deliver to their mothers the purest happiness there is. The intense elation that accompanies childbirth is unmatched by any other event in a

woman's life. It's better than great sex, more moving than first love, more satisfying than winning a Nobel Prize or an Academy Award. . . . When they are stripped bare, facing the day of judgment women confess that they value their children more than another or anything else on earth.

(pp. 39–40)

From the moment the first baby arrives, the new mother and her partner are deluged with new challenges. Every relationship is altered. Such changes are bound to be stressful. Some mothers say that the arrival of the infant deepens the friendship aspect of their marriage, particularly if their spouses are active fathers and nurturing partners.[12] However, Lerner (1998) cautioned that for most couples, the arrival of the new baby is not likely to help the marriage; having a baby is supposed to be a joyful event, so that it is easy to underestimate the crisis faced by the new parents.

Parenthood is often considered as a rite of passage into adulthood. Yet resentment or fear of the irreversible changes set in motion by this life experience is likely to co-occur (Doss, Rhodes, Stanley, & Markman, 2009; Trad, 1991). Although the new mother may be thrilled by the birth of the child, most express some ambivalence, loss of freedom, longing for a less complicated life or some other more negative feeling about being a parent (Condon & Dunn, 1988; Spinelli et al., 2016). These feelings can be especially confusing given the intensity of longing the mother might have experienced for a baby. Fear, anger and grief around lack of freedom and lack of control are some of the emotions that women are reluctant to express, because they often feel that they are alone in these feelings and that they are socially unacceptable.

Postpartum "blues"[13] in the first few weeks after delivery are experienced by half of new mothers, generally spontaneously waning by the end of the second week after birth. If symptoms persist for several months and become more intense, it would be important to seek professional help. The prevalence of maternal depression is about 25% at 1 month, decreasing to 15% by the time the child is 3 years of age (Wang, Wu, Anderson & Florence, 2011).[14] Lack of social support, marital discord, a history of depression, a lack of internalized role models and difficult infant temperament are significant factors (Harris, 2002). Having postpartum depressive symptoms during one pregnancy increases the risk of having them during a subsequent pregnancy (Schetter, Saxbe, Cheadle, & Guardino, 2016). Maternal depression can be harmful to infant psychological development, disrupting attachment and even affecting developmental milestones (Shaver & Cassidy, 2016). Relationships with patients are also likely to be less than optimal. Therapists who are breastfeeding will be comforted to know that moderate manifestations of this disorder are responsive to non-pharmacological interventions (Clay, 2006).

At the same time, many women acknowledge their pleasure in providing happiness for another (Leahy-Warren & McCarthy, 2011). This is often in contrast to their own childhood discontent (Stern, 1998). Winnicott (1965) went even further to suggest that "at the earliest stages the infant and the maternal care belong to each other and cannot be disentangled" (p. 39). Many women experience a position of power as they transition from "being a single, circumscribed, self-contained organism to reproducing herself and her love object in a child who will from then on remain an object to this child—different from any other earlier or later" (Bibring et al., 1961, p. 17). The mother in a psychological state of reverie is sensitively attuned to and empathic with her child's needs, blurring her own boundaries with her baby's. Lerner (1998), in describing her work with patients, provided a good description of this intense ambivalence that mothers experience related to their infants:

> I hear about the intensity of feelings an infant can evoke from blind rage, to numbness and boredom, to overwhelming love and tenderness. I hear from mothers who tell me they wanted to throw their crying baby out the window—when the crying wouldn't stop, and also from these same mothers, that if anything really bad ever happened to their baby they couldn't see going on living. I hear about the fierce protectiveness: the intensity mothers feel about keeping their children healthy and safe and the unbearable pain that comes when they learn they can't.
>
> (pp. 42–43)

The confluence of biological, psychological and familial changes results in periods of intense emotional distress. In a study by Leifer (1977), more than two-thirds of the women experienced modest to extreme negative emotion; most felt that it was more intense and they were more labile than prior to the child's birth (Campbell, 1989). For primiparous women, the anxiety experienced seems to be focused on adequate mothering. In *The Mother Dance*, Lerner put it succinctly:

> Mothers know when their mothering is being judged, and it is understandable that we can get paranoid about it. When a child becomes the focus of negative attention, the mother may experience a complex mix of feelings that are difficult to unravel: guilt for one's actual parental shortcomings (we all have them), shame and embarrassment about how one's mothering is being perceived, anger at the child for "causing" the mother to look bad, resentment at others who are being judgmental, and worry about the child's problems. This confusing tangle of emotions blocks the mother from gathering her resources and approaching the problem in a calm solution-oriented way.
>
> (p. 81)

Toward the end of the second month, this anxiety concerning adequate care of the baby often is replaced by boredom of the routine and emotional constriction (Leifer, 1977). About two-thirds of the mothers in the study thought that being a parent was more stressful than they envisioned. This may in part be the result of less realistic expectations of the primiparous mother compared to the multiparous mother, and is probably exacerbated by a more traumatic delivery (Condon & Dunn, 1988; Delmore-Ko, Pancer, Hunsberger, & Pratt, 2000).

Many new mothers sense a shift in their reactions to their own mothers, revisiting, renegotiating and redefining themselves in terms of their own mothers as models. There is often a new respect for them, which often co-occurs with a parallel positive feeling about their childhood. One therapist put it this way:

Vignette 2.7
I've always had a great deal of respect for my mother. There were, however, many things that annoyed me and that I vowed never to do with my own children. They were small things, like she was always late to pick me up anywhere and I was always so embarrassed at how messy our house was. But now, I wonder how she ever did all that she did. I have one infant and some days I can't seem to get myself showered or the house picked up. She had five children and always managed to get dressed and make meals for us. I feel guilty that as an adolescent I was always telling her how she could do it better. I wonder how I will take it when my daughter does the same thing to me. Will I be tolerant like my mother or annoyed and guilt provoking?

It is not unusual for these new identifications to show an admixture of guilt, ambivalence and resentment (Bibring, Dwyer, Huntington, & Valenstein, 1961). It is clear from this example that the new tasks demanded of her as a mother gave her a different perspective on her own mother and their relationship. Mixed feelings about her mother are replaced with a more peaceful and respectful relationship. Concomitantly, there is often the development of feelings of competence and effectiveness as an adult that generalize to other aspects of her identity. The new mother experiences a heightened status that gives her a position of power not previously felt (Ballou, 1978).

Body image often resurfaces as a concern of the postpartum mother (Ebil, Senkud, Basara, Saglam, & Gezer, 2012). This concern is both superficial and symbolic. At a more superficial level, the issue of body image surfaces as the once pregnant therapist contemplates returning to work. Many are surprised at how slowly their previous shape and weight are regained, with dissatisfaction and self-blame contributing to weight retention (Phillips, King, & Skouteris, 2014). At the symbolic level, the new mother who has spent a little less than a year carrying this life within her must adjust to the feeling of emptiness and loss where the baby had been. This involves the final reconciliation that the baby, once an intimate part of her body, has become a separate being, with his or her own feelings, motivations and intentions (Ballou, 1978). In addition to the hormonal fluctuation that may be wreaking havoc on the new mother's emotional system, the "loss" of the fetal attachment can create a feeling of depression and acute grief.

Technical Implications and Considerations: Anticipation of Returning to Professional Life

If a therapist denies her struggle over balancing her professional and mothering role, unaware of her conflict between working more to prove her professional competence and working less to prove her maternal adequacy, she may actively encourage her female patients struggling with similar issues toward one side of the conflict or the other without appreciating that her advice has less to do with her patients' circumstances and reflects her own conflicts.

Although plans to return to the professional setting have long been made, returning to work and how much to work continue to be areas of conflict and anxiety for the new mother. It is a difficult decision to make in advance because the new mother's vision of herself may be different than the pregnant therapist's self-image. Many a therapist has been startled by fluctuating images of her identities as a professional mother. Both psychological and financial factors impact on a therapist's decision to return. In our survey of group therapists, many therapists were surprised by their feelings toward their clients while on maternity leave. Some missed them and were curious about the details of their lives. Others maintained some contact with coworkers or co-leaders, but were less curious about the progress of their patients being that they were completely absorbed by their neonate. Some therapists felt pressure to return when they did not want to, whereas a few regretted their decision not to return to their previous position.

Assessing Childcare Needs

As the mother prepares to physically leave her baby, more frequently than not with a caregiver outside the family, high levels of anxiety and turmoil are bound to be generated. At a practical level, the importance in obtaining safe and comfortable childcare arrangements cannot be underappreciated. Every new mother worries whether her baby will be safe, feel lonely, cry without her, or love the childcare worker more than her. Every mother is different, and so too will be her inclination to return to practice. However, if her anxiety reaches intolerable proportions, good therapy may not be possible, and the new mother should allow herself the freedom to reassess either her return date or the quantity of work to which she will return. The mother may also be responding to invisible pressures from her background and present social context without conscious awareness. In part, the attenuation of this anxiety is based on the working through of the social pressures she experiences and further evolution of the separation individuation process (Trad, 1991).

The mother's ability to return to work requires her to successfully feel attached to the child and yet perceive him or her as a separate individual who "delights in his response to her, a response which enhances her sense of him as separate and yet involved with her" (Ballou, 1978, p. 407). Many therapists return to work around the third month postpartum, which is often the period of mother–child mutuality. The mother's ability to feel competent in this interaction is based on the degree to which she felt adequately mothered and the extent to which the reconciliation of her relationship with her mother provides her with a model of a mutually satisfying and interactive relationship (Ballou, 1978). This step is one of many in a lifelong process in which the mother must continually adjust to the child's push toward individuality (Trad, 1990).

Arranging childcare involves a frank discussion with one's partner, not only about the particulars of childcare but even the responsibility of arranging for it. Having children seems to transition the couple into the more stereotyped gender roles and division of labor (Katz-Wise, Priess, & Hyde, 2010), a shift that is more dramatic if the couple has more than one child. Lerner (1998) has noted that "we act as if it's the woman's job to figure out child care" (p. 69). In general, mothers are more involved with childcare arrangements even if both partners work equally. The mother often feels more guilty about leaving her baby and at the same time may feel more confident in her judgment of people in terms of picking a childcare arrangement (Lerner, 1998).

With regard to assessing one's needs for childcare, a therapist must be particularly concerned about the stability of arrangements during her therapy hours. If the child is in day care, what will occur if the child is sick and is not able to attend the center (almost certain during the first year of day care)? If the child is cared for by a sitter, what will happen to the therapist's patients when the sitter calls out sick or does not show up at the last minute? Who will stay home? What other resources are available, and how able is the new mother to utilize them? The willingness of the mother-therapist to readily assume that she needs to answer and solve these problems alone may set the stage for lifelong, culturally sanctioned familial patterns that she may later come to resent. Parents who develop a broad network of support can lessen the disruptive effects of occasional childcare instability.

PREPARING TO RETURN

It is important to begin preparation for the return to therapy several weeks in advance. First is the issue of dress. Chances are the new mother's body has not returned to its previous figure, and the thought of wearing maternity clothes sickens most new mothers. Nothing is more uncomfortable than wearing clothes that are too tight. This irritant will serve as a low-voltage electric shock that keeps the therapist's energies focused on her bodily state and secondarily on her infant who she is already missing, rather than on her patients.

Second, we advise taking at least two trips to the office prior to the first official day back. The first may occur 2 to 4 weeks after the baby's birth and could involve a jaunt to the office with the new baby for colleagues to meet and admire. This will give the new mother a chance to reassess early on her inclinations to return to work. The second trip should occur without the baby (leaving the baby with the babysitter, relative or a childcare worker who will be caring for the child) and should essentially be a "dry run." At a practical level, the trip should include preparing your office for your return, reading mail, contacting patients and touching base with coworkers or colleagues. At an emotional level, it will enable the new mother-therapist to begin to experience emotionally and practically the integration of her dual roles and to begin working through separation from her baby.

REDISTRIBUTION OF HOUSEHOLD RESPONSIBILITIES

A baby complicates one's professional and home life exponentially. In addition to childcare responsibilities and professional life, household chores loom large. What often happens is that while the new mother is at home, she assumes many of the household and childcare responsibilities. This pattern becomes petrified over time, as deep-seated cultural expectations of mothers remaining at home and fathers' jobs taking priority seep into even the most previously egalitarian relationships. However, with her return to the workforce, the new mother-therapist cannot continue to be the sole administrator of the household chores, as the additional responsibilities alter what constitutes a fair distribution of labor in the household. Anticipating and discussing these gendered expectations prior to beginning work outside the home with a spouse can aid in the redistribution of task assignments and can ease re-entry back to professional life.

Returning to Professional Life

The Phenomenon: Managing Work and Home

Although, the number of mothers returning to work has steadily increased since the 1970s, little has been written about the new mother's experience as she returns to her previous position. There is also little agreement as to whether combining parenting and employment is stressful or serves as buffer for the psychological stress experienced by new mothers, thereby improving self-esteem (Miller, 1996).

Reactions to returning to work widely vary. There is likely to be an admixture of desire, relief, guilt, anxiety, fear and dread in returning to a predictable reality in which one is accomplished. Many therapists report clouded thinking, feeling physically drained and having high levels of distractibility (Waldman, 2003; Zackson, 2012). They express great anxiety about managing both work and home. Others report feeling sharper and more active, vacillating between feelings of exhilaration and exhaustion. One therapist described it as

> feeling like I am in nether nether land, drained by the household chores and demands of my child, I worry and miss my baby while attending these endless and boring administrative meetings. I love and want to be with my

child, and at the same time envious of my colleagues who have freedom to attend the Friday dinner and evening lecture with a famous psychoanalyst.

Initially, the therapist may fear that her therapeutic abilities have deteriorated with the coming of the baby and her "preoccupation" with him or her. She fears that patients will view her differently both physically and psychically. She experiences the struggle between her loss of connection to her baby and at the same time her lack of complete commitment to her patients. At the same time, returning to work may enhance self-esteem and the stability of one's identity and attenuate fears regarding clinical acumen. In fact, for many women work becomes a safe and more relaxing haven than home (Hochschild, 1997). Gradually, however, as the therapist assimilates and accommodates to the dual role integration, she may find herself less over-involved, more able to set limits and confront patients, and have greater comfort with patients' knowledge of some personal aspects of the therapist and greater sensitivity to parental concerns of patients. She may also be able to tolerate frustration in her work without experiencing personal frustration.

Motherhood widens the scope of one's personal experience, and in doing so may sensitize the therapist to the conflicts and complexities of parent–child interactions and problems (Bashe, 1989; Fenster et al., 1986). Waldman (2003) provides a poignant example:

> A., a man in his mid-forties, had been in weekly individual treatment for several years. He presented with a life-long depression. . . . A has become increasingly frustrated with me as I have become frustrated with him. This has manifested in my effort to get the focus off his children and spouse and onto him. This shift has led him to occasionally tell me that he feels I am not "validating him" enough. When he says this, he quickly follows it up by saying that he knows I cannot ever validate him enough, no one can. . . . I found myself gazing at his face, a familiar moment that brought me to thoughts of my child. It was only then that I realized that A yearned for the wholly positive mirroring that he had never received and that I felt with my child. . . . Understanding on such a visceral level A's need has helped me be more compassionate toward him.
>
> (pp. 57–58)

Many report an enriched sense of satisfaction and improved functioning at work, associated with their new status and a recognition of the mutual influence that occurs between therapist and patient (Bassen, 1988; Saakvitne, 2000). Some therapists described significant positive long-term changes in the way they approached their work and patients. They report a greater depth of understanding, more attunement to the affective elements in the relationship, increased ability to resonate with patients and greater authenticity (Waldman, 2003).

For other therapists, change was in the direction of a decreased internal pull to be nurturing; they felt less of a need to be over-involved and over-identified with their patients; they felt more neutral. They reported being more active and self-assured in the sessions (Zackson, 2012). They also felt that their personal experience with pregnancy and parenting had enabled them to become more comfortable and more able to empathize with their patients' issues of pregnancy and parenthood. One therapist said, "I was more sensitive to the failure of the maternal–child relationship." There is an increased humility around the "expertise" of parenting; the new mother recognizes that her own behaviors are now sometimes shamefully similar to the behaviors of parents that she had previously condemned.

Managing distraction is easier for some therapists, especially if they can compartmentalize their roles. Zackson (2012) captures the extreme in a therapist's first session back from leave:

> The first time was very hard but even the first day I found that when I was with the patient I had forgotten about the rest of my life. I forgot I had a child. I forgot I was married. I was just there thinking about what was going on and then. . . . I was "oh my God, I suddenly forgot. For the first time since she was born I forgot about her."
>
> (p. 81)

Zackson relates this to a lessening of maternal preoccupation.

Unresolved issues around separation individuation and professional identity enter the therapist's work with the patient. For example, the loss of the baby from the mother's body may result in the therapist's attempting to fill the void symbolically with patient substitutes (Balsam, 1974). One way this may manifest itself is that the therapist may find that she feels the urge to squash patients' efforts toward independence when it might not be appropriate to foster them, as in the following vignette.

Vignette 2.8

My first day back to the office, a young woman whom I had been seeing for 6 months announced that she had done well during my absence and felt that she did not need to continue therapy. I felt a panic, anxious about my professional skills, worried about my financial status, irritated that I had given up the exclusive relationship with my child to return, and deflated because I did not feel needed by my patients. I tried to control these feelings, but found myself sifting through her account of her life since our last session for indications that this desire to discontinue was an acting out of her conflicts around independence. This line of thinking may not have been inappropriate except that I knew these other feelings trumped a more considered view of whether she should stay in treatment. Because my own feelings seemed too overwhelming to sift through, I was not able to dispassionately explore her request and she terminated therapy that day.

Another way in which unresolved separation/individuation issues may manifest themselves is in the therapist's fantasies that her baby is experiencing overwhelming loneliness or crying all the time without her. Or the therapist could experience unshakable guilt that she is shortchanging her child (Balsam, 1974). Although it is hard to deny that the baby will experience a loss of familiar and loving arms, such preoccupations are likely to be the therapist's projection of her own loss of the child. A therapist may attempt to manage these feelings by engaging in nurturing behaviors that go beyond what a patient may require. Here is an example.

Vignette 2.9

Prior to my maternity leave, I maintained a 50-minute hour with a 10-minute break between sessions to reflect, write notes, use the bathroom, and return phone calls. I occasionally went over when a patient was in the middle of what seemed like important material or when an unresolved crisis had occurred, but almost never went into the next patient's hour. When I returned from my maternity leave it seemed like seeing patients was very hectic and there seemed never enough time to return all the calls or write notes and I resented spending time at the end of my day to finish notes and calls when I wanted to get home to my baby. When I examined the situation, I noticed that I was consistently using my 10-minute break to finish up with patients. Sometimes I was even running over into the next hour. My patients seemed more helpless than usual and I felt pressure to provide more. I realized that this was probably coming more from me than them. When I stopped doing this, they didn't seem to fall apart any more than usual.

A therapist may also more directly respond to this loss by feeling depressed or having few emotional resources to manage her patients. In fact, the rates of depression for mothers of 1- to 2-year-olds is twice as high as for other mothers (Rubenstein, 1998). Rubenstein's theory is that mothers sacrifice more than fathers do and that these sacrifices have a psychic cost. In the previous case, the therapist may feel annoyed with patients who take up too much time and react to them by pushing them away prematurely (Balsam, 1974). One therapist recalled that she felt that she could not tolerate the same needy behaviors in her patients with borderline personality disorders that she had previously permitted, especially when they required time outside the sessions. It seems like the new mother needs to reconcile herself to the fact that she has multiple caregiving roles that compete for her attention.

Another common reaction of therapists on return to work is difficulty in maintaining empathic attunement due to an affective spillover of personal satisfaction. This may take the form of feeling elated and powerful, capable of handling most anything or any type of problem such as a difficult, suicidal or chronic patient without a thorough appreciation of the therapeutic dilemmas or extra time required to treat such an individual. It can also take the form of an insensitivity for the patient's problems (e.g., how can they be so depressed when life has wonderful things to offer?). It may also take the form of annoyance with a patient or an intolerance for the patient still struggling with the same issues or conflict that he or she had prior to the therapist's maternity leave. The following vignette has some of these features.

Vignette 2.10

Initially when I went back to work, I had little tolerance for patients who seemed to obsess endlessly about their problems. I had this one male patient who presented as being somewhat unhappy in his marriage but could not decide whether to stay or leave. He had been married 25 years to a woman who had a borderline personality and who frequently threatened suicide, had fits of rage, etc. However, he had raised a family with her, and had never left despite claiming to want to do so. Before my maternity leave we had explored his passivity and self-esteem. Upon my return, I felt little empathy for his plight. I maintained a rather hedonistic stance, with a personal view that life had too many things to offer to be unhappy. He left therapy soon after I returned, deciding at least temporarily to remain with his wife. I heard from a colleague a few years later that he felt that I had been pressuring him too much to leave. I recognize only in retrospect my lack of sensitivity for this man. I had a similar reaction to a male patient who was pursuing a divorce and trying to decide whether to pursue custody of his 3-year-old daughter because he felt that his wife was very narcissistic and would use the daughter for her own gratification. It was a very messy divorce and seemed (and was) a no-win situation for him. In retrospect he was in a tremendous amount of pain, but I was unable to help him explore because I was high on life. I also see now that I may have been so threatened by these two situations. I denied the reality of their conflicts and was insensitive to their struggles.

Although it may not be possible or even necessary to hide one's enthusiasm about having a baby, it is essential that one be able to maintain empathic attunement to the patient's plight. If not, the result will be similar to what happened in the preceding example, where the therapist was not able to work with these patients' conflicts, even at a very superficial level. As the therapist implies, she may have used denial because of her own anxieties about the future of her own marriage.

Another fantasy that may interfere with the therapist's work is her fear that her baby may come to recognize, prefer or even love the childcare worker over her. Balsam (1974) described how this impacted the therapy.

[A therapist] was seeing a long-standing patient after her absence during which another therapist had cared for the patient without incident. . . . When she found herself saying "were you ever as angry at Dr. X as you are with me." . . . The most recent activated acute situation of this sort was rivalry between her and the babysitter regarding the baby's love. After her reflections the burden of proof was not placed on the patient.

(pp. 286–287)

This fear can be exacerbated if, on her maternity leave, she lost any patients to a substitute therapist, or in the group situation, if the group seems happily ensconced with the co-therapist on her return. Perhaps the therapist in the earlier vignette who had difficulty examining whether the patient was truly ready to leave was dealing with this fear that her child could get along without her.

Guilt and Worry

New mothers spend an enormous amount to time and energy both at home and at the office worrying and feeling guilty. Despite feminist efforts, many new mothers are vulnerable to inordinate amounts of self-blame for their children's problems, even when they themselves are overworked and/or without a supportive network. This may in part be because mothers are generally more involved in their children's lives at an early age (Lerner, 1998). When worrying becomes excessive, it keeps the new mother from thinking about other worrisome things in her life such as ailing parents. Lerner (1998) offered this advice:

on my worst days, my worry can reach such extremes that I can only conclude that I'm entirely unfit to be a parent. So I call my best friend, who tells me that she, too, is entirely unfit to be a parent, as we all are. This reminder makes me feel much better. . . . Every mother has a certain amount of "worry energy" to disperse into the world, and a child is an excellent, almost unavoidable, lightning rod for it. . . . If you must worry (and most of us must), rotate your anxious concerns among family members, rather than letting the full weight of your worry envelop and settle on one child like a fog.

(pp. 89–97)

Guilt is a common emotion. It often centers around loyalty. Commonly, the therapist experiences guilt that her personal life has a now more central role than previously, and she is often less flexible when patients need to reschedule, but at the same time often needs to alter her own schedule to accommodate childcare (baby's illness, doctor appointments, etc.). However, the therapist can also feel guilty that she is shortchanging her child and that she is enjoying her return to work. Balsam described a therapist's response to the realization that she had been engaged with an interesting patient and had momentarily forgotten her baby.

One therapist was with an interesting patient who was telling her in a lively way the events during her absence. An opportunity had arisen for him to go to China as a translator for a few months. . . . so engaging was his description. A few moments later she realized that she had missed the vital ending. Momentarily she had tuned out in shock realizing that for the first time she had forgotten her infant at home . . . she asked him to explain it again. He was annoyed, said that she was not as "with it as usual."

(Balsam, 1974, p. 287)

Guilt over divided loyalties also may lead to an over-nurturing attitude toward patients or a tendency to not encourage a patient to explore issues of separation from therapy in order to reassure oneself of professional competence.

Technical Considerations and Implications for Intervention

The therapist faces an array of decisions at this time.

Providing Information About the Baby and Childbirth

On the therapist's return, some patients are intensely curious about the baby and pepper the first sessions with initial personal questions. For other patients, there is a remarkable dearth of interest. They seem to want to deny the existence of the baby and the previous 9 months' intrusion and resume the "exclusive" dyadic relationship. Such patients' behavior can actually be a disappointment to the therapist (Fuller, 1987). It is a good idea to anticipate some of the personal questions that patients may ask on returning and develop ideas on how to respond to them. Some therapists perceive questions to be intrusive and demanding. Some have a greater desire to reveal more. Most therapists provide some information about the baby—mostly sex, name, weight, general health and date of birth (Bashe, 1989; Fuller, 1987). Some therapists vary their revelations depending on the patient and reason for the question. For many analytical therapists, much of the actual information disclosed is secondary to the meaning of their patients' curiosities. Decisions on how much to reveal on a case-by-case basis may best be handled by consulting colleagues and talking to one's own therapist and supervisors. When considering personal revelations, a good procedure to follow is to question potential benefit versus possible harm. A corollary to this is to ask what gratification the therapist may be experiencing with regard to personal revelations. Most therapists who had previously experienced a pregnancy felt that it was easier to handle the questions the second time around (Bashe, 1989).

Scheduling and Availability

Professional and personal development at this stage involves the challenge of balancing the timelessness of the mothering role with the structure and commitment of the 45- to 50-minute hour (Bashe, 1989). It also involves a clear understanding of one's priorities and how these impact on one's capabilities of managing and caring for patients. The new mother must fit her professional schedule to her personal responsibilities at home. Although the pregnancy stage has passed, this task and resulting changes may continue to kindle patients' concerns regarding the therapist's commitment to and the patient's identification with the baby (Bashe, 1989). The first issue to be addressed is with regard to the therapist's professional time commitment. There are alarming trends nationally about how much mothers and fathers are working. National surveys suggest that of parents who work, only 4% of men and 13% women worked less than 40 hours a week (Hochschild, 1997). Even if a therapist is willing to put in the same amount of time that she did prior to her pregnancy, the hours may be different. For example, one new mother/therapist told us that she intended to limit her day hours so that her husband could be at home to care for their child while she worked, thereby limiting the hours that a sitter would be employed. This was problematic for some of her geriatric patients, who preferred to travel during the day.

Many therapists report that their new responsibilities do not afford them the same flexibility in scheduling patients that they previously had had. New patients might be best served by being referred elsewhere. Ongoing patients might be more severely affected because they can experience this lack of flexibility and reluctance to reschedule missed appointments as an attenuation in commitment to them. For example, one therapist attempted to rearrange patients so that she could be off with her children on a school holiday. For one long-term patient, this represented a clear demotion in status. The initial exploration focused on physical availability. Eventually, discussion led to a productive exploring of her displacement as the only and favorite child, although much acting out and anger had to be tolerated initially.

Many therapists experience anxiety and conflict about how available they need to be or should be for their patients. Guilt at not being available for patients and annoyance around the attention that patients require are not uncommon. Van Niel (1993) reported,

> I detected my obvious weariness at one point when I found myself doing things I do not ordinarily do. I was so frustrated with the depressed patients that I actually began to make an appointment for one of them with an adjunctive therapeutic practitioner, a job counselor. Again with supervision, I realized that at that particular time I had unresolved dependency conflicts of my own, and with adequate support and more rest these feelings gradually subsided.
>
> (p. 132)

These feelings, too, often parallel worries about being a good-enough mother. Focusing intensely on availability with patients may be covering up the same worry on the home front. Worry and guilt about home commitments may be a cover for worry and guilt about work issues.

Handling Last-Minute Cancellations

Last-minute cancellations potentially pose problems for therapist mothers. Even today, women end up with the brunt of the childcare responsibilities, and it is frequently the mother who must cancel her patients to take a sick child to the doctor or rearrange her schedule to take children to the dentist or school functions. Narcissistic patients often have a great deal of difficulty tolerating these disruptions in treatment. The question emerges as to whether and how much to reveal to the patient regarding the reality of the situation. The following vignette illustrates this point.

Vignette 2.11

My 3-year-old son, who had been relatively healthy, came down with a series of illnesses, a high fever, an ear infection, the measles and so on. He was in day care so that over the course of a 2-month period, I had to cancel and/or rearrange many days of patients to care for him. For one divorced narcissistic professional woman that I had been seeing for several months, I had to cancel one and rearrange two appointments at the last minute. For the first two, I told her that a family emergency required that I change the schedule. When she came in after the third change, she announced that she was firing me, stating that she worked 60 hours a week and could not tolerate what appeared to be my disrespect for her incredibly busy schedule. I tried to explore her anger, hurt and insult, but she stuck with the realities of the situation. I did not further explain what happened and did not know whether I should have or whether the reality of the appointment changes were simply too narcissistically injuring and could not be worked through at this early point in her treatment. Had I anticipated that my son would be so ill that spring, I may have been able to anticipate this narcissistic patient's reactions and either alerted her to this possibility and/or encouraged her to pursue other treatment options. She was very angry and I debated whether I should mention why I had to cancel at the last minute. She left treatment and I heard from a colleague who knew her that she did not pursue further treatment.

This example portrays the impossibility of the therapist's anticipating the vicissitudes of childhood illnesses. If the therapist had some history with a sick child, she could have indicated so at the commencement of treatment, which would have allowed the patient the choice of pursuing treatment elsewhere or adapting to the possibility that the therapist is likely to occasionally rearrange or cancel appointments. This not being the case, should the therapist have detailed more of her reasons for canceling and rescheduling? Does knowing the actual reality make it more difficult for the patient to feel and express her anger toward the therapist's unavailability? In this particular case, given the inability of the therapist to predict future cancellations, it may have been just as wise to allow the patient the option to find treatment elsewhere. Unfortunately, the patient did not pursue treatment, and we have to wonder the extent to which the patient's experience with this therapist colored her willingness to make an emotional investment in treatment again. The need to be respectful of a patient's right to an explanation must carefully be weighed against the extent that it will hinder exploration of its meaning, and possible therapeutic gain that can be accomplished by exploring the meaning. For more disturbed patients, a more specific explanation may help with the reality that the cancellation is not related to their behavior or being.

The First Hour After the Treatment Interruption

Not all patients will return to treatment. In addition, some will return only briefly, often to be reassured that the therapist is well and/or available. Some of these patients will have discovered in the hiatus that they can and desire to manage their affairs themselves. However, many therapists feel that the abrupt termination is most likely related to unresolved issues around the therapist's pregnancy. Although little can be done about those who do not return, for those who do, listening and addressing unresolved pregnancy issues is important so that the latter type of termination can be averted.

If another therapist or emergency backup was used during the therapist's maternity leave, this too may have important meaning to the patient and so should be discussed as needed on the patient's return. This topic is often difficult for the therapist to broach because of her own feelings concerning another therapist satisfactorily meeting the patient's needs. These feelings can range from possessiveness and guilt to relief or worry over the loss of patients to this other therapist. Here is a vignette from an advanced resident psychiatrist about how the interim coverage and patient issues collided. It also revisits the issue of acceptance of gifts

Vignette 2.12

For a year I had been working weekly with a middle-aged, single, childless, depressed female patient in an supportive expressive psychotherapy and medication management when I became pregnant. I arranged for another therapist to see her weekly for 2 months until I returned from maternity leave. Upon my return, the patient reported that she had been doing well. Toward the end of the session she requested that she remain with the new therapist and that I continue to see her monthly for medication monitoring. I initially thought it was a good idea as I was a trainee leaving in a year. Our sessions continued but the sessions began to take on the characteristic of two buddies chatting and she would end with, "now you take care of that baby." After 4 months the weekly therapist took a 2-month planned leave and I agreed to cover for her increasing our monthly medication sessions if necessary. While the therapist was on vacation, the patient came into the session bringing a gift for the baby, which was a baby bangle with an elephant on it. I told her that the clinic had a policy of not accepting gifts. She stated that it wasn't a gift that she had found it around the house as she was cleaning up. As she got up to leave she asked whether she could switch back to therapy with me. The session ended, the next already scheduled in a month. I did not know how to handle the gift and request.

In supervision, the background of the patient was explored in more detail. This patient was a product of a very young single mother and was raised by her grandmother. When the patient was an adolescent, her mother had matured and had another girl. Her mother raised her sister. The patient had reported that she had tried to develop a relationship with her mother and would bring her gifts, but it seemed that the mother always favored the new child. She was both hurt and angry by the mother's rejection. When the mother was ill, the patient quit her good paying job, moved in and cared for her until her death. On rare occasions when the sister visited, she felt like an outsider when they were together. The therapist reported that the patient could not easily express anger and it seemed to emerge in the form of depression. After the mother's death, the patient was not able to find another job for years, partially due to the unresolved mourning process and moderate depressive symptoms. The therapist recognized in retrospect how her maternity leave replayed for the patient the lost mother. The patient was angry at the therapist for abandoning her, but could not express it, only in the form of requesting a change in therapists. This seemed like an attempt to find a stable mother. The "you care for that baby" was both an acceptable cultural response, but also reaction formation for the jealousy and envy of attention that she felt that her new little sister (therapist's baby) was receiving. The second therapist left and the patient felt abandoned once again. Her baby gift paralleled her gifts aimed at winning her mother's affections.

Although patients' references to and questions about the baby and the therapist could be somewhat controlled or avoided while on maternity leave, hiding from this once the therapist has returned to practice is not possible. However, the therapist now has the luxury to explore the meaning behind these questions and subsequent actions. That is, are some questions fueled by concern or obligation or significant unconscious and conscious related experiences (Clarkson, 1980)? Understanding patients' motivations for these actions, questions can aid in deciding whether and how much information to provide. As is mentioned in Chapter 6, disclosure is more appropriate with children and adolescents (Fenster et al., 1986). Fenster et al. (1986) felt that some self-disclosure regarding the therapist's plans for managing both a career and being a mother might be helpful for two reasons. First, it assures patients that she is available to them while she is in the office. And second, it may provide a much needed model for female patients concerning combining and managing a career and home life.

Some patients request to see the baby. Although some therapists that we interviewed granted their patients' requests, most did not make an effort to show the baby to their patients. We feel that this is an instance in which the meaning of the request ought to be more fully explored and therapist self-evaluation must be pursued to determine whether such a display will be overly gratifying or wounding for either the therapist or patient.[15]

Ongoing Negotiation and Improvisation of the Home/Work Balance

It is important to realize that the career/home balance is a fluid and evolving process. The result of dealing with and improvising around the practical aspects of her life both at home and at work further define the therapist's identities as both a mother and a therapist. At a practical level the therapist/mother must decide how much to work outside the home. When combining home and work, trends of time allocation from the 1960s to 2000 indicate that both men and women are working longer hours, and these hours are coming from leisure time. This decline in free time is sharper for women than for men (Sayer, Bianchi, & Robinson, 2004). Working either full- or part-time has its pros and cons. Although part-time mothers often feel excluded from organizational advancement, interpersonal connections and skill development opportunities, they also report greater satisfaction at home, with their jobs, and with their children (Higgins, Duxbury, & Johnson, 2000). Even returning to work "full-time" in an organizational setting has sometimes put women on the "mommy track" because of their commitments to children and home (Schwartz, 1989). About 15% of mothers report their perceptions of discrimination such as being paid less or denied a promotion (Crowley & Kolenikov, 2014). Each therapist/mother's personal circumstances will influence the evolution of her professional and home commitment and identity. It is clear, however, that for most mothers (unlike fathers), it is a perennial balancing act with priority going toward the family (Kaufman & Uhlenberg, 2000). Many therapists' desire to work and concomitant work schedules evolve over time. Thus, depending on their perceived family needs, some go from part-time to full-time when children go to school. Whereas others reverse this pattern, feeling that their children need them more as they enter school and are exposed to peer pressures and school requirements. Luckily, many therapists, unlike women in more male-dominated professions, often have the capability of adjusting to these reassessed needs over time. However, some thought ought to be given to this possible need for reassessment and rearrangement as she agrees to take on some of the longer-term, more difficult patients.

As time goes on, the "bliss" of babyhood fades into more frequent unresolved quarrels with children and spouse. Oftentimes the desire to have a fuller professional life comes from the feeling that home life is chaotic, depleting, and without a break (Hochschild, 1997). This may in part be the result of mothers feeling constantly on-call for other family members (Larson, Richards, & Perry-Jenkins, 1994). Sociological data suggest that for women who work outside the home, only one-third of their husbands do more housework and childcare to compensate, whereas the rest do the same or less (Hochschild, 1997). The fathers' participation in household and childcare tasks is determined more by their gender-related beliefs about these things (i.e., who should stay home when a child is sick) than by their time availability or their resource contribution to the household (Minnotte, 2016). Although in principle, most couples agree that childcare responsibilities should be shared in some way, only a small proportion agree that household chores should be shared. Furthermore, parents disagree about their contribution to childcare and household chores. Mothers see themselves as taking the majority of responsibility, whereas fathers feel that they do share at appropriate levels in these tasks (Chong & Mickelson, 2016). This perception has not changed over the past three decades (Hiller & Philliber, 1986).

Moreover, mothers' perceptions of the fairness in the sharing arrangement mediates their levels of relationship satisfaction; such mediation does not occur with fathers (Chong & Mickelson, 2016).

Such a pattern can be renegotiated with a spouse for redistribution of the household chores and is well worth the effort. Men and women collaborate in forming and maintaining gender-specific roles, and so changes usually do not happen as the sole decision of the woman (Thompson & Walker, 1989). Those couples who do share in the responsibilities do seem to feel more satisfied with their home life (Stevens, Kiger, & Riley, 2001).[16] The continuing negotiation of this balance is particularly important, as there is evidence that the balance and the symbolic meaning that women attach to their work has implications for their psychological health, relationships with children and spouse, and the division of labor within the family. Those mothers who are ambivalent about their involvement with their professional work are suffering from greater amounts of depression and feel overloaded by their responsibilities than those who feel more at peace with the balance they enact (Perry-Jenkins, Seery, & Crouter, 1992). However, even for these couples, mothers take more responsibility than do fathers (Hochschild, 1989). Generally, when spouses do participate in household chores, they are the "nicer" chores, such as going to the zoo rather than cleaning the bathrooms (Blumberg & Coleman, 1989), and their tasks are generally undertaken more intermittently (e.g., mowing the lawn) than the daily tasks of cooking and cleaning (Lachance-Grzela & Bouchard, 2010).

As demands of home become greater, many therapists find themselves further isolated by the 50-minute hour. Collaboration and socialization with colleagues and friends ameliorate professional isolation and an emotionally draining home life. These contacts are likely to reduce isolation and lift spirits (Hochschild, 1997). Some therapists find solace in connecting with others who are struggling with similar circumstances. This can take the form of emphasizing certain aspects of their identities. For instance, they may get together regularly or intermittently for a light-hearted chat over coffee or a serious discussion of clinical issues. In writing this book, we would frequently meet to work together while our children, approximately the same age, would play together. This arrangement was tremendously affirming as intellectual questions, thoughts and writing were interwoven with emotional support and reassurance concerning our anguish over "family" growing pains.

General Recommendations

1. What works best for the therapist, her family and career takes place in a context of ambiguous and shifting cultural definitions of what is considered acceptable. Many therapists struggle in isolation, anxious that their thoughts or their situation is abnormal. They are not aware of the many relational resources that might be available to them. It is our recommendation that reduction of this isolation is important for the maintenance of adequate self-esteem and good mental health. Although each therapist/mother must negotiate her identity balance, the consensual validation from compeers and mentors should not be underestimated.

2. In this chapter, we have repeatedly noted that complex decision making takes place at each stage along the pregnant mother's journey and postpregnancy. We counsel that considering possible solutions to problems well in advance of their implementation supports the best decision as does taking into account as many relevant factors as possible. Among such factors are the length of the therapeutic relationship, the severity of the patient's difficulties, the therapist's social, financial and other resources, and the broader treatment environment.

Notes

1. Progesterone, which has a sedative effect, rises during pregnancy. Glucocorticoids, which are not thought to produce memory impairment, also rise during pregnancy (Gross & Pattison, 2007)
2. Although it is not particularly relevant in the context of our discussion here, we do believe that if the therapist had explored the patient's associations that it would not have necessarily led to the patient's questioning the therapist's pregnancy status. Such a discussion is more likely to lead to exploration of the patient's more personal material. This is taken up in the next section.
3. The Centers for Disease Control and Prevention (2015) reported that birth defects occur in 3% of all babies. Birth defects are the leading case of infant deaths, accounting for 20% of all infant deaths.
4. A screening ultrasound and blood test at 10–13 weeks screens for several chromosomal defects such as Down syndrome and other disorders such as those with cardiac problems. This test catches about 85% of those screened and as a 5% false positive rate (American Pregnancy Association, http://americanpregnancy.org/prenatal-testing/first-trimester-screen/). *Chorionic villus sampling (CVS)* is a diagnostic test that is performed 10–13 weeks of pregnancy to determine whether or not a baby has a normal number of chromosomes (46) and for birth defects like Down syndrome, trisomy 18, trisomy 13, and some other chromosome abnormalities. CVS is generally performed by inserting a needle through a mother's abdomen or cervix into the

placenta. A small piece of the placenta is then removed and sent to the laboratory for genetic testing. A blood test for neural defects needs to be administered separately in the second trimester. In amniocentesis, a diagnostic test that is performed at 15–18 weeks, a needle is inserted through the abdomen into the amniotic fluid where the fetus is floating. It can be used to determine both chromosomal number and abnormality as well as neural tube defects. Both tests require about a half a day of time. (http://nfwh.nm.org/genetic-screening-and-testing-during-pregnancy.html)

5. In Chapter 7, we discuss the special issues of disclosure of the pregnancy created when the therapist is a member of a nontraditional family.

6. Pre-pregnancy of body image is a strong predictor of how women handle their changing shape with pregnancy (Skouteris, Carr, Wetheim, Paxton, & Duncombe, 2005).

7. For some pregnant women, deciding whether or not to have an amniocentesis is a stressor, and can be a source of tension in relationships.

8. Relatively new research suggests that there is an increasing level of oxytocin through the pregnancy and after birth. This not only improves memory and learning but is also partly responsible for the intense connection to the growing fetus and newborn. The increase in oxytocin could also heighten the therapist's attention to the affective components of their relationship to their patients, which are often reported by therapists.

9. See footnote 8 regarding oxytocin.

10. Skype and Google Hangout are not HIPPA-compliant platforms. There are a few free ones that are, however. Therapists would need to check state licensing laws as well as insurance carriers to know whether these services are within state guidelines and could be reimbursed by insurance companies if her practice allows for it.

11. A question to think about is whether you would spontaneously (or in response to a query) offer the name and sex of your partner or spouse. If not, why would you see this as different?

12. Our reading of the literature and interviews has led us to think about the pregnant therapist and new mother as predominantly a heterosexual one who is married to the father of her baby. We do acknowledge that there are hosts of other arrangements that we have not addressed here, such as pregnant lesbian therapists and those women who are not married to the father of their baby, but do so briefly in Chapter 7. We wish to be inclusive of them if our writing seems to apply. Obviously this is an area for more detailed study.

13. Characterized by mild irritability, depressed mood and anxiety (Grigoriadis & Romans, 2006)

14. More severe forms of the disorder, postpartum psychosis have only 0.1%–0.4% prevalence and usually require hospitalization (Sit, Rothschild & Wisner, 2006).

15. In order to gain some clarity from the therapists' point of view on the reasoning behind this question, therapists might consider whether a demand to be shown the therapist's spouse or partner would receive the same answer. If not, how is this different?

16. Regardless of the actual number of actual hours a partner helps out, the perception of the therapist/mother of how helpful her partner is seems significant.

CHAPTER 3

Patients' Reactions to
Therapists' Pregnancies

A therapist's pregnancy is likely to precipitate in patients' myriad thoughts, feelings, impulses and behavior. Although some reactions can be observed across a wide range of patients, others are quite particular to the individual. They have their roots in multiple sources. One source is those facets of reality that are introduced by the pregnancy. For example, learning that the therapeutic work will be interrupted for several months while the therapist is on maternity leave can easily engender frustration, worry and irritation. The patient's anxiety may be evoked through the realization that at any moment, the therapist might need to take a sabbatical due to complications with the pregnancy (McWilliams, 1980). These reactions are all understandable, do not bespeak necessarily of any pathology and might well point to healthy sectors of the patient's personality. Still other reactions are due to the therapist's way of handling her pregnancy. For example, a therapist who denies a pregnancy that is evident to the patient is likely to induce bewilderment in that patient. Whether the client's reaction is due to the situation the therapist is presenting to the client or how she is handling the situation she presents, it can be understood as in the domain of the real relationship (Weiner & Bornstein, 2009). Other reactions may be rooted in early conflict or deprivation. For example, the therapist's pregnancy may bring to the surface the client's longing for a more attuned caregiver, the lack of which may have contributed greatly to the client's current difficulty. This category corresponds to the early psychoanalytic conceptualization of transference (Frosch, 2002). Freud wrote in conjunction with the Dora case, "a whole series of psychological experiences are revived, not as belonging to the past, but as applying to the person of the physician at the present moment" (1905, p. 116). The relationship itself, co-constructed by patient and therapist over time, is also a force in shaping the patient's response to the pregnancy. For example, if the patient and client have had ruptures in the relationship that were never healed fully, if a sense of fragility exists within the dyad, then the specter of negotiating this very new situation may be daunting to both parties.

Many, if not most, responses will not be uniquely attributable to one category or another but will be a blending of different factors. For example, particular responses may be connected to the client's history of trauma, but the form that it takes might be shaped by the culture of the relationship. A client may be envious of the therapist's baby because of early deprivation but also be able to talk about this painful feeling with words because verbal exploration is so well established in the therapy relationship.

In this chapter, we explain not only the range of reactions patients have but also their multiple roots. The former is important to help therapist to know what to anticipate. The latter is key in helping the therapist make a correct attribution of the foundation of the client's response. All of this information is useful only insofar as it informs the therapist's responses. Therefore, in the latter part of the chapter, we consider how the therapist's appraisal of patient's reactions can lead to the development of effective lines of intervention.

Understanding the Patient's Responses

The therapist's pregnancy provides an ever-changing, multidimensional context for the client's work. Therapists can facilitate this work by recognizing the multiplicity of factors shaping the patient's response to the therapist at any point of the pregnancy and weighing those factors. Therapists might ask themselves whether the client's reactions concern the realities posed by the pregnancy, the client's own dynamics, the therapist's reactions to aspects of the pregnancy, or the culture of the relationship. At least four benefits accrue from recognizing the complexity of patient responses to their therapists' pregnancies, that is, the interplay of those elements that brought the patient into the treatment and those reflecting the real relationship.

1. **The therapist is able to strengthen the therapeutic alliance through the demonstration of respect and empathy.** The client's willingness to collaborate with the therapist is predicated on his or her sense that the therapist both respects and understands him or her. Respect and empathy are conveyed the therapist appropriately acknowledges the real relationship, even when other conflictual elements might be present. Consider the following vignette.

   Vignette 3.1
   After 2 months of analysis, Alice is told that her analyst is pregnant. She also learns that the analyst will be taking a 6-month sabbatical from her work. At the outset of the treatment, Alice had been given no hint by the analyst that an interruption was likely or even possible. Alice experiences and expresses anger over being confronted with the decision of whether to continue with the analyst after a long hiatus or to transfer to someone new. She expresses the opinion that the analyst had an obligation to tell her of her circumstance before the commencement of the analysis.

In this vignette, the patient poses a legitimate issue related to informed consent. The patient had a reasonable belief that if the analyst were aware that the work would be disrupted for an extended period at a fairly early point in treatment, she should either refrain from taking new patients, or reveal the likelihood of the disruption. Additionally, the patient was at minimum likely to be denied gains. Were the analyst to interpret the patient's response rather than to acknowledge its legitimacy, it would convey disrespect of the patient. It would suggest that the analyst did not need to give the patient information that might affect the patient's decision to enter treatment with that analyst.

Sometimes, clients' behaviors that are rooted in the real relationship might be embedded in the principles that guide social interaction in a given culture (Tinsley & Melman, 2003). McCluskey (2016) uses Hochschild's (1997) concept of *feeling rules* to capture societal prescriptions for how one must feel in particular circumstances. McCluskey avers that a pregnancy is a circumstance that requires particular feelings on the part of those interacting with the pregnant woman. Cultural norms also include rules for interactions with pregnant women. Expressions of solicitude and concern as well as expressions of congratulations are common (Wolfe, 2013). Suppose at the beginning of the therapist's ninth month of pregnancy, the client asks, "How are you feeling?" This response can be understood in multiple ways. It may be due to an emotional factor such as the client's long-standing worry about parental fragility. However, frequently, such a response will be no more than the client's observance of a social norm—like many others in the therapist's life, the client may be wishing her well. The therapist's unreflectively assuming it is the former rather than the latter diminishes the humanity of the patient and thereby lessens the potential of the treatment to enhance the client's well-being. Conversely, as Hjalmarsson (2005) noted,

> the clients' real relationship with and conception of a therapist serves as the most effective breeding ground for a clients' transference feelings and reactions. The pregnant state in the therapist is a particularly powerful example of how the real relationship between client and therapist exists on parallel lines with the maturation of transference.
>
> (pp. 10–11)

2. **The therapist can offer input that validates and strengthens the patient's capacity to test reality.** This benefit again pertains to the therapist's recognition of what aspects of patient–therapist interactions pertain to the real relationship versus those relevant to the goals of treatment. It is especially crucial for those clients who have difficulties with reality testing. By acknowledging that a perception, interpretation or judgment is justified, the therapist engages the patient in the meta-cognitive activity of discernment, that is, the enterprise of figuring out what perceptions fit what is occurring in the

relationship and what perceptions do not. Patients' confidence in reality testing is bolstered and their willingness to look at this function further is strengthened by the knowledge that the difficulty with social perceptions is delimited (and hence, addressable) rather than pervasive.

3. **The therapist can recognize therapeutic opportunities.** When the therapist can see that something in the client's response is not rooted in the real relationship, then, the pregnancy has served as a stimulus for work. Requiring particular discernment are those occasions when the patient forms a response that either is justified by the therapist's behavior, or is consistent with social convention, but in both cases, has facets that bear investigation. Such a circumstance requires that the therapist acknowledge the reality-based piece while encouraging examination of those pieces pointing to the patient's dynamics. The following vignette illustrates the intermingling of reality-based and dynamically based components in a client's response and the sensitive responding it required of the therapist.

Vignette 3.2

Two months previously, a therapist told Beverly about her pregnancy. The therapist had been seeing Beverly for several years. Initially, Beverly had offered words of congratulations. The therapist accepted with appreciation the patient's well wishes, but also made an attempt to explore the patient's initial reactions. These latter efforts did not prove fruitful. Somehow, Beverly managed to refocus her attention on the therapist's likely reactions to her pregnancy rather than Beverly's own.

As the pregnancy progressed, problems arose. The therapist needed to submit to repeated diagnostic procedures, all of which were stressful in that they revealed whether or not the pregnancy was viable. Although the therapist would have liked to have freed herself from her commitments to her patients on these days, she felt unable to do so primarily because of the economic consequences of cancelling appointments. She came into these appointments feeling haggard and looking wan. Whereas her other patients appeared to be only dimly aware of the enormity of her physical discomfort and emotional distress, Beverly was uncannily sensitive to both. She made small talk in the sessions punctuated by some delicately proffered inquiries into the therapist's condition. When the therapist pointed out to Beverly that she seemed to be skimming the surface, Beverly revealed a deliberate effort to protect the therapist. Beverly said the therapist's discomfort and agitation were apparent to her. She assumed it had to do with the therapist's pregnancy and she certainly was going to avoid anything to make matters worse for the therapist.

After recovering from her surprise, the therapist recognized the connection between Beverly's solicitous response to her and the heroic caretaking Beverly had performed for her grandmother when she was a girl of only 7 years old. Her constant availability to the ailing grandparent had led her to give up many of the enjoyments of her age group, such as cavorting outside with her friends after school. However, such sacrifices had enabled her to achieve a special position in her parents' esteem relative to two younger and two older siblings. Eventually, both therapist and Beverly were able to see within the context of their relationship how Beverly denied so many needs in order to preserve this source of self-esteem and identity.

In this example, Beverly's response to the therapist was intimately connected to the appearance and behavior of the therapist. Not only was the pregnancy a powerful stimulus, but so too were the therapist's pregnancy-related manifestations. Moreover, Beverly's view of the therapist as being in a state of need was accurate and perceptive. However, if the therapist were to proceed as if nothing was to be learned about Beverly because her reactions were reality-based, she would miss a great deal. The fact that Beverly was so attuned and responsive to the therapist's condition reveals a great deal about her, and thereby provides a wealth of material for her increased self-understanding.

Many of the phenomena that emerge in the therapeutic relationship have this character. The therapist provides a collection of stimuli for the patient's response but the intensity and manner in which the patient responds relates to the patient's concerns and conflicts. In this way, the patient's response to the pregnancy provides a route to the patient's increased self-awareness. Dismissing the patient's reactions as being due simply to the failure of the therapist to be a blank screen is to miss much of interpretive value.

4. **The therapist can plan productively for the later stages of pregnancy and the maternity leave.** As we see in the following vignette, the client's reaction to the therapist's pregnancy may provide some indication of how the client is likely to respond to ensuing events including the birth of the baby and the maternity leave.

Vignette 3.3

A therapist was not surprised when Mark, a schizoid patient in cognitive-behavioral therapy, told her that he was looking forward to her maternity leave as an opportunity to learn to cope with his problems on his own. He had reacted this way to prior anticipated interruptions in the therapy due to therapist vacations. During these breaks, Mark's functioning consistently deteriorated so significantly that he could barely care for himself. Recognizing that Mark's response to the impending separation was a counterdependent defensive reaction, the therapist set up a bevy of resources for the patient to tap during her absence. For example, she planned to have a series of phone check-ins with him.

Had this therapist assessed Mark's response differently, had she seen his optimistic perspective on her impending departure as a realistic non-defensive response, she would have planned the separation differently. She might have provided Mark with fewer supports and prior to the break, and would have focused more intensively on how he might summon his own resources during her absence.

Given the likely complexity of patients' reactions to their therapists' pregnancies, how might the therapist disentangle the various elements in order to realize the benefits listed earlier? The simple answer is, "by paying attention." Noticing the nuances of the patient's reactions and how those reactions align with the client's background and the history of the therapeutic relationship can help the therapist recognize what type of intervention might be appropriate. Beyond this careful observation, two sets of clues can illumine the meanings of patient reactions. The first is the structure of the patient's response and the second is its content or thematic properties.

Structure of the Patient's Response

When the therapist is trying to discern the basis for a patient's response to her pregnancy—whether it derives from reality factors, dynamics of the patient, or both—that therapist does well to keep in mind that the patient's reaction might be direct or indirect. A direct reaction occurs when the patient is aware of, and gives expression to, some facet of his or her response to the pregnancy. For example, Alice in Vignette 3.1 provided a direct expression of her anger concerning the therapist's communication of an hiatus in the treatment.

Although emotional responses based on the real relationship tend to be direct, not all direct responses are realistic, as we see in the following vignette.

> **Vignette 3.4**
> Laila had been in psychodynamic therapy for 1 year when the therapist revealed to her that she was pregnant and would have the baby in 3 months. The therapist indicated further that she would not be able to see Laila for a period of 1 month. The patient first expressed shock and proceeded to comment that the therapist did not look pregnant, leading the therapist to wonder if the patient questioned her truthfulness. In the weeks that followed, Laila slowly admitted that the therapist did look somewhat pregnant. However, she increasingly focused on what she saw as a remarkable contrast: the therapist had successfully become pregnant at a time when she, Laila, was struggling with fertility problems. Eventually, she crystallized her conviction that the therapist had become pregnant in order to evoke envy in, and achieve victory over, the patient. Laila expressed considerable ire toward the therapist for having taken this step and indicated that this development was the most recent in a long series of hurts her therapist had inflicted on her.

Although Laila had direct access to her anger, her delusional belief that the therapist became pregnant as a hostile gesture toward her was clearly a transference-driven response. The therapist might explore with Laila whether believing that the therapist had sinisterly planned her pregnancy spared her from an emotion such as the pain of grappling with sadness over her suspected infertility and her envy of the therapist.

In some circumstances, it might be unclear whether the patient's response has any foundation in the concerns and conflicts that brought the patient into therapy. Recognizing potentially diagnostic features of the patient's response might assist the therapist. As Penn (1986) noted, reactions to the therapist's pregnancy that have a transferential character have their underpinnings in events that occurred early in the patient's life. Because they are frequently embedded within the personality of the individual and developed in regard to a historical rather than a contemporary situation, they have a quality of rigidity. These response patterns have a readiness to occur across a range of circumstances, often regardless of their appropriateness. Also telltale is their inappropriate intensity, often being too high or too low for what the situation demands. These reactions frequently have dominion over the person and rarely share the affective stage with other feeling states. Consequently, when under the sway of such an element, the individual fails to show the rich array of reactions that healthy individuals typically have in relation to complex events.

The value of indirect responses is that they frequently point to driving forces in the client's behavior or experience that have some dynamic significance. The indirectness of the manifestation usually entails the exertion of a defensive effort against some psychological element the pregnancy has stimulated. The element itself might not have any pathological status. The defensive effort against it merely suggests that the element itself cannot be comfortably integrated into the fabric of the broader personality structure. Furthermore, some of the means of indirect expression have substantial costs to the person and may jeopardize the individual's functioning outside of therapy. Examples are provided in the section that follows. For these reasons, it is important to recognize when a given reaction inside or outside of therapy is tied to the pregnancy; it can then be the object of understanding and intervention using the tools available to the therapist depending on her theoretical orientation.

In the sections that follow, examples of types of indirect responses are provided.

Acting Out

Rather than articulate a reaction to the therapist's pregnancy, the patient may express it through behavioral manifestations outside of the treatment. Consider the following vignette.

Vignette 3.5

The week after the therapist announced her pregnancy in a family therapy session, Naomi, the teenage daughter, confessed that she had had unprotected sex with a young man she met, and was now terrified that she might be pregnant. The family occupied itself with this distressing situation for several weeks. The therapist noticed that no mention was made of her pregnancy, and she felt inhibited in making an inquiry about their reactions out of a concern that she appears unduly self-involved.

This example is consistent with the common observation of clinicians that the patient's discovery of the therapist's pregnancy frequently precipitates episodes of acting out (see Tinsley & Mellman, 2003, for additional examples). In such instances, the patient's acting out can serve a number of functions. First, it prevents the appearance of disturbing emotional elements both in the patient's awareness and in the therapy sessions themselves (Cole, 1980). Perhaps the family members had feelings of anger, envy or both toward the therapist, and the panic engendered by the daughter's situation provided an effective camouflage for them. Sometimes, a motive exists to keep the direct expression of feelings out of the sessions themselves to protect the pregnant therapist, who might be seen as fragile (Hartwell-Walker, 2016; McGourty, 2013; Tinsley & Mellman, 2003; Wolfe, 2013). Given that the therapist now has special worries about this family, the acting out serves a function of punishing the therapist for having added to the family members' distress. Also, to the extent that Naomi admires the therapist, her opportunity to be like her in this most salient way would be gratifying to Naomi. Finally, the therapist's pregnancy may have stimulated in not only Naomi, but also other family members, the longing for a baby. Such a wish could be directly gratified by Naomi's sexual activity.

In some cases, the acting out constitutes an opportunity for the emergence of psychological elements that previously had not entered the therapeutic field. Miller (1992) describes her play therapy with children during her pregnancy, and how generally, the stimulus of her pregnancy expedited her work with them. She shares the case of David, a four-and-a-half-year-old boy who for the first time in treatment revealed the close connection between his oppositionality and feelings of helplessness and sadness, the clear provocation for which seemed to be her upcoming maternity leave.

The topic of acting out was one of the major early focuses in research on the pregnant therapist. Berman (1975), who performed the earliest systematic investigation, studied the patients of nine female psychiatrists during both the last 6 months of their pregnancies and a 6-month control period. Therapists participated in an unstructured interview and completed a behavioral checklist to reflect the frequency of suicide attempts, violent behaviors toward the therapist or others, precipitous terminations, unplanned or unexpected pregnancies, or sudden marriages. Behavioral disturbances were classified as major or minor. Berman found that the patients of the pregnant therapists did show increased acting out relative to other periods. The most common form of acting out was dropping out of therapy prematurely. Suicide attempts and unplanned pregnancies also occurred. However, importantly, most incidents of acting out (for example, brief episodes of substance abuse or the failure to use contraceptives) were minor.

Later investigations yielded findings consistent with Berman's observation of increased acting out during pregnancy. Fenster (1983) found that 77% of the therapists in her sample had one or more patients who terminated either during pregnancy or afterward, and many of the therapists attributed these terminations to the pregnancy. Bassen's 13 analysts found acting out to be extremely common during pregnancy. Four of the 13 analysts had at least one patient who had become pregnant or had impregnated someone during the analysts' pregnancies or maternity leaves. Bassen does not, however, provide evidence that all of these events constitute acting out. Therapists also reported increases in missed sessions, tardiness and late or incorrect payment for sessions. Only 2 of the 13 analysts reported no acting out at all. For most of the analysts, the acting out was present in only a minority of their cases; yet, one analyst reported losing three out of four of her cases. Katzman's (1993) study of 24 bulimic women also revealed considerable acting out: "17% of the ongoing clients at least reported late or missed menstrual periods; three became 'accidentally' pregnant; two reported instances of 'forgetting' to use birth control and one woman reporting binging 'until her belly felt pregnant'" (p. 26). Wolfe (2013) interviewed 13 therapists who were currently or recently pregnant and found evidence of more frequent boundary crossings, such as making comments about the therapist's body (e.g., suggesting the therapist looks good for a pregnant woman) or trying to touch the therapist's body. Warren, Crowley, Olivardia and Schoen (2008) interviewed 43 professionals who treat eating-disordered patients, and found that most of them had received commentaries on their appearance during their pregnancies.

In all of these studies, what we do not know are the contributions of the therapists in the co-constructed therapy relationships. Does pregnancy alter the therapist's sensitivity or manner of a response in a way that might promote acting out? Zackson (2012), for example, hypothesizes that some premature terminations during pregnancy might be attributable to the therapist's own difficulty in talking about her pregnancy. Ultimately, both therapist and patient contributions will need to be studied—especially as they interact with one another to produce specific outcomes—to fully account for the acting-out phenomena that frequently emerges during pregnancy.

Increased Resistance

When patients show an increase in resistance upon having heard of the therapist's pregnancy, it is very likely that the resistance relates to issues activated by the pregnancy. By 'resistance' we are referring to the inability of the patient to make progress toward his or her therapeutic goals; the patient is "stuck." Why does the patient resist? The most obvious answer is that he or she is seeking to avoid addressing thoughts, feelings, urges, fantasies and other psychological elements that are unacceptable to the self. And yet, resistance is not entirely attributable to the client's dynamics. Patients' resistance to the full exploration of their reactions emerges from a broader social context of pronatalism, which is the placement of a high value upon procreation. Although pronatalism exists within most western societies, it has not been embraced for all times. Rather, it has its roots within the Victorian era, when gender roles—men going to work and women remaining home to tend to children—became solidified (Lovett, 2007). A pronatalist position requires than an unflaggingly positive attitude be assumed in relation to a pregnancy and a pregnant woman. Within this framework, anger or any form of negativity has no place within the interaction.

Increased resistance takes many forms. Bassen (1988) catalogued the observations of 13 analysts of patient resistance in the following way:

> lack of extreme delay in recognition that the analyst was pregnant, conscious withholding of responses, insistence that positive or negative feelings about the pregnancy were realistic and not subject to analysis, adhering to one set of responses to ward off others, feelings in the transference (such as the adoption of a counterdependent stand or responding as if the only impact was the separation involved in the analyst's maternity leave), denial that the pregnancy had any meaning to the patient, various forms of acting out and the inability to see that certain associations, behaviors, and/or feelings toward the analyst were a response to her pregnancy.
>
> (p. 283)

Bassen's therapists perceived patients as exaggerating their own customary defenses in response to their therapists' pregnancies.

Increased resistance is much more common in some populations than others. For example, Fenster's (1983) therapists observed that, generally, children and adolescents are more resistive than adults, and men are more resistive than women. Katzman (1993), in examining the progress notes of eating-disordered patients, found that defensiveness might be associated with length of time in therapy and the degree of maturation of the relationship. Longer-term patients were more likely than newer patients to express more caution about the therapist's pregnancy. Possibly newer patients had an insufficient fund of experience with the questions to know what types of questions about herself she would brook.

Some patients exhibit indifference to the therapist's pregnancy, and the therapist may be tempted to interpret this non-reaction as defensiveness. However, as Rosen (1989, p. 26) writes, "It is important . . . to guard against making an event which is highly significant for the therapist disproportionately significant for the client." As suggested in the beginning of this chapter, some patients may respond to the pregnancy primarily within the real relationship. Other patients may have reactions activated by neither the real nor the therapeutic relationship. In other words, the therapist's pregnancy may be a matter of true indifference to some patients. Fortunately, cues are available to assist the therapist to discriminate between defensiveness and indifference. As is seen in the next chapter, pregnant therapists frequently have the worry that their own preoccupation with the pregnancy leads them to perceive the patient as reacting to the pregnancy when he or she might not be. Given this common anxiety, it is important that the therapist have cues to determine whether a reaction is a response specific to the pregnancy.

A major cue is whether the patient's behavior in treatment changes as he or she is increasingly confronted with knowledge and manifestations of the therapist's pregnancy. Consider the following vignette:

Vignette 3.6
Trevor was in his fifth month of treatment. His style was to talk in a loud and barely interruptible way about his work difficulties and to point out how others were to blame for them. He appeared to lack the slightest awareness of, or interest in, the therapist's reactions. On one occasion, he was oblivious to the therapist's fit of sneezing. In learning of the therapist's pregnancy, his response was consistent with all of his earlier responses to her: He took it in passing. His single response was the question: "How long will you be out?" When the therapist responded, "A month," he nodded and went on to another topic.

Trevor's behavior probably was not a specific defensive response to the therapist's pregnancy per se but rather a manifestation of his general level of interpersonal relatedness. He lacked sufficient connection to other people to have a particular response to some dimension of, or event in, others' lives. On the other hand, had the disregard of the therapist been a rather new behavior or at least one that varied in intensity from the past, then the likelihood that he was responding to the therapist's new circumstance would have increased.

Symbolic Expressions

One phenomenon associated with the therapist's pregnancy is the broadening of the transference or the emergence of themes that previously had been given little expression in treatment. Oftentimes, however, these new themes will initially appear in a symbolic or derivative form. That is, the material produced by the patient will be a disguised expression of some psychological element. Typically, the disguise serves a defensive function, in that it spares the individual creating the disguise from the direct awareness of the element, as is illustrated in the following vignette:

Vignette 3.7
An inpatient therapist resumed psychotherapy with Zachary, a man with whom she had worked during two prior hospitalizations. Her appearance

during this hospitalization was markedly different, in that she was almost 8 months pregnant. Zachary came into the hospital because of the intensification of his usual obsessive concerns about damaging his family members. However, on the commencement of his work with the therapist, his worries seemed to shift to a disturbing preoccupation with the sexual lives of the women on his unit. He found himself trying to overhear their conversations and engaging in other clandestine activities to make discoveries about their sexual involvements. The therapist recognizes that Zachary's focus on the female members' sexual involvements was a disguised manifestation of his interest in the therapist's sexual life.

Spence (1973) recorded one patient's utterances from the time that the patient began treatment with the pregnant therapist until the patient directly articulated some recognition of the pregnancy. Spence found that when the patient produced derivatives associated with the pregnancy, she (the patient) was seemed least inclined to approach the therapist about her condition. The association served the function of creating a disguise and a means for containing the anxiety associated with the therapist's pregnancy.

Common Themes

Although many themes might emerge in relation to the therapist's pregnancy, three have particular salience: (a) symbiosis and separation; (b) envy and competition; and (c) sexuality and jealousy. The direct or symbolic prominence of these themes suggests the presence of conflict, trauma or disturbed early relationships, or any combination of the preceding. The objectives of the treatment will determine whether these elements are explored, or the depth of their exploration. However, the therapist's awareness of what has been activated for the patient will enhance her attunement, even if a particular theme is not explicitly discussed.

Symbiosis and Separation

Patients' conflicts related to separation from early caregivers often emerge with prominence during the therapist's pregnancy (Bassen, 1988; Cole, 1980; Tonon, Romani, & Grossi, 2012; Wolfe, 2013). Indeed, the pregnancy does in reality present the patient with a set of losses and thereby invites the patient to relive earlier experiences associated with loss and separation.

Prominent among the types of losses the patient confronts is the psychological and even physical availability of the therapist (Raphael-Leff, 2004). To grasp the kind of unavailability patients might experience, consider the following therapist's words:

> As I sat with my patient, I realized that for the past 10 minutes, I had no idea what she was talking about. I had been entirely focused on my baby's kicks and wiggles. This wasn't the first time I had been so lost in a session.

This therapist is not alone in her inward focusing. Overwhelmingly, therapists have echoed her sentiments in describing their own self-absorption and pre-occupation with the baby during pregnancy. Some therapists talk about being distracted by unpleasant sensations such as nausea during pregnancy. According to Shaw and Breckenridge (2014), therapists they interviewed reported that "managing their bodily experience and sensations took attention and care as well as managing the relationships" (p. 147). Whether patients can directly sense the therapist's lessened focus on him or her, or simply infer it based upon the therapist's status, they are likely to respond with anxiety, irritation, sadness, or another negatively toned feeling. These feelings are likely to be intensified if the therapist's self-preoccupation re-evokes memories of their mothers' pregnancies and accompanying deepened levels of self-absorption (see Balsam, 2012, for further discussion of the body image of the mother as it emerges in treatment).

Other losses also accompany the therapist's pregnancy. The patient loses the therapist temporarily or permanently as she departs on maternity leave. McCluskey's (2016) patients did not realize that her pregnancy meant that she would need to leave them, at least for a period. Such unawareness suggests that patients might exercise denial in relation to the loss, requiring the therapist to deal with the upcoming reality explicitly and early. When the therapist returns, she may restrict her work schedule and her availability by telephone (Turkel, 1993). On a less practical, more intrapsychic level, any fantasy of having an exclusive relationship with the therapist is held up to the bright glare of reality. The patient might now lose a sense of merger with the therapist via the recognition that the therapist is a separate person (Zackson, 2012). As Penn (1986) noted, the pregnancy challenges the unspoken conviction that the totality of the therapist's being is for the self. All of these losses easily provoke awareness that the patient is separate from the therapist. The pregnancy, the patient can easily realize, is the result of an event that the therapist has willed (in contrast to an involuntary event such as physical illness). Consequently, the patient more readily sees it as an active abandonment (Chiaramonte, 1986).

To a patient who is seeking an unalloyed sense of union with the therapist in order to address a developmental need, the awareness of separateness from the therapist gives rise to an array of disturbing feelings. Patients fear what catastrophes might ensue given the therapist's lessened availability during the pregnancy and absence during the maternity leave. Whereas some patients fear external harms ("I was sure something bad would happen"), others focus on internal dangers ("I thought I might go crazy"). For some patients, rage over the abandonment is the dominant affect. For others, sadness over the loss of the idealized therapist who would never disappoint the patient in this way is prominent (Penn, 1986). Guilt or shame may be intense as patients wonder what they might have done to cause this loss.

Given that these feelings—sadness, rage, fear, guilt and so on—are painful ones from which a patient might wish to recoil, their stimulation often evokes a defensive response. As Lax (1969) first observed, individuals might respond to this separation crisis through a regressive identification with both the therapist and the therapist's child. Through this identification, the patient is able to entertain the fantasy of symbiotic merger with the idealized mother figure. For example, a patient of one of the authors had had a long course of treatment during which she talked about many serious inadequacies in the ways in which her mother parented her. When the therapist became pregnant, she recognized how she was creating for the patient a repetition of many of the early abandonments she had experienced. While the therapist was pregnant, the patient was unable to focus on the parallels. Instead, she recalled a mother who was far more loving than the one she had described earlier in treatment. At the same time, she became very actively involved in the pleasurable fantasy of having a baby herself. However, as a single parent, and as someone who would not embark on a reckless course of action, it was unlikely that the fantasy would be made real in the short run. Nonetheless, summoning both the notion of a baby for whom she could care and of her own idealized mother, she was able to feel at one with a figure who would not deprive, disappoint, or abandon her. Any separation anxiety that she felt in relation to the therapist's pregnancy was supplanted by an oceanic euphoria.

As noted previously, patients' acting out during their therapists' pregnancies occurs quite regularly. The patient's identification with the therapist is one mechanism underlying the acting out. By engaging in unprotected sex and by becoming pregnant, the patient is able to identify fully with the therapist in her role as mother, carrying within her physical and psychic boundaries a child who is at once a symbol of the therapist's child and a symbol of the patient herself. At the same time that she is symbolically merging with the therapist, the patient is replacing the therapist through her baby. He or she is also diminishing felt vulnerability by becoming self-sufficient. Because the merger occurs internally, the patient protects the self from external losses, such as the loss of the therapist. The patient is thereby liberated from the need for relationships—real or internalized (Jackel, 1966). As Zackson (2012) points out, the patient is essentially substituting the wish to be a baby with the desire to have a baby.

Rather than acting out, some patients find the means to strengthen their identification with the therapist within the bounds of the relationship itself. For example, one therapist told us that when she was pregnant,

> my patients acted as if they could not get enough of me. Unlike earlier, they rarely missed a session and were never late. After the baby came and I went back to work, they resumed their old habits of coming late and canceling.

Surveying eating-disorder patients, Vandereycken and DeKerf (2010) found that by identifying with the pregnant therapist, respondents achieved a more favorable view of womanhood. Patients also fortify their identifications through the use of their customary defense mechanisms, the successful use of which spares them from a conscious experience of separation anxiety stimulated by the therapist's pregnancy. Mandy, in the following vignette, illustrates the use of a complex defensive repertoire to diminish separation anxiety:

Vignette 3.8
Upon becoming aware of the pregnancy, Mandy exhibited extreme solicitude. She was preoccupied by how "adorable" the therapist looked in her maternity clothes. At the same time, however, the therapist appeared very fragile to her, a perception that was in contrast with the consensual opinion that the therapist looked quite robust. She responded to this perception with frequent inquiries about the therapist's health. The caretaking effort was similar to that in which she had engaged with her mother after the birth of her sister. The mother had become quite depressed, and Mandy, only a young child herself, had attempted to relieve her mother of the difficulties by taking upon herself most caregiver responsibilities for the younger sibling. To do so, Mandy needed to summon reaction formation in relation to her anger toward her mother for having given birth, an event that led to the mother's unavailability. At that time, her parents and extended family members dubbed her "mommy's little helper." This moniker was a source of self-esteem as well as a community support for her use of reaction formation against loss. She summoned that role in response to any major separation challenge in her later life.

As Penn (1986) observed, individuals who have had early experiences of abandonment leading to difficulties in negotiating the development of tasks of separation-individuation often in their response to the therapist's pregnancy, use defenses that parallel those used in the early situation. Patients do so because, to some extent, the original defenses did have adaptive value. For instance, Mandy was somewhat able to prop up her own mother by becoming a mother to her. More importantly, however, she was able to identify with her mother's reception of emotional supplies and thereby to gain sustenance for herself. As Chodorow (1999) notes, for women, identification with the mother runs deeply and comes to the fore during critical life transitions such as a birth. Although identification with mother is a natural phenomenon, it can also be used for defensive purposes, as in Mandy's case. So, too, in the therapy relationship was she able to glean emotional resources by buoying up the therapist and then by identifying with the therapist's position of having received care. However, she embellished upon her work with her mother. The patient denied her anger in both situations. By using reaction formation, she was able to view the therapist as "adorable" and make her into a perfect object of caretaking. The "split" in her image of the therapist as "adorable" but fragile belied her anger; she feared her unconscious fantasized aggressive responses might damage her therapist. Hence, through use of not only identification, but also idealization, she created, at least transiently, the state of symbiotic bliss for which she longed.

Hence, the regressive swing to a state of fantasized symbiotic merger, which many patients undergo, has the immediate positive consequence of restoring or promoting a sense of well-being. Yet, for many, the fusion fantasy is difficult to sustain, as so many of the events involving the pregnancy progressively involve further experiences of the patient separating from the therapist. Most patients, despite their best defensive efforts, have some experience of loss vis-à-vis the pregnant therapist. Ulanov (1973) saw this sequence of abandonment anxiety, fusion fantasy and rejection of the fusion fantasy as providing the patient with a critical opportunity for growth. According to Ulanov, whereas the therapist's pregnancy does not create the fusion fantasy, it does activate and expose it for examination. Ulanov observed that, particularly for female patients, this fantasy is often latent throughout the course of treatment. With the inescapable recognition that the therapist has an infant (fetus), the patient is given the experiential base to abandon the fantasy of being the therapist's infant. In so doing, the patient is helped to complete the important developmental task of gaining sufficient separation from the maternal figure to be able to construct a truly independent identity. As with the therapist, such separation is achieved while maintaining connection. Hence, the pregnancy of the therapist leads, in Ulanov's language, to a rebirth in the life of the patient: the self is reborn, but in a new and healthier form.

Envy and Competition

The pregnancy of the therapist provides an exceptional opportunity for the stimulation of envy in the patient (Dyson & King, 2008; Rogers, 1994; Skaife, 2012), and this opportunity is multi-faceted. Patient's envy can be directed at the baby (or fetus), the therapist or both figures. Although a husband, wife (in the context of a lesbian relationship) or partner (in the context of a co-habitation situation) can be the object of envy, usually such figures are associated with the affect state of jealousy, which is discussed in the next section.

Envy of the Therapist's Baby

The baby is a potent stimulus for the patient's envy—that is, the patient experiences envy of the infant's position vis-à-vis the therapist (Adelson, 1995; McGourty, 2013; Wiesenthal, 2008). As noted previously, the patient uses a regressive wish to be fused with the therapist as a defense against separation anxiety. An aspect of this wish is that the patient is in the infant position, passively receiving all necessary emotional nutrients from an idealized maternal figure. It is the increasingly visible presence of the real infant that helps to expose the unreality of the patient's wish. At the same time, the infant is the fantasized recipient of all that for which the patient longs but cannot have. Unsurprisingly, then, patients can express extreme levels of anger toward the fetus in the form of a passive wish that it be harmed, an active desire to harm it, or both at different times. Such communications are most common in a highly disturbed population (Herrin, 2001). Of course, these expressions are quite frightening to therapists, so much so that some have been forced to discontinue their work with particular patients. This anger may be terrifying to the patient (Wedderkopp, 1990), particularly if he or she is unable to discriminate between verbalizing and acting out a feeling. The patient may attempt to diminish the fear of his or her aggression by punctuating hostile expressions with moments of solicitous concern about the baby's well-being. One of the authors of this book observed this contrast in an inpatient group. A particularly low-functioning group member talked about her fervent hope that the therapist would miscarry. As if this had not been said, another member proceeded to suggest that the therapist would be more comfortable if she raised her legs.

Envy rarely occurs alone. Based on the patient's developmental history, the envy toward the therapist's baby will have different accompanying emotions. For example, some patients will be struck with the insufficiency of their own parental figures by imagining the superior parenting of the therapist. In such an instance, the envy is likely to be mixed with disappointment and resentment. Other patients will be more active in fantasizing the eventual characteristics of the infant that will make the infant more compelling or endearing to the patient than the patient. Concretizing the infant may suggest that the infant more clearly has the role of a sibling, the person who will be the comparative standard for the self. It may inspire the patient to become the embodiment of the good patient in order to "best" the rival infant. The patient might also compete by becoming exceedingly needy, thereby securing, at least on a fantasy level, more attention than the infant is receiving.

An example by Underwood and Underwood (1976) speaks to the good use to which the patient's awareness of envy can be put. They described a hospitalized male patient who had murdered two male strangers and had attempted the murder of a woman. An insanity defense led to his acquittal. His work in therapy led to his awareness of having envy and resentment toward the therapist's unborn baby. He linked these emotions to his rivalrous feelings toward his stepbrothers. He realized, too, that the two men he shot symbolized the murder of his stepbrothers and that the woman he murdered represented his mother.

Envy of the Therapist

The therapist is also a major target of the patient's envy, an emotion that has many possible aspects. The patient might be envious of the therapist's sexuality, a contemporary manifestation of the little girl's envy of her mother's capacity to be sexually gratified (Ellman, 2000). For some patients, the envy may have a general character—the therapist's having something contrasts painfully with the patient's sense of deprivation (Tonon, Romani, & Grossi, 2012). For other patients, the envy is more specific: the therapist has that for which the patient longs—a baby (Katzman, 1993; Wolfe, 2013). For those women experiencing significant fertility problems, a reality component to this wish exists. One of our interviewees, who was running a group for women with fertility problems, found that many of the women in her group became solicitous of her during her pregnancy, which the therapist experienced as a defense against their envy. For some, the envy may not be of the baby but of the pregnancy itself. Mann (2014) writes about the tendency of severely traumatized individuals to look to pregnancy as an opportunity for self-repair.

Like patients who have contended with fertility issues, patients who have had losses of children are likely to experience the envy more intensely. Birth parents whose children were adopted or patients struggling with fertility problems might feel envy and other negative reactions more acutely, depending upon their individual circumstances. Wiesenthal (2008) describes the case of a woman who became pregnant during therapy and expressed ambivalence about having a child. This patient had an abortion prior to learning about her therapist's pregnancy. Even though the patient congratulated the therapist, she expressed anger and missed subsequent sessions. The therapist reached out to the patient and the patient did return to treatment. Although the patient explored themes related to abandonment, it might also have been the case that the therapist's pregnancy activated that part of her that did want to proceed with the pregnancy.

This wish to have a baby is not limited to female clients. Men, too, can envy the fact that the therapist is having a baby or that the therapist is capable of having a baby, unlike himself (Diamond, 1992). The wish to have a baby does not require a great deal of maturation. This wish seems to exist on a pre-oedipal level for boys and girls (Chasseguet-Smirgel, 1984). Parens (1990) observed that both boys and girls who are approximately 14 months old show comparable levels of nurturant activity in relation to babies and dolls. Their behaviors suggest an identification with the mother's maternal activities. However, girls and boys begin to depart from one another sometime around the third year, when the interest of little girls increases and that of little boys diminishes with regard to nurturant activities.

In addition to the tendency to nurture, toddlers have been observed to pass through a period of intense genital curiosity and exhibit an interest in experiencing genital sensations that are necessarily different for girls and boys. Observations of very young children's interest in both nurturance and genital activity have led to the postulation of the existence of a pre-oedipal genital phase (Kestenberg, 1982), which has been termed the inner-genital phase. It is conceptualized as a forerunner to a developmental line of parenting. This developmental line has been studied primarily in children who have been assumed to be cisgendered (that is, where the gender assignment matches the gender). The empirical study of transgender children, whose gender identities do not match their assigned gender, would be very important, particularly given the young age at which children discern their gender identities (Moller, Schreier, & Romer, 2009).

Although envy of the therapist's success in bearing a child is quite common across different populations, it is by no means invariable. Certainly, part of the variability is created by the different extents to which the wish to have a child has been gratified in the patient's life. The authors have noticed in their own practices those individuals who are actively involved in parenting young children or who have had great fulfillment as parents are not especially envious of the therapist during pregnancy. However, for some patients, envy arises as a significant force even when the patient does not seem to have experienced any particular deprivation in the realm of childbearing or childrearing.

In our own experience and in reports of our interviewees, female patients seem to admit to stronger reactions to the pregnancy of the therapist than male patients. Generally, envy figures prominently in these reactions. Such direct expression of envy was seen in the vignette in which Laila imagined that the therapist had gotten pregnant merely to spite her. Yet, other female patients will be more similar to their male counterparts in exhibiting little responsiveness to the therapist's status. They may notice it relatively late and proceed to act as if it were a matter of little consequence to them. For these manifestly unreactive individuals, any affect that is associated with disapprobation such as envy will be subject to disavowal. Although the reasons for this atypical pattern of response are various, in many instances, this reaction is due to an impediment in the female patient's identification with her mother (Diamond, 1992; Lax, 1969), as is seen in the following vignette:

Vignette 3.9

Sherry gave no clue of noticing the therapist's pregnancy and so the therapist informed her of it at the end of the fifth month. Her response was polite, congratulatory, but largely, indifferent. Shortly thereafter, Sherry showed a rather sudden interest in her own career. She sent out a salvo of applications and began interviewing at a furious pace. In her sessions, she spoke excitedly of her interviews, making comparisons of her different opportunities while expressing dissatisfaction over her current job, where she, according to her, was not able to "get ahead." As the pregnancy advanced, Sherry expressed some incredulity that the therapist could continue to manage the professional and personal aspects of her life, with a hint that the therapist's being fettered by the latter was to the therapist's misfortune. Sherry described her mother as a narcissistic person, who, as Sherry was growing up, competed with her in whatever area Sherry involved herself at the moment. Whether in painting, cooking, or horseback riding, Sherry's accomplishments were followed by her mother's intense pursuit of recognition in those very areas. Her mother presented her own efforts as motivated by the wish to be Sherry's buddy, to share her interests.

The relationship between Sherry and her mother entailed an identificatory failure. Because of the mother's need to be the recipient of narcissistic supplies, the mother's engagement in maternal activities was extremely limited and her maternal identity was weak. Sherry's effort was always carve out for herself some area on which her mother could not encroach. Within therapy, Sherry responded similarly by establishing a clear differentiation between herself and the therapist, as the therapist's role as mother was underscored by the pregnancy.

In this case, Sherry was not able to experience envy until she had addressed her identificatory problems with her mother sufficiently to be able to establish an identification with the therapist as a woman. In fact, this step was not taken until well after the therapist had returned from her maternity leave. In this case, and in other cases (e.g., Al-Mateen, 1991) described in the literature, the crucial work in the patient's treatment did not occur during the therapist's pregnancy itself. Some patients need the security of having the therapist back from the maternity leave and available in the foreseeable future to engage in certain types of work. Other patients might benefit from the increased understanding of patients therapists see as bringing to their work (Zackson, 2012). For Sherry, the pregnancy enabled the flowering of critical themes whose identification and eventual (postpartum) exploration enhanced the patient's well-being immeasurably.

Sexuality and Jealousy

When the therapist announces her pregnancy to the patient, she presents the patient with two pieces of reality that are especially provocative. The first is that she is a sexual being, a person who engages in sexual activity (Penn, 1986; Turkey, 1993; Zackson, 2012). In this age of assisted reproductive technology, the possibility exists that the therapist's pregnancy did not result from intercourse. Although some patients may consider this pregnancy trajectory, any pregnancy is nonetheless likely to be evocative of the mother–father representation. As Silverman (2001, p. 49) writes, "Pregnancy is psychically linked to heterosexual sex." At some later time, the patient may learn—through the therapist's intentional disclosure or some other means—that the therapist resides in some other family configuration. This discovery will prompt another set of reactions, depending upon the patient's own situation and dynamic issues. For example, a newspaper announcement of the birth may reveal that the therapist's baby has two mothers, leading the patient to infer that the therapist is in a lesbian relationship. Silverman (2001) documents a case in which a heterosexual patient's exploring the possibility of the therapist's lesbian identity led to the deepening of the therapeutic relationship.

Patients are likely to be unsettled, to varying extents, by their realization of the therapist's status as a sexual being. Up until this point, their defenses might have enabled them to regard the therapist as asexual, someone whose relationships for all intents and purposes are restricted to the confines of the therapy space and perhaps to the patient himself or herself. While in some cases the patient will continue to exert himself or herself even in the face of a discrepant reality, in others the patient will incorporate the new information into his or her schema of the therapist. The perception of the therapist as a sexual being may stimulate, or lead to the intensification of, an erotic transference, especially in male patients (Fenster, 1983; Pielack, 1989). The following vignette, contributed by one of our interviewees, illustrates this phenomenon:

Vignette 3.10
In the last trimester of my pregnancy, one of the members of my outpatient psychotherapy group realized that he'd been waiting for years to have sex with me. Once I got pregnant, he got in touch with it. For years, he was complaining that nothing was happening in treatment and he acted out a lot. . . . The group helped him to talk about it.

Sexual feelings may be expressed directly, as in this case, or indirectly (i.e., through derivatives). As an illustration of the latter, Pielack (1989) discussed the case of an adolescent male who became preoccupied with the physical characteristics of the ideal female during his therapist's pregnancy. Some patients may find sexual impulses toward the therapist to be so threatening that they express them neither directly nor derivatively and become more defensive than during other periods of the treatment. That is, the patient may be less inclined than usual to reveal anything of an erotic nature as it pertains to the therapist—or, in some cases, to anyone else. Whether the patient responds directly, indirectly or not at all, valuable information is frequently obtained during this period about the patient's attitudes toward sexuality.

Jealousy is another feeling stimulated by the therapist's pregnancy: it is evoked by the patient's awareness of the therapist's engagement in an intimate relationship outside of the treatment. In this context, we are using Klein's (1975) distinction between envy and jealousy. Whereas envy is a feeling arising in a dyadic situation, jealousy requires three players. From a psychodynamic perspective, the prominent emergence of jealousy in response to the therapist's pregnancy generally points to the activation of Oedipal issues. The patient becomes the child, who realizes that either from the girl's perspective, only the mother can be impregnated by the father, or from the boy's, only the father can impregnate the mother. These notions are likely less applicable to gay and lesbian children. Instead, as Goldsmith (2001) and Isay (1996) posit, the homosexual child may have, during the Oedipal period, an attraction to the same-sex parent. Although the child's position in the Oedipal situation may later affect the texture of the patient's affective response—for example, whether the patient feels a rivalry with the pregnant therapist—still in both heterosexual and non-heterosexual relationships, room for jealousy exists.

Some patients, particularly those with a history of sexual trauma, might experience knowledge of the therapist's outside relations as akin to witnessing a primal scene, an event of being excessively stimulated by parental figures. Upon this discovery, the boundaries that once created a sense of safety in the therapy relationship might no longer be perceptible. In order to re-establish them, the patient may attempt to cross other boundaries, such as asking the therapist highly personal questions about the pregnancy, thereby forcing the therapist to set limits

(Uyehara et al., 1995). One of our interviewees described a psychotherapy group she led in which the members were, for the first time, discussing her pregnancy, albeit in a very delicate fashion. One male member who spoke very infrequently blurted out the question, "Are you going to have the child naturally?" The therapist was stunned, as were the other group members, and his comment had the effect of suppressing the discussion altogether. The therapist reflected that unconsciously, the achievement of this end might have been his motive. Had the therapist been fully aware of the member's anxiety, she could have empathized with it in a way that woul 9d have helped the patient look at the significance of his question and even reality test whether the important boundaries of the group had truly dissolved. For other patients, witnessing the primal scene might constitute a gratification of the patient's voyeuristic impulses, a gratification that may or may not meet with disapproval from the patient's superego.

The patient's jealousy, from psychodynamic and non-psychodynamic per-spectives, may not be most accurately or productively understood within an Oedipal or primal scene framework. Instead, the therapist may choose to work with the more experience–near formulation of the patient's being shut out—a third wheel—in another's exclusive relationship. Most major theoret-ical orientations provide the therapist with assistance in understanding the patient's jealousy and helping him or her to address it. For example, within cognitive-behavioral therapy, jealousy is understood as "angry, agitated worry" over a threat to a valued relationship (Leahy & Tirch, 2008, p. 19). Within this framework, the perceived threat, particularly for individuals whose experiences of jealousy are intense and frequent, is associated with emotional schema such as "I will always be alone" or "I am a worthless person" or "I am a bad person for feeling jealousy." The cognitive-behavioral approach provides a plenitude of strategies such as helping members to tolerate uncertainty in relationships—an uncertainty that they believe their jealous worry may eradicate—through such techniques as validating the feeling while inquiring about its extremity, increas-ing tolerance of uncertainty in relationships, mindfulness and examining the emotional schemas linked to the jealousy, to name a few (Leahy & Tirch, 2008).

Practical Implications

- During pregnancy, therapists might encounter patient reactions that are more intense than at any other time in treatment. Therapists who can recognize the likelihood of strong reactions are likely to be better situated to respond to those reactions with empathy and attunement.
- Therapists must keep in mind that these reactions, whether intense or mild, have many roots, including the real relationship and the concerns and con-flicts that bring the patient to treatment.
- Distinguishing the type of reaction the patient is having aids the therapist in using the reaction and its analysis to nurture the patient's growth because it enables the therapist to plan potentially helpful interventions.

- Therapists can distinguish between various types of patient reactions by attention to the structure of the patient's response and the thematic content.
- Therapists are well served by welcoming the client's expressions of feelings and thoughts about the pregnancy. As Ellman (2011) notes, the therapist can have a chilling effect on client's communication if she takes a highly non-disclosive (and possibly self-protective) stance vis-à-vis the pregnancy, specifically, and her person, in general.

CHAPTER 4

Therapist Reactions

In tandem with the discussion of patients' transferences to alterations in the therapeutic frame, we now explore the pregnant therapist's reactions to the changing therapeutic process. Consider these two contrasting examples. In the following vignette, we find a therapist whose sanguine perspective might have led her to overlook some important patient reactions.

Vignette 4.1

One therapist reported that she had had a wonderful pregnancy. She had been extremely excited about having a baby and could not recall any negative reactions that her patients had while she was pregnant the year before. As she saw it, her outpatients were extremely supportive of her pregnancy. None had overtly expressed anger, envy, jealousy, or fear of her abandonment. Despite a few cancellations on her part, patients had an unusually good show rate during her pregnancy. Almost all of them had brought gifts for the baby and several times she had gotten some good advice from them about childcare matters both before and after the baby was born. She had noticed, however, that after she returned from a 4-week leave, her cancellation rate significantly increased, and that this trend continued until most of these patients left treatment and she had a significant infusion of new referrals.

This therapist's description is not unique. Other therapists have reported that their patients were "politely pleased" or articulated a rather shallow, positive socially acceptable acknowledgment of the pregnancy. Some even claimed that their patients appeared unaware of their pregnancies (Lax, 1969). Indeed, it has been suggested by others that therapists and patients reflect societal norms and may have a propensity toward denial of pregnancy and its multiple effects (McCoyd, 2009).[1] The following vignette provides an interesting contrast.

Vignette 4.2

A trainee, 8 months pregnant, approached her supervisor in the hallway with a frantic request for emergency supervision. On inquiry, the trainee desired the supervisor to transfer a particular male client to another therapist because she felt that she and her unborn baby were in danger. The supervisor was somewhat surprised. A few weeks ago that trainee had decided that 2 weeks after her delivery, she would come in weekly to see this client, although she was going to take a 12-week leave from seeing her other clients. At the time of her decision she felt that a 12-week hiatus from treatment would seriously impact their psychodynamic work together.

Further exploration revealed that the male client, in twice-weekly psychodynamic psychotherapy, had a dream in which a woman drowned her baby in a bathtub with the help of another little boy. His first association was to acknowledge a desire to visit the therapist at her home after the baby was born, as he lived in a nearby apartment complex. The therapist was extremely unnerved by this dream and the indirect uncharacteristic expression of aggression by this patient, a sensitive student in the helping professions who had no history of violence. Her anxiety prevented her from obtaining further associations to the dream. She had assumed the dream indicated that this client may not be able to contain his aggression and might physically harm her in the session. Thus, she was requesting permanent transfer of the client who had been in treatment with her for 2 years. She wondered if she and her husband should move. She expressed worry that the patient might attempt to visit her home after the baby was born.

On examination, the trainee was able to recognize deviations in her usual technique (e.g., neglecting to obtain further associations) and was able to link this to her "surprise" at the material presented by this client. Although she agreed to continue to see this client and could intellectually put her fears into a more realistic perspective, she remained somewhat uneasy, fearing harm to her baby. The supervisor found this especially interesting, given that the year before she had appeared to be undaunted by violent patients on a locked ward.

These contrasting examples, extremes on a continuum of therapist responsivity to patients' reactions, are not atypical of therapists' reported experiences during pregnancy. As we have seen in the prior chapter, patients often can have intense and primitive responses to the pregnancy or patients can claim to have no feelings at all. Just as our patients can have a multitude of emotions about the pregnancy, so too can the pregnancy create special feelings for the therapist that are sociologically and psychodynamically determined (McCoyd, 2009; Nadelson et al., 1974). These internal processes need to be acknowledged and understood, especially as they impact the therapeutic relationship. If the pregnant therapist is not aware of the effect that the pregnancy has not only on her patients, but also on her own psychology, as in the first example, she will fail to enter both psychologies into her equation of hearing, understanding and responding to her patients' concerns as they unfold during the pregnancy.

Not unlike the pregnant therapist in the second example, she may misinterpret the material that patients present to be solely a manifestation of their personal issues, and not consider the possibility that the material may be related to her own influence on the therapeutic process (Nadelson et al., 1974). Thus, she may make therapeutic decisions based on her own personal issues that may be outside her awareness. Patients may have intense reactions at a time in the therapist's professional life when she has the most difficulty processing and responding to them (Chiaramont, 1986). Even therapists with a great deal of skill might have particular blind spots around pregnancy due to the unique issues surrounding it. As Whyte (2004a) indicates, if the therapist

> can negotiate the challenges to her own pre-existing equilibrium which pregnancy confronts her with, she will be better placed to address the stormy period in therapy which her pregnancy is likely to provoke in her patients, and some therapeutic gains can be made over this phase of the analysis.

> (p. 6)

In this chapter, the therapist's conscious and unconscious feelings, impulses and fantasies experienced both during the pregnancy and on return to clinical work, and the effects of these psychological contents on the treatment relationships, are examined. The chapter consists of four sections. The first section focuses briefly on the importance of the therapist's understanding of the impact that a pregnancy has on her own psychology and that of her patients. This awareness is critical across theoretical orientations and models of intervention. Chapter 2 provides background for this section. The second section examines commonly reported therapists' reactions in response to both reality-based and transference-based patient reactions that can impede the therapist's understanding of her patient if left unchecked. Since the previous edition, a number of therapists have reported upon their countertransferential responses (Baum, 2010; Raphael-Leff, 2004; Suchet, 2004; Whyte, 2004d; Wolfe, 2013). The third section explores the therapist's recognition of her reactions as critically linked to the transference and how an awareness of the former can be used to identify and better understand the latter. Finally, recommendations are suggested to aid the pregnant therapist in recognizing her particular sensitivities to her patients' reactions.

The Influences That the Therapist's Psychology and Life Changes Have on the Therapeutic Process

The therapist's feelings toward the patient and the therapy are omnipresent throughout the life of the therapeutic relationship regardless of the therapist's personal circumstances. They exist whether they are the result of specific historic events in the therapist's past life, or the reactivation of early conflicts provoked by the therapist's psychic balance disturbance due to a changing life circumstance, or to the realities presented by the patient. The therapist's response to any physiological, psychological and/or social changes can create psychological stress and impact her functioning within the therapeutic setting.

In pregnancy, not only must the therapist manage emotionally her own changing state, but also her potentially heightened reactions to the patient's intense responses (Penn, 1986). The stress of trying to manage both may further compromise her usual effectiveness. Indeed, many authors have acknowledged that pregnancy heightened and intensified their own personal reaction to the therapeutic setting (Bassen, 1988; Lax, 1969; Penn, 1986). When an aspect of reality stimulates painful reactions in the patient, countertransference may be more defensive, and sorting out transference from reality-based perceptions is difficult (Dewald, 1982, 1994). The therapist's awareness of a gradually increasing intrusion of her pregnancy into the therapeutic field, coupled with an intensification of patient's transference, is likely to exacerbate the therapist's stress level. This is especially clear in the second example of the therapist who became terrified by the patient's reactions to her pregnancy. At a time when the therapist is overburdened with her own emotional changes, teasing out the subtle interplay of the patient's reality and transference from her own intense countertransference may feel almost impossible.

For this reason, we consider all the perceptions, emotions and responses to the therapeutic situation to be countertransference reactions. This includes those reactions that are primarily provoked by the client's contributions and those that emerge more directly from the therapist, whether emanating from hormonal fluctuations, physiological changes, unresolved intrapsychic conflicts or social role uncertainty. Although it can be useful to identify those countertransference elements provoked by the client and those more directly emanating from the therapist, we see countertransference as a phenomenon co-created by the therapist's past conflicts and present circumstances, and by the patient's own conflicts and reactions (Tyson, 1986). We view these reactions as an inevitable, inherent characteristic of the therapeutic milieu for the pregnant therapist rather than an exceptional phenomenon.

Therapists in general, even under ideal circumstances, often have a great deal of uneasiness acknowledging and are hesitant to speak openly with supervisors and colleagues about their countertransference and its impact on their clinical work (Bienen, 1990). This is particularly true when feelings are negative. The intimate nature of pregnancy, its initial secrecy, and increased self-awareness and vulnerability can exacerbate this difficulty (Fenster et al., 1986). Despite the well-respected professional literature suggesting the importance of understanding one's reactions in relation to the therapeutic process, there remains a deep-seated notion that the therapist should not feel anything beyond an interest in and a consistently mild benevolence toward patients (Loewald, 1986; Tyson, 1986). Yet, therapy is a relationship between two people, both of whom, because they are human, have feelings; patients are encouraged to have their inner thoughts unfold in therapy, while the therapist must subordinate hers to the therapeutic task.

Countertransference left unchecked can interfere and have harmful effects on the therapeutic process. The therapy in the second example might have fallen prey to unchecked countertransference if the therapist had not had some recognition of the intensity of her emotion and sought supervision. The recognition and acknowledgment of countertransference, therefore, is essential to guard against its unwanted intrusion into the therapists' interpretation of the therapeutic reality. Countertransference thought of in this way cautions the therapist to be vigilant of its influence in order to avoid distorted perceptions and ensuing therapeutic errors, thus optimizing the projective screen (Lax, 1969).

To the degree that the therapist understands the impact that the pregnancy has on her psychology, she can understand its bearing on the treatment situation. The therapist's reactions to this burgeoning life situation, as with all other personal life circumstances, is only partly the result of the actual event (Dewald, 1994). The therapist's personality, her unresolved internal conflicts, the style in which she adaptively or defensively organizes and manages her perceptions, present life circumstances and supports will collectively influence her response to her pregnancy and therefore potentially affect the therapy. However, countertransference viewed exclusively in this way encourages the therapist to strive for minimal reaction to the patient (Lax, 1969). This prohibition can result in guilt and shame, particularly when the therapist has an intense reaction to the patient (Imber, 1990). This attitude discourages therapists from scrutinizing their own responses, given that the acknowledgment of negative feelings about the therapy can potentially reveal narcissistically wounding realizations about one's competence in one's life work. This may be particularly true of the pregnant therapist, whose changing physiological status already may precipitate an emotional disequilibrium.

The recognition of countertransference is important for more than just avoidance of misjudgments and errors. As Heimann (1950) pointed out in a classic paper, countertransference is an "instrument of research into the patient's unconscious" (p. 82). That is, a true appreciation of the existence and intensity of the patient's unacknowledged negative feelings about the therapist's pregnancy can only be attained by the therapist's awareness of her own negative feelings, such as envy and hatred. The recognition of these emotions in herself "may at times give the most meaningful understanding of what is central in the patient's chaotic expression" (Kernberg, 1965, p. 40). Thus countertransference understood and used as a "clinical instrument of perception" (Tyson, 1986, p. 266) can have a constructive and creative potential for the therapy. Perhaps if the therapist in the first example had been more tolerant of her own repertoire of negative affects toward the pregnancy, she could have more easily identified these in her clients and aided in the articulation rather than the acting out of them. Learning to recognize and acknowledge countertransference can enable the therapist to use it as an emotional guidepost alerting her of the important relational dynamics and transferences. Learning to sensitively and intuitively use one's countertransference perceptions adds a valuable tool to the therapist's palette.

This view of countertransference is consistent with our view of distinguishing transferential and reality-based patient reactions discussed in Chapter 3. Some therapists' reactions are attributable to patient dynamics, some to her own dynamics, but most are a combination in the process that occurs between them. Given this, most countertransference reactions have some instructive value vis-a-vis the patient.

This chapter is aimed at helping therapists recognize and acknowledge common countertransference issues of professional identify, discomfort with personal disclosure, issues of sexuality, fear of patients' negative reactions, and issues of loss and abandonment that can occur throughout the pregnancy and once the therapy has resumed. Through examples we suggest how these reactions may operate to enhance or intrude on this unique clinical situation. If the therapist can be more aware of her own changing states and long-standing internal conflicts, she will be more available and attuned to her clients' issues as they evolve and manifest themselves during her pregnancy. We see this perspective as consistent with the view of transference that we embraced in Chapter 3, in which we distinguish between transferential and reality-based reactions.

Pregnancy: A Time of Professional and Personal Identity Reorganization

The first pregnancy ushers in a new developmental phase and a new role. The constellation of roles that previously organized a woman's life—wife/partner, daughter, friend, professional—will continue to compete for her energies and loyalty as this newly burgeoning life within her begins to assert its presence. In order for a woman to take the developmental step toward motherhood, she must modify her identity and sense of self by reexamining, reprioritizing and integrating her former roles to accommodate this new maternal role (Ballou, 1978; Fallon & Brabender, 2012).

The biological childbearing timetable frequently coincides with the formative and often intense period of career building for the psychotherapist (Turkel, 1993). Whether it be the first few critical years of an academic position or position on a treatment team in a mental health setting, or the initial phases of networking and building a private practice, the psychotherapist has considerable emotional investment in the development and consolidation of a professional competence. Just as the therapist begins to solidify her professional identity, the inception of a pregnancy challenges the primacy of her intense focus on professional goals, creating an emotional upheaval and a state of flux for the therapist's role identification. Thus, to traverse this developmental step, the pregnant therapist must learn to blend family and career roles at a personal level while continuing to differentiate and separate these same roles at a professional level (Fenster et al., 1986). As Paluszny and Posnanski (1971) expressed, the pregnant therapist is "existing in two worlds simultaneously" (p. 274). These loyalty conflicts of both mother and therapist permeate her world all through the pregnancy and long after she returns to work; they will be reflected in how she organizes her professional activities and responsibilities as well as her personal ones (Anderson, 1994). The therapist's concern and often intense anxiety about how the professional and maternal roles will co-exist, complement, or interfere with each other is not uncommon (Pielack, 1989).

Questions such as: "Can I be both a good mother and a competent therapist?"; "Will I have to give up caring for my patient 'children' in order to give my real child good enough care?"; "Can I handle the demanding schedule and logistical challenges of being both a psychotherapist and caring for a child?" confront her current defenses and role identifications (Nadelson et al., 1974). These anxieties continue to simmer throughout pregnancy. Despite careful planning and reading, it is very difficult to anticipate the effect that the birth of a child will have on both personal and professional life, until one is ensconced in the experience. Professional and personal identities are challenged throughout the pregnancy and often well into the postpartum period, as the therapist grapples with issues of self-definition and self-worth while attempting to take up simultaneously her roles as mother and therapist.

Many more professionals are returning to work full-time after the pregnancy, and this may be different from their mothers or teachers. Thus identity and role must be negotiated without the benefit of a maternal role model who remained home full-time, at least until children entered school (Laughlin, 2011). Often the previous generation of mothers had a familial caregiver available. Thus, in returning to training, teaching or practice after the child is born, emulous of a different life choice than her own mother, the modern-day psychotherapist most likely deviates from her childhood role model and cultural norm of the stay-at-home mother (Uyehara et al., 1995). In addition, following the trend of most working mothers as described early on by Hochschild (1989) in *The Second Shift*, she will likely continue to perform a significant portion of the household and childcare duties even if she continues full-time employment outside the home (Almeida, Maggs, & Galambos, 1993; Baxter, Hewitt, & Haynes, 2008; Bianchi, Sayer, Milkie, & Robinson, 2012; Deutsch, 2001; Shelton, 1992). At a practical level, the proportionately higher cost and decreased availability of affordable and responsible childcare workers compared to the previous generation makes the endeavor to accomplish both roles adequately an imposing undertaking. Thus, the pregnant therapist must wrestle with a sense of having discarded a childhood cultural ideal of motherhood in the face of attenuated household aids to support this divergence from previous generations (Uyehara et al., 1995). An aspect of this period is the pregnant woman's beginning reconstruction of her relationship with her partner (typically the father) of a co-parenting relationship. For the working woman, the father's own level of involvement affects enormously the mother's ability to fulfill both roles to her own satisfaction (Deutsch, 2001). To the extent that the pregnant woman obtains a sense during pregnancy that her spouse is not going to be as substantially present as she had hoped or as he might be, her conflict over her dual responsibilities is intensified (Hochschild, 1989).

This professional–personal crisis occurs most intensely in the primiparous therapist. Although in subsequent pregnancies, the therapist having experienced pregnancy and childbirth may be somewhat at peace with her professional–personal blend, the demands and complexities of a larger family will require some adjustment to her previously found compromise (Fenster et al., 1986; McGarty, 1988; Pielack, 1989). In fact, a number of our interviewees reported a greater ease in dealing with the demands of work during pregnancy and the demands of pregnancy during work with their second and subsequent pregnancy relative to the first.

Each therapist manages this developmental crisis differently, experiencing her own unique kaleidoscopic combination of anxieties with her previous intrapsychic constellation determining the way in which she responds to these changes. Common manifestations of how the pregnant therapist manages the professional–personal identity conflict are denial of her physical state, anxiety and guilt that she is doing an inadequate job in both the personal and professional sphere, and anger at those in the environment who have failed to make special accommodations for her.

Denial that the pregnancy has an impact on one's life and therapy is not an uncommon response for first-time professional mothers (Nadelson et al., 1974; Naparstek, 1976). These therapists attempt to maintain a business-as-usual stance. When working in an institution, the administration and sometimes co-workers collude with this by expecting the therapist to continue at the same pace prior to the pregnancy, such as taking night call or seeing patients well into the evening. (See Chapter 11 for a further discussion of the pregnant therapist's relationship to colleagues.) Pregnant therapists, similar to therapists dealing with illness and disability, often use counterdependent mechanisms to manage their anxieties (Dewald, 1994). This may be particularly true for those therapists who have entered long training programs that preselected them for traits not considered part of the traditional female repertoire, such as strength, assertiveness and independence (Goz, 1973).

Her open acknowledgment of the impact of her physiological changes on her stamina is an admission that she is not a superwoman; she might perceive her curiosities and questions about it as an assault on her competence and omnipotent fantasies that may falsely underlie her professional confidence. Through a parallel process, the lack of an open, collegial discussion is likely to be recreated in the therapeutic situation. For the psychoanalytically oriented therapist, this feeling of deviance can be especially intense, if it is seen as a violation of the professional ideal of anonymity. As is discussed in Chapter 11, the institutional disregard of the presence of a woman's pregnancy gives the message that it is unacceptable.

In the following vignette, an analytically oriented therapist gave us a powerful example of the therapist's use of denial of the impact that the pregnancy had on her, how it interfered with the therapy session, and how it perhaps continued to have long-term effects on the patient's career path.

Vignette 4.3

It was toward the end of my first trimester. At the time in addition to my full-time position at psychiatric hospital, I had a 12-hour a week practice that I usually began at 6 p.m. and concluded at 10 p.m. three days a week. The most disturbing physical symptoms during my pregnancy were nausea and sleepiness, predominantly in the first 5 months. I could not keep my eyes open, and was often so nauseated that I felt the room spinning. Often in the evening, I felt so tired that I felt as if I was experiencing depersonalization. This one particular evening, I breathed a sigh of relief as I began my last patient. I was tired and nauseated. It was hard for me to focus on the patient's words. Suddenly I felt that I was not going to keep whatever was in my stomach. With as much composure as I could muster, I excused myself and quickly exited to the bathroom down the hall in the office suite. I closed my office door behind me with hope that sound would not travel. I vomited. I took a mouthful of water, spit it out and looked in the mirror to make certain none of the fragments of my late afternoon snack were visible on my face or clothes and quickly returned to the session. I took my seat and remained silent. My patient was silently looking at the floor. Finally after about 30 seconds she asked me if I wished to stop the session. I asked her about her thoughts and she stated, "You're obviously sick." I shook my head and asked her about her feelings about my possibly being sick and what it might mean to her (the patient didn't know at the time that I was pregnant). She was silent a while longer and then stated that she was having a difficult time concentrating. The session continued with fits and starts including topics about her husband, work, her mother-in-law without much substance to each. At one point she stated that she thought I might be angry at her. We explored the possibility that she might be angry with me. One of the themes that had come up in prior sessions and continued in the next session was her desire to change her career and become a therapist.

In the next session, she stated that she had been thinking about it and wondered whether she would be able to do all the studying required. In later sessions, she eventually gave up on the idea of being a therapist, saying that she wasn't certain that she could really listen to others' problems. At the time, I felt that I had adhered to the analytic principles and not let the early months of my pregnancy affect this therapy. I felt a little embarrassed at this incident and was irritated with my body for not being cooperative with a strict analytic stance—not to have your personal life interfere with therapy. Looking back on it with this particular patient, I think that I unconsciously might have been annoyed that she had called attention to my diminished capacity to be with her in the session when I felt so sick. She challenged my feeling that I could do it all—be both a good mother and good therapist. I think that part of the patient's eventual rejection of her desire to be a therapist had to do with my inability to recognize that I was struggling with my own identity. I think that her saying that she couldn't listen to others and couldn't devote the studying time was because she felt that she could not sacrifice her own health for her patients, something that I shouldn't have been doing either! Who'd want to be a therapist if allowances can't be made when you are truly sick? I was not able to help her deal with her professional identity issues; I was too sick and wouldn't admit it.

We focus our discussion of this vignette more on the way in which it illustrates how the pregnancy can be seen as an intrusion or technical difficulty for those who rigidly subscribe to a blank screen analytic approach. The strict compartmentalization between professional and personal life that is the *modus operandi* for many therapists is not possible as the pregnancy progresses. As Waldman (2003) suggests, "The therapist should not hide behind the cloak of transference when she in fact has brought the circumstance into the treatment room in a way highly unusual for dynamic treatment" (p. 53). This therapist may have masked her countertransference by adhering to the "strict analytic stance" (Freedman, 1956). She recognized neither her personal–professional struggle nor her resulting anger, even when the patient pointed it out to her. Instead, she attempted to explore the patient's anger that was probably present as well, but was not as salient for the patient at the time.

As we see from this example, if the therapist is not aware of her own anger, then she may assume that it is the exclusive province of her patient. Likewise, if the therapist cannot acknowledge her own identity crisis, she may not be able to help her patients resolve their identity crises. This therapist's stoic stance and belief of adherence to the analytic frame feeds her omnipotent fantasies and camouflages her discomfort with her own increasing physical limitations and the emotional demands that pregnancy brings. Instead she blames herself for an uncooperative body. Uncomfortable with her own personal needs, the therapist may have perceived the option of discontinuing the session or moving it to another time as self-indulgent. Facing her nausea and fatigue realistically and allowing for needs unique to her altered bodily state, she may have equated her identification as a pregnant woman as being an inadequate therapist (Goz, 1973). Recognition of the countertransference aspects of the incident gave the therapist an opportunity to work through her professional identity issues and to explore what was so painful about accepting that she, too, is human.[2]

When a therapist denies her needs, she may counterphobically agree to even more assignments, an increased case load or more demanding patients to prove her competency (Baum, 2010; McCluskey, 2016). The following vignette offers just one of many examples that one psychologist told us happened to her in her fifth month of pregnancy.

Vignette 4.4
I agreed to take a forensic testing, which was not part of my regular practice. Perhaps I reasoned that this would be a quick and easy one. I could possibly

do more of this after the baby was born, and didn't want my referral source to think that I wasn't interested in referrals even if I was 5 months pregnant and growing steadily by the day! The reporting requirements of the case dragged on into the ninth month. I had to put in many additional evenings working on the reports. I felt overworked, taken advantage of and irritable, which affected my ability to efficiently complete the report. I felt guilty that I had taken so long to complete the case and depressed that I had to invest considerably more effort to attain my usual clarity in thinking and writing.

This therapist's desire to reassure herself of her continued professional competence backfired, leaving her depressed and facing a perceived failure. The therapist retrospectively acknowledged that she had not recognized her own internal conflicts over balancing her professional and personal commitment.

In the following vignette, the therapist was clearly more aware of the continued value of professional activities, yet was still unable to achieve a satisfying balance:

Vignette 4.5
At the end of my seventh month, I conducted a 2-day Rorschach workshop. I was exhausted and could not enjoy a baby shower thrown for me at the end of the second day. Yet, I enjoyed the admiration of the workshop participants who were incredulous that I would take on such a feat so far into my pregnancy. I felt indomitable.

In each of these examples, the therapists had difficulty acknowledging their own humanness and vulnerability, a problem not unique to pregnant therapists (Ulman, 2001). For a therapist to deal effectively with her patients and their intense feelings, she must accept that her physical and emotional state may require special consideration and alteration in the therapeutic situation (Anderson, 1994).

A variety of factors may bear on women's ways of resolving work-parenting tensions. Therapists in the prior vignettes gained a great deal of self-esteem by their professional activities; they may be reluctant to divest themselves of some professional activities because they may anticipate that their mothering role may not provide as much or the same type of gratification. This perception may be related to their experiences in their family of origin or may be impacted by the reported experiences of their pregnant friends and colleagues. They may perceive that society still defines women in terms of childcare activities, and so they need to assert their professional self, lest it die.

Perlman (1986) provided the following interesting example of how her own unconscious rejection of the mothering role played out with this difficult case.

The countertransference feeling that threaded its way throughout this case was whether or not I wanted the patient to be my baby. The major issue for her all along had been whether or not she was wanted. For me to provide a therapeutic environment for her to be able to really understand her and provide her with the proper emotional communication, I needed to want her i.e. to want to conceive her, carry her within my body, deliver her and then nurture her after birth. However, the most prevalent feeling she tended to evoke in me was one of irritability, sometimes escalating into a feeling of wanting to get rid of her. The irritability was dominant in the pre-pregnancy period; the feeling of wanting to get rid of her developed during the time of my pregnancy. These feelings came from two sources. One, the objective countertransference she induced in me was one of not really wanting her. She behaved in a whiny, cranky, critical way that evoked feelings in me that she reported her mother felt toward her. The other source came from my own past. I had grown up believing that bearing, delivering and raising a child was primarily an aggravating experience. This patient was behaving like a colicky baby, which caused me to be annoyed with her. I had believed that all infants were equally frustrating and draining, and therefore brought a great deal of ambivalence to the situation from my own history. I had the idea to some extent that getting pregnant and having a baby meant giving up my life to a parasite who would not provide any gratification. I was resistant not only to having her as my baby; I was resistant (or ambivalent) about the idea of having any baby. Initially, I had difficulty with the interpretation, suggested by the control analyst, that the patient was experiencing my pregnancy when she kept feeling that her abortion had been incomplete and that she was still pregnant. I felt that if I gave her this interpretation she would find it bizarre and ridiculous, especially because she had a tendency to be constricted in her facility with fantasy and scoffed at "unrealistic" ideas. She was always asking to know the facts. It was striking therefore that when the interpretation was presented to the patient (in spite of my reservations) she immediately latched onto the idea, was fascinated with it, picked up on it, played with it and expanded it. It was this dramatic acceptance of the interpretation by the patient that in part helped me to realize that the reservations had really been mine. I was reluctant to make this suggestion to her because I myself was experiencing ambivalence about being pregnant. It was not until I was able to make this interpretation to the patient that I was able to become pregnant.

(pp. 98–99)

Related to the fear that mothering will be less gratifying than professional activities is the understandable fear of inadequacy in the mothering role; whereas work activities are familiar, the new activities of mothering for the primiparous therapist are not. It is natural for women to seek refuge in activities that may bring reliable affirmation versus those areas in which one's views are untested. Perhaps lack of predictability also creates anxiety in the soon-to-be mother. These therapists may need reassurance in their new mothering role.

For some, the inability to come to a reasonable compromise of mothering and professional activities is influenced by the comparisons of themselves to others, including male colleagues and intimates. Grossman, in her interviews of pregnant therapists, quoted one therapist as saying,

> It's a very male orientation what working and being valued and being valuable in the workplace has to do with the amount of time you put in. But it still feels to me that I'm putzing around and I'm not particularly serious if I'm only working half time.
>
> (Grossman, 1990, p. 73)

For others, maintenance of one's identity and self-esteem requires doing things better than their male colleagues. The fantasy of managing professional activities fully and at the same time being an involved mother is a way to achieve more than the men in our lives and more than the mothers who raised us full-time.

As can be seen from the previous examples, issues surrounding the professional–personal role integration must be addressed both during the pregnancy and after childbirth if the therapist is to enjoy her new role and be an effective therapist. Part of the successful juggling is learning to cope with the inevitable and ongoing tension between the two roles. One of Grossman's pregnant therapists aptly describes this tension:

> I can't decide whether I should take the time to take notes after a session or rush home to the baby to see if he's alright. I feel so split all of the time. Nothing that I do somehow feels quite right. It's hard to find a way to integrate it all.
>
> (Grossman, 1990, p. 73)

Often therapists feel that they are doing inadequate work in both spheres (Uyehara et al., 1995). One of the authors had the fantasy that she might sidestep the entire dilemma by continuing exactly the same way with her clients and decreasing the amount of sleeping time. Those omnipotent fantasies of "having and doing it all," each without impacting the other, begin to erode as fatigue and nausea of the first trimester emerge.

At the same time that many pregnant therapists struggle to let go of professional commitments and activities, some pregnant therapists desire to abandon their professional activities almost entirely to have a more exclusive relationship with their infants. These have rarely been captured in the literature because these therapists are even less likely than ones who return to practice to take to the time to write about their experiences, given that their newfound balance is tilted primarily toward their new mothering role. Moreover, they are less likely to be available as participants in research studies on mothers who are therapists. Perlman (1986) made the point that many of us attribute pressure for women to leave their professional lives and remain at home to our spouses' demands and even to the needs of our children. However, this attribution fails to acknowledge that the pregnant therapist may want this for herself.

Some of the therapists in the earlier vignettes may have taken on too much work in order to establish an identity different from their own mothers' choices. Professional overload at this time may also disguise a wish to assume a purely maternal identity. That is, by taking on more than they could realistically handle, they could "prove" to themselves that they cannot work and take care of an infant and "must" make a choice.

Even if the therapist wishes to maintain significant professional activities after childbirth, it is important for the therapist not to deny her own wishes for an exclusive relationship with her baby. A therapist who is uncomfortable with this wish may find it manifested in annoyance with her patients when they fail to take her circumstance into consideration. For example, a therapist reported feeling vexed when a patient made emergency calls to her several times late in the evening. She thought, "How could the patient not realize that a ringing phone would wake up the baby?" By expecting the patient to intuit her situation, she avoided the guilt that might occur if she were to set a limit.

Sexuality

Before the pregnancy, the female therapist operates within the professional realm in much the same way as her male confreres. Benedek (1973) hypothesized that pregnancy for the therapist was a taboo subject because it represented an aspect of sexuality. With her capacity for childbearing realized, her gender and sexual status are potentially catapulted into vivid focus. It is in this realm of sexuality that a therapist may be uncertain about what to tell her patients about herself and her life. If the therapist is comfortable with these feelings, she can use her gender and these life events in the service of productive exploration with her patients (McGarty, 1988). If she is uncomfortable with her own sexuality or with the exposure of this intimate aspect of her life, she may be particularly troubled when patients focus on the physical changes of pregnancy.[3] The following vignette describes a supervisory session with a pregnant trainee who, after presenting the session, wanted to know what "should" be said when patients referenced her sexuality.

Vignette 4.6
A permanent staff group therapist in a day hospital setting asked a very competent advanced psychiatry resident to co-lead a group. She was approximately 12 weeks pregnant when she began group. Although the resident had informed some of her fellow residents of her pregnancy, she was uncertain whether staff or patients knew. During her second session, a bipolar male patient with borderline features and gender identity issues asked her "quite out of the blue," "are you a virgin?" This resident had a very young appearance and was quite small in stature. The pregnant resident

looked quite stunned and her face became flushed. There was an awkward silence before her co-therapist, a seasoned group leader familiar with the patients stated, "You don't have to answer that." The patient laughed and apologetically said that he was joking. However, after that, the patient remained quiet for the rest of the group, somewhat withdrawn.

In exploring the incident during supervision, the therapist considered what she would have said if she had not been pregnant. She stated that she would have investigated what the meaning of his knowing this information would be. The supervisor then asked her why she would not have said the same thing in this instance. The therapist replied that in 2 months the patient would know the answer, and it was uncomfortable for her to think that he soon would know the answer. The therapist encouraged the therapist to explore other patients for whom she might have felt a similar discomfort. She was able to acknowledge that her response was gender related. Had the patient been a female, she would have not felt so embarrassed. She said, "I feel embarrassed that he will know I did it at least once."

Although there is probably little debate about the therapist's response to the question posed here by the patient, it is sometimes difficult for the pregnant therapist to ascertain what to reveal to a patient about herself. The therapist potentially missed a good opportunity to explore possible fears of gender identity or sexual competence. This resident, with a little help, was quite aware of her own discomfort and embarrassment around her "spoiled image" and issues of sexuality particularly with regard to her male patients. Like this student, many therapists report anxiety from expectations of disapproval for their overt display of sexuality (Bashe, 1989; Fenster et al., 1986). This anxiety might be even greater for older therapists, given that a delayed pregnancy is often greeted with amusement and other condescending reactions rather than the customary positive expressions (Gross & Pattison, 2007).

As discussed in the previous chapter, some therapists feel that their male patients have greater avoidance in dealing with the pregnancy than their female counterparts—they recognize the pregnancy later, talk and explore less specifically about the pregnancy, and act out more than their female counterparts (Fenster et al., 1986). Other therapists, however, report an increase in sexual material presented (Bashe, 1989; Pielack, 1989). Almost universally, the pregnant therapists found it more difficult to work with male patients in relation to the pregnancy (Walls, 2002). Naparstek (1976) found that many therapists readily acknowledge that they overlooked cues or underestimated their male patients' responses. The reported lack of responsiveness from male patients around the issue of pregnancy may in part be patients' sensitivity to their female therapists' discomfort with sexuality (Bashe, 1959; Fenster et al., 1986; Naparstek, 1976). The therapist's response, too, may be to withdraw from this exposure, as she may unwittingly underestimate the role that her pregnancy may have on her patients. This discomfort may result in neglecting the exploration of subtle transference displays.

Indeed, pregnancy infers the possibility of a sexually active woman; this realization can function as a lightning rod for the erotic transference that can precipitate transferential storms. This may be true when patients are severely disturbed (Walls, 2002). It is not uncommon for therapists to report difficulties in managing the increase in erotic transference, as Cullen-Drill (1994) did in her experience with her client's development of an erotic transference.

> His sexual fantasies involving me made me anxious because it was the first time I had experienced an intense erotic transference by a client and because I was so obviously pregnant. I felt uncomfortable hearing that he spent time thinking about me in his sexual fantasies between sessions. Some of my discomfort undoubtedly was related to my own conflicts about the compatibility of sexuality and motherhood. Undoubtedly, societal and cultural attitudes that frequently inhibit the sexuality of mothers contribute as well. My own discomfort made it more difficult for me to interpret his sexual attraction to me as unresolved oedipal strivings.
>
> (p. 11)

Common even for very skilled therapists in response to discomfort with sexuality is the interpretation of non-sexual aspects of the transference, such as the patient's reactions to the hiatus in therapy. Another defense against interpreting an erotic transference is viewing the interpretation of the transferential material as premature, even when it is quite clearly present (Goldberger et al., 2003).

To Disclose or Not to Disclose, and Other Issues of Privacy

Pregnancy is an event that cannot be obscured behind one's professional countenance. The physical changes of the unfolding pregnancy preclude therapists' opacity around this event. Questions such as how to understand and handle patients' interests in the therapist as a real person arise. Is the therapist's neutrality compromised, and "tolerance for the transference disturbed," as some have suggested? (Schwartz & Silver, 1990). Or can the event and patients' interests and responses to it be treated comfortably, as any other curiosity? Are there any therapeutic benefits to be acquired through more personal disclosures as patients' responses are actively explored? (Rubin, 1980). Or, based on the notion that the therapist's own issues should not intrude in the patient's struggles, should therapists' answers be limited to minimal information with the focus entirely on the patient's fantasies, as some of the literature on illness in the therapist has posited? (Abend, 1982, 1986; Councilman & Alonso, 1993; Dewald, 1982, 1994). Perhaps such exploration should even be more actively discouraged? Answers to these questions for each therapist regarding their personal disclosures are most heavily influenced by theoretical orientation and stance regarding transparency. There are likely to be divergent views on what and how much to reveal about one's pregnancy, with the humanists advocating more disclosure as patients' interests and needs dictate, and psychodynamically oriented therapists focusing more heavily on the meaning of the events to patients rather than the reality. However, even strict, traditional psychodynamic therapists report experiencing an internal and external push to self-disclose (Comeau, 1987; Fenster et al., 1986; Gerson, 1996; Leibowitz, 1996).

Regardless of where the therapist falls on the disclosure continuum, whether and how to directly answer patients' ostensible concerns about the pregnancy and at the same time attend to the layered meanings of this important event in the therapeutic interaction remains perplexing. Therapists' personal reactions and patients' unique responses to the pregnancy are intertwined with the "real" or non-transference patient–therapist interactions, such that even the most seasoned therapists and their supervisors struggle to tease apart these components and find the most optimal therapeutic responses (Bassen, 1988; Bienen, 1990). The scarcity of solid supervisory guidelines, pressure from the patient to gratify their curiosity, and the therapist's own internal press will likely result in enactments and countertransferential responses, either in the direction of revealing too much information or not providing enough information.

With sensitivity to theoretical diversity and recognition of the range of acceptable therapist transparency, we attempt to support the principle that disclosures should be made only with the patients' best interests in mind. Examples and instances in which therapists' disclosures were based primarily on the therapist's needs rather than on the patient's needs will be presented. These center on disclosing more than might otherwise be helpful and revealing less than might otherwise be indicated.

Self-Disclosure: When Is It Too Much?

Several studies have noted that self-disclosure among pregnant therapists increases relative to the pregnancy (Wolfe, 2013; Zackson, 2012). The therapist may disclose more than might otherwise be indicated for many reasons. We discuss three reasons that a therapist either may reveal more than is therapeutically indicated or does so prematurely: inability to contain personal excitement or exhibitionistic needs; therapist–patient role reversal emanating from desire for sympathy or wish to deflect anger; or guilt from having excluded patients from aspects of this event.

The Therapist's Excitement

Important events in a therapist's life require personal processing-—processing the day's activities—both the significant and mundane, through the matrix of unresolved conflicts and the prism of internalized relationships. Finding such an outlet for processing is often difficult for the pregnant therapist who spends her days listening to others and is exhausted by evening. Without such an outlet, it is particularly easy to understand how excitement or pride around the pregnancy can leak into the therapy hour (Fenster et al., 1986). There are some patients we "just like as people and in a way it would be fun to tell them more" (Bashe, 1989, p. 111). This uncontained desire to share is most likely to occur around achieving some new state or acquiring some new information (discovering that one is pregnant, or receiving normal amniocentesis results, discovering the baby's gender and so on). Cullen-Drill (1994) gives us this example in her therapy with Marie, a depressed, anxious widow treated for severe anxiety and depression who had been transferred from another clinician who left the agency when Cullen-Drill was 13 weeks pregnant.

> Since we were just beginning our work together I decided to tell her about my pregnancy. Her response was, "Are you going to leave, too, and I'll have to get someone else?" I remember feeling startled at her lack of enthusiasm for my good news, and realized that I probably told her too soon more from my own desire to spread the good news than to prepare her for changes that would ensue. . . . Learning of my pregnancy recalled her painful feelings of abandonment, separation and sibling rivalry.
>
> (p. 9)

In this example, Cullen-Drill became aware that old traumas reawakened by current stimulus events can form potent transference reactions even from the outset of treatment. Although some have recommended that new patients be told of the pregnancy from the commencement of treatment, Cullen-Drill recognized that in this case her revelation was more to gratify her own preoccupations than to aid her patient. However, perhaps her self-criticisms of the premature disclosure were somewhat harsh and could be viewed as projective identification with the therapist's enthusiasm for the pregnancy, signaling for Marie an earlier replication of her mother's shift in energies toward her younger sister.

Even when we attempt to follow analytic guidelines, the subtleties of behavior can easily relay our underlying feelings. We know from the literature on the therapist's illness, it is easy to unknowingly facilitate our patients' acquisition of knowledge of our personal state (Schwartz & Silver, 1990; van Dam, 1987). Consider the following vignette.

Vignette 4.7

I found out that I was pregnant at the 2-month mark. Although I had not gained any weight, my breast size jumped up two notches and I achieved a temporary sabbatical from my flat-chested natural state. Although I did not need to buy maternity clothes and I did not want to, I bought several dresses that accentuated my breast size. Several of my female patients noticed, but they did not mention it at the time. They reported in retrospect that this marked the time when they thought that I might be pregnant. One female patient who was also flat-chested some weeks later began talking about being envious of me because of my seemingly perfect life. We did not get too far then, because I was unaware of what had provoked the competition between us and had focused on other things such as having completed my training (she was still in school) and her envy of "my perfect marriage" (she was having marital difficulties). Those differences existed, but were not the most salient for her at the time. Although she did mention something about me having a perfect body, I did not pick up on it because I was not ready to reveal my pregnant state. I put this patient in a difficult spot, because in retrospect I wanted to celebrate my new status but was unwilling to openly reveal it. I don't know what I could have done because I was unaware of the impact of my changing wardrobes, except to confine my new clothes to weekend use. What I had completely "forgotten," from my previous history gathering, was that this patient had had a late pregnancy miscarriage and had significant residual unresolved grief. After my pregnancy was over, she became depressed and I, more alert to her and less to my own preoccupations, was able to help her deal with this more directly.

In this example, the therapist is aware of her own revel in her altered physical state (e.g., her enlarged breasts), which she enjoyed and even bought new clothes to accentuate. It is likely that this patient recognized the therapist's enlarged breasts, perhaps initially because of her sensitivity toward her own small breasts. She, however, could only address her observation indirectly by expressing her envy at her therapist's perfect life and mentioned her "perfect body." This is derivative of what was the more unmentionable—her envy of what was an unconscious recognition of the therapist's pregnancy. The patient, who perhaps wanted to be a good patient, judged that the therapist was not ready to address this deeper concern directly, and so mentions it more indirectly. Her pain and loss were too great, her depression too deep and she could only go further when the therapist was more attuned to her grief. Following the return to work after the pregnancy, the therapist was in a much better position to be empathic to her patient's pain. The therapist, more secure in her personal situation, no longer had to defend against the anxieties of miscarriage. This patient was quite sensitive to the therapist's state. Had the patient attempted to address this lack of attunement at the time of the preceding interaction, she may have experienced further frustration and may have been forced to abandon her image of her sensitive and empathic therapist.

Role Reversal

Abend (1982) asserted that the revelation of information about an illness can sometimes be motivated by a desire for sympathy or a deflection of anger. The pregnant therapist can likewise be motivated. Although specific disclosures may evoke sympathy or deflect anger, increasing and ongoing personal disclosures have the gradual and cumulative effect of reversing roles. As McCluskey (2016) wrote, "The therapist's pregnancy can be evocative of that need for a sense of the maternal in all people and it can be a chance for the client to feel more included" (p. 7). Goz (1973) provides an interesting example of this phenomenon. Both Goz and her patient were pregnant, with her patient being 4 months ahead of her. During the pregnancy, she reported her patient's expression of pleasure at their similar states and a mutual sharing of experiences (e.g., mood swings, physical discomforts). After the birth of the patient's child and before the birth of Goz's child, her patient spoke of her childbirth and new mother feelings "in the manner of a teacher talking to a student" (Goz, 1973). In discussion of this "reversal," the patient expressed pleasure that she could return support and share knowledge; in contrast to her tentative style, it boosted her self-confidence, to feel herself an expert. At the same time, she felt guilty and pushy for asserting herself and "overstepping" her bounds. Although Goz felt that although this patient realized considerable benefit from the dual pregnancies, the increased personal disclosures may have contributed to her lack of diligence in exploring the patient's resistance to dealing with the therapist's pregnancy (particularly because the patient's pregnancy was unwanted).

In the following vignette, both the deflection of the patients' anger and the desire for sympathy can be seen, as a role reversal occurs when the therapist reveals her pregnancy and loss of one of the two fetuses.

Vignette 4.8
I kept the information of my pregnancy from the group way beyond when I told other people. . . . I worried that they would feel abandoned or that they would abandon me. I just somehow couldn't deal with any anger that they might have. Before I told the group I felt non-disclosing. I had a certain amount of guilt of having my clients disclose and knowing that I was holding back from them. . . . I did share with individuals and couples that I had two embryos, but not with the group. I had been to the doctor earlier in the afternoon. The doctor told me I had lost one of the embryos and I wanted to shoot myself and I felt so sad. I went to the group right after this. I could not really think of anything else. It was at that time that I shared it with the group that I was pregnant and that I had lost an embryo. It was really strange, telling them that sorrowful thing wasn't hard for me, but telling them that I was pregnant was hard. The group responded compassionately.

In this dramatic example, the therapist experiences anxiety over disclosure of the pregnancy to the group. The therapist feels guilty at having excluded them and at the same time fearful of the group's response, anticipating that they may abandon her or be angry with her. This example reveals how information about the pregnancy (or loss) can deflect the potential anger that may have been present if the therapist simply disclosed her pregnancy either in this group or earlier. It also illustrates the difficulty that can occur if the therapist has sessions directly after visits with the obstetrician. Such residual stimulation, of course, could be present for both positive and negative events. Also, the therapist's personal struggles distracted her from exploring what it was about this particular group that made her reluctant to disclose the pregnancy initially.

Guilt

This therapist also mentioned her guilt over excluding her patients when they are revealing of themselves. This was particularly difficult for her before their discovery of her pregnancy. As with the previous therapist, some therapists deal with the guilt about excluding patients from knowledge about the pregnancy by revealing more than they might otherwise reveal after the delivery. Bassen (1988) reported that several of the analysts whom she interviewed felt discomfort initially when their pregnancy had not yet been disclosed to their patients. Similarly, most analysts in her study felt the same exclusionary guilt in dealing with their patients' questions subsequent to their delivery. This exclusionary guilt may have been the basis for many analysts' very intense reactions and subsequent difficulty in dealing with female patients who were intrusive and demanding in response to the pregnancy. Exclusionary guilt may also be the basis for postpregnancy practices articulated in the literature, such as the endorsement of providing birth announcements (Penn, 1986). The unilateral distribution of birth announcements without respect for the uniqueness and unique vulnerabilities of each patient potentially undermines the therapeutic process. Similarly, Fenster et al. (1986) discussed disclosure as allowing patients to feel included in their therapists' pregnancy and its potential for strengthening the real relationship. Yet, the reality of the therapist's pregnancy is one of exclusion, particularly during maternity leave.

Other non-verbal forms of disclosure might occur, such as moving your office to one's home—not uncommon for many therapists after maternity leave. Such changes can have a negative impact on patients if they are not anticipated prior to their implementation. Gerson (1996) wrote about the effect her move to a home office had on her patient, Sara.

> Sara, the patient who had left analysis accusing me of acting in self-interest with her, returned to analysis six months later saying that the sudden change in my boundaries had been terrifying. She said the change replicated her family, where we knew there had been no boundaries. Her mother treated her like a chum and her father like a desired girlfriend. Although I had certainly understood her family enmeshment, I had not appreciated how much she needed to see me as rigidly non-revealing. This assured her that our boundaries would be maintained and that I would be different from her family.
>
> (p. 64)

In this case, Sara returned to treatment and was able to articulate her transferences, and thus work them through.

Senior therapists differ markedly on the extent of disclosures that emphasize the real relationship and the therapist's life cycle—an acknowledgment of the humanness and vulnerability of the therapist and thus, the patient. They assert that disclosure allows for role modeling and identification. Yet, why is this event considered any different for the therapist than other significant life event, such as getting married, being elected to a valued office or losing a significant person? Would a therapist be as likely to send a marriage announcement? For a therapist who has the urge to disclose more than she might feel comfortable revealing in other circumstances, exploration of one's motivations seems essential. For instance, guilt about having more, fear of envy and so on can be powerful motivators to alter one's style and level of disclosure.

Revealing Less Than Might Otherwise Be Empathic

Pregnancy violates anonymity. In other instances where the therapist's private affairs potentially impact the therapy, such as the therapist's illness, many advocate keeping information to a minimum (Abend, 1982, 1986). Although similar, the therapist's illness may not be quite analogous to a pregnancy, because in the former there may be little if any visible evidence of the therapist's state to the patient. Although some acknowledgment is necessary, there may be no other minimum disclosure required. Yet there may be times when maintaining the analytic stance provides a much-needed mask for the therapist's uncomfortable feelings. Examples of this are not abundant for two reasons. First, pregnant therapists report that their pregnancy pushes them into a more disclosing relationship. The example presented earlier in this chapter with the therapist vomiting and attempting to continue the session without comment may come closest to it. Second, because little disclosure is the norm, there is likely to be less agreement that non-disclosure is a therapeutic error. However, ignoring derivative material because one is not ready or comfortable in openly dealing with the patients' questions and concerns about the pregnancy may involve countertransferential elements. There are at least three reasons why the therapist is likely to disclose less than might be considered therapeutic: the therapist's denial of the effects that the pregnancy might have on her patient; her discomfort with the invasion of her privacy; and her protection of her unborn child. We discuss these in the sections that follow.

Denial of the Pregnancy's Impact on the Patient

The therapist's failure to introduce or discuss the pregnancy may result from her denial of its effects on her patient. This denial may emanate from many sources, including anxiety about its impact on her own life, its effect on issues of professional identity and competence, viability of the fetus, and cues from colleagues (e.g., Butts et al., 1979, Mariotti, 1993). Denial of its impact potentially protects the therapist from viewing herself as vulnerable, as Gerson's (1996) example illustrates.

> Louisa was the only patient who expressed worry about my physical health, apart from the viability of my pregnancy. I understood her worry then as related to her anxiety about abandonment associated with her termination. I interpreted this to her. She responded by correcting my interpretation, saying that she had a human concern about me, just as she would with a friend. Much later, I was able to understand my quick interpretation as, at least in part, reflecting my own denial of my physical vulnerability.
>
> (p. 60)

Gerson's patient expressed concern (with an implicit question) about her health. Rather than acknowledge the real relationship and consider disclosure, Gerson chose to interpret it. Although she was likely correct in her interpretation, the direction chosen was driven by denial of vulnerability as well.

Denial of the pregnancy's effect on patients may protect the therapist from the guilt she would otherwise experience if she views herself as pursuing her personal desires for a family without considering how it might intrude upon the therapy (Cullington-Roberts, 2004; McGarty, 1988). She anticipates that her pregnancy will have negative consequences on her patients. Therapists acknowledging the possible negative impact that the pregnancy may have on patients may feel that therapy is less than the ideal that a male colleague might provide. Numerous examples of denial are presented in the previous section. McGarty (1988) provided an example of how her denial precipitated an occurrence of acting out.

> A week after I delivered, she showed up at the office door of my home . . . she insisted on coming into the office to have a stack of insurance forms signed then and there. In a latter session, she told me her fantasy had been that I could have brought the baby into the office and done the forms while I nursed him. During the pregnancy the patient had expressed very few feelings about the pregnancy itself or my unavailability following the birth. I believe her visit to the office was an enactment of these feelings. On reflection. I tried to minimize the impact of my first pregnancy on myself and the patient. I tried also to make my gender much more peripheral than it in fact was . . .
>
> I believe that my patients' different behavior during my second pregnancy was partly a function of my doing things differently. I announced the second pregnancy earlier to anyone who had not noticed it and also announced the date I would stop work much earlier . . . and talked a good deal more in supervision about the plans I was making. In subsequent pregnancies many women find they are more focused on the children they have and plans for them, rather than on changes in themselves. My own

experience in listening to my older son's reactions to my pregnancy and thought of a new baby helped give me a vivid perspective for my patients who were struggling with these issues.

(p. 687)

The therapist's guilt and denial or minimization may increase the potential for patient acting out. What is not verbalized will be enacted (Baum & Herring, 1975). As McGarty's experience and others report, primiparous therapists utilize more denial during their first pregnancies, whereas in subsequent pregnancies, the therapist is more comfortable handling both the reality of pregnancy and childbirth as well as the diverse meanings to their patients (Nadelson et al., 1974; Naparstek, 1976).

Therapist's Desire for Privacy and Discomfort With Disclosure

For many therapists who reveal little about their personal lives, pregnancy may be the first piece of private information that the therapist must openly and actively acknowledge to her patients. Initially, this sudden required exposure of personal information and the patient's concomitant curiosity may be quite disconcerting, feeling like an invasion of privacy (Ulman, 2001). Thus, some therapists may find themselves keeping this information from patients for as long as possible. The therapist's desire to keep the pregnancy private may be subtly communicated to her patient, so that patient's dawning awareness may be attributed to other things (Uyehara et al., 1995). For example, a patient, when told of the therapist's pregnancy at the sixth month, said that she had been aware that the therapist looked heavier, but was uncertain whether the therapist was pregnant or gaining weight and did not want to embarrass the therapist if it was the latter. The therapist recognized with the help of her own therapist that it had been her desire not to discuss it with the patient both because of her discomfort with the invasion of privacy and also the exposure and uneasiness of her changing body shape. What the pregnant therapist became aware of only later was the patient's projection of embarrassment onto the therapist: this patient was acutely sensitive to her own body issues, worrying about the effect of gaining a single pound at times. This speaks to the more general issue that therapists cannot help their patients with conflicts that they as therapists cannot acknowledge in themselves.

Sometimes the discomfort is more specifically related to the potential consequences of the pregnancy and desire to have those events remain private. Haber (1992) revealed her own anxieties about patients' recognition of the pregnancy before the results of the amniocentesis were available at 16 weeks.

I was concerned about patients finding out before that time. If for any reason I had to make a decision to terminate the pregnancy, I did not want to share this with patients. . . . None of my patients noticed. . . . attributed this to my unspoken wish. Although I struggled over when and how to tell patients about the pregnancy, I did not hesitate to tell prospective new patients about the pregnancy and I referred them to other practitioners.

(pp. 26–27)

Haber articulated what most pregnant women fear—that patients will discover or want to know about the pregnancy before the therapist considers it a viable one. This is often the first time that the pregnant therapist experiences her exposure and vulnerability.

Increasing self-disclosure provides patients with an opportunity to be more giving to their therapist (Wolfe, 2013). Although some therapists are comfortable and even appreciative of being the "object" of concern, as patients express curiosity, interest and concern about health, the baby, plans and so on, some therapists are uncomfortable with this role reversal (Guy, Guy, & Liaboe, 1986). The following vignette reveals this discomfort:

Vignette 4.9

I was 8 months pregnant, feeling like a beached whale. As we sat down, I uncharacteristically plopped down with a sigh. My patient in a sympathetic way asked me if I was worn out as it was later in the afternoon. I was embarrassed that it was so obvious and that she was aware of it. I knew that my reaction had multiple meanings to her but could only feebly explore them because I was too preoccupied with my own exposure. Looking back on it, I was very uncomfortable with the switch in roles.

This vignette and the one concerning the therapist who vomited are similar in terms of the lack of disclosure. Both therapists felt vulnerable about the information that would be gleaned from them and were uncomfortable with their patients' mothering efforts.

Another not infrequent reaction by therapists is to attempt to reverse the reversal by becoming more protective of their patients (Bashe, 1989). Our therapist in the next vignette described it this way.

Vignette 4.10

I received a lot of mothering. It felt good to be taken care of. But my authority was lost and the boundaries were skewed. In private practice, they were always concerned about me. I felt uncomfortable at times with their advice. Caretaking played itself out. For example, parents would park their cars in different spaces so someone could walk out to my car at the end of an evening group. I became more maternal. I melted when these kids would come into the room. I had Erikson on my mind the whole pregnancy, thinking about issues of trust and mistrust. I felt I could not enjoy myself as a woman. I had to say, "don't worry, I will get a sub for when I'm gone."

This therapist openly expresses the ambivalence that she experienced with her patients' caring responses. At one level she acknowledged that she enjoyed the "mothering." Yet, at the same time, she felt that it diminished her authority, her ability to maintain boundaries and perhaps her efficacy. She expressed discomfort with the advice. Perhaps the mutual mothering response that it invoked in her was partly defensive, as a way to distance herself from her patients mothering her.

Fear of the patient's aggression (the result of anger or envy) and the ensuing desire to protect oneself and one's child may be another reason for therapists desiring to limit disclosure. The more general topic of this fear will be covered in the next section. Lax (1969) described how the analysts that she interviewed did not disclose their pregnancies and felt that their patients did not know. These analysts began to knit blankets or embroider large table coverings, hiding their pregnant bodies under their handiwork. Lax speculated that these pregnant analysts were unconsciously afraid of being robbed; they coped with these infantile fantasies by hiding their unborn babies. One therapist told us that she had purchased a new house with the intent to turn one of the rooms into an office. She had begun seeing patients there. However, after the baby was born, she decided not to use the space as an office; she worried that patients would glean information about the baby and her family that may induce jealousy or envy. She feared that patients may "see" or hear her child and that it would intrude into the therapy session. She acknowledged that she could not tolerate her patients' anger or jealousy toward her child, an insight that she came to much later when discussing this with her colleagues.

It can be difficult to hear derivative material if an expecting therapist feels a need to protect her born or unborn child. Etchegoyen (1993) described how her unconscious need to protect her baby from attack prevented her from understanding her patients' material. Although many therapists are willing to allow themselves to be objects of patients' intense emotional reactions, they are much more reluctant to have their children (born or unborn) be in this arena. A natural inclination to want to protect one's children makes it more difficult to handle attacks against them with equanimity (McGarty, 1988). McGarty provided this example:

> The patient arrived one day in a furious state, announcing she had just seen my 3-year-old walking with his sitter and had thoughts of killing him. Even though I did not actually consider her dangerous, I felt my whole body tense. A thought flashed through my mind, "I really don't need to do this work." As I thought my way from my reaction, I understand more clearly the fear that had been aroused in her by my pregnancy. She had verbalized one of my worst fears. My silent thought was precisely her worst fear—that I would be more concerned with my children and not be interested in treating her anymore.
>
> (p. 688)

This example provides an excellent illustration of a more pervasive issue that begins in pregnancy, but continues throughout motherhood. Through a process of projective identification, this patient's hostile verbalizations encouraged the therapist to entertain thoughts of the "rejecting" mother. In that interface between the real and the countertransference, most pregnant therapists make various assessments to commence, continue or terminate with patients who present countertransference difficulties of this sort during pregnancy and motherhood.

In summary, sometimes disclosing information and encouraging patients to discuss the pregnancy can impede the therapy. At other times, withholding information about the pregnancy and discouraging patients from discussing the pregnancy (either overtly or covertly) can detour therapy. Ultimately, the therapist needs to be attuned to her own countertransference and understand the context and meaning of the therapeutic interaction. Through this lens she must ultimately evaluate the pros and cons of disclosing information about the pregnancy and baby.

Managing Patients' Negative Emotions

One of the most common countertransference problems during pregnancy is the discomfort with patients' negative emotions; its counterpart also can involve an uneasiness with one's own negative reactions. Although troubling for the non-pregnant therapist, several factors during pregnancy conspire to exacerbate this difficulty. First, the intrusion of the pregnancy, potential alterations in frame and the realities of a therapy hiatus increase the potential for negative patient reactions. Pregnancy, as a stimulus, calls up from the unconscious primitive emotions. The capacity to comprehend and contain these negative emotions requires a healthy understanding and working through of one's own childhood experiences and difficulties, particularly those involving sibling rivalry (Walls, 2002). Second, in order for the therapist to fully comprehend the intensity of the patient's negative feelings and aid him or her in understanding them, it may be necessary for the therapist to experience in the present a similar or concordant countertransference (Racker, 1972); the pregnant therapist may find that intense negative feelings, such as hatred or envy, or destructive fantasies, are particularly difficult to tolerate in herself and her patients because of an overall increased sense of emotional and physical vulnerability and uncertainty of her capabilities (Nadelson et al., 1974; Ulman, 2001). However, she also may not be able to recognize these repressed or warded off intense negative feelings in her patients, because she is unable to tolerate the corresponding feelings in herself (Imber, 1990). This intolerance may exist because it is at odds with the burgeoning psychological/biological maternal and nurturing qualities needed to protect the developing fetus.

Therapists may be very vigilant in their awareness of negative reactions to pregnancy and recognize the importance of pursuing these affects. At the same time, many acknowledge difficulty in doing so and admit that they may be less diligent in fully exploring them (Bashe, 1989; Goz, 1973). They report feeling burdened by these negative thoughts and some therapists even acknowledge resentment toward some of their patients spoiling their joyful experience (e.g., "It was a little bit like raining on my parade," Bashe, 1989, p. 72).

Our survey of group therapists indicates that patients' anger around issues of abandonment and envy toward the fetus are the most common and difficult for them to manage (Fallon & Brabender, 2003). The literature seems to support these findings (Bashe, 1989; Bassen, 1988; Fenster et al., 1986; Gavin, 1994; Imber, 1990). Otherwise attuned and competent therapists often fail to pick up on how envy and abandonment are enacted in and outside the session.

Anger and Aggression

Therapists report a wide array of angry and aggressive behaviors expressed in response to the pregnancy. The extent to which anger and aggression are overtly expressed by the patient and heard by the therapist depends on the patient's dynamic constellation and the therapist's intrapsychic makeup, as well as her clinical acumen in exploring, containing and working through these negative feelings.

Some therapists report little overt expression of anger toward them or their baby. Although we are in no way discounting patient temperament, this lack of expression may be the result of the therapist's decreased ability to hear patients' angry thoughts. Fluctuating attunement to patients' reactions may be influenced by preoccupations with health and the baby's well-being and other anxieties. "Cooperative" patients collude with their therapists in their efforts to withdraw from threatening aspects of patients' feelings. This dynamic of cooperation in the face of one's usual intrusive and demanding style is usually only temporary behavior. Depending on how this "cooperative" attitude is attended to, it can be very damaging to the therapeutic relationship, with the patient experiencing the lack of safety and tolerance in relation to these negative affects, or it can be growth promoting, as patients begin to recognize that they can respond to the needs of others and that they are capable of caregiving behavior.

Other therapists can consciously acknowledge their vulnerability to patients' anger and avoidance (Toomey, 2011; Wolfe, 2013). Bashe (1989) indicated that her therapists reported difficulty listening to more primitive material and stories that involved health of babies and crib death. They acknowledged that they felt vulnerable and felt a temptation not to pursue these negative affects. One of her therapists described it this way: "It's a time when you don't want to particularly be the focus of someone's rage. Oftentimes where for all I logically believe that people's angry feelings can't hurt my baby I just feel sometimes enough of this" (Bashe, 1989, p. 72). For example, one therapist, in response to a patient's expression of murderous wishes toward her fetus, exclaimed, "You don't mean that"[4] (Bassen, 1988). Supervisors are particularly useful in helping self-reflective therapists to retrospectively and non-judgmentally analyze their material. For example, one of Bassen's therapists reported that she consciously refrained from dealing with derivative material related to the pregnancy until she was certain that she had a healthy, viable fetus. Bassen provided us with a second similar example regarding an analyst who moved to a larger house shortly after her pregnancy and reported that this event elicited much more envy and hostility than her pregnancy had. This therapist related it in part to lack of her countertransference around the move and did not feel the need to make it up to patients as she had with her pregnancy (Bassen, 1988). In this case, patients may have felt safer in expressing their anger and envy of a new house rather than a new baby.

Another potential countertransference response to therapist anxieties concerning expression of aggression and hostility is to present oneself as a victim. Gavin (1994) provides a good example. She explained that her late announcement of her pregnancy status was in part her fear of being a bad mother and her patients' anger and hostility, which, she recognized in retrospect, revealed her unresolved feelings of sibling rivalry, parental abandonment, envy and childhood rage. Once she was able to resolve some of these issues, she was able to tell the group. Below is the session in which she introduced her pregnancy.

> The group centered on . . . feeling that men are more powerful, whereas women are struggling to cope with their "dirty parts," unclean genitals, periods starting. . . . I felt that I was being drawn into a collusive alliance with the women. I too became woman-the-victim rather than an equal partner in my choice to become pregnant. As a victim I was more tolerable than as a possible depriving abandoning powerful mother. . . . As I have my own early childhood experience of emotional abandonment, leaving me feeling unsupported and isolated, I was thrown into powerful emotions of my own. . . . The strong parallels between my early life and that of many of the group members made me very available and receptive to their experiences, but it also meant that I had to work hard to retain my function as therapist/ container and not slip into becoming a group member. . . . At a countertransference level . . . I deserved to be punished for my poor mothering of the group. I felt that as I had so clearly experienced poor mothering myself my treachery towards the group was doubled. I felt my own lack of early mothering might mean that I could not provide this for others, a most painful dilemma. . . . As I began to accept internally that it was possible to relive the pain of early abandonment, to integrate it into my adult life, but not be destroyed by it and to integrate ambivalent feelings about mother and being mothered, these feelings were mirrored in the experiences of the group.
>
> (pp. 67–70)

This very rich description has many interesting facets. Gavin recognized how her fears of patients' anger and then expression of concern as well as her own childhood traumas of abandonment impeded the progress of the group; after she was able to acknowledge them, the group was able to follow suit. Also, not uncommon is her self-flagellating statements in which she felt she "deserved to be punished for her poor mothering." Guilt over her choice of her baby over the group may figure prominently into the psychology of her self-deprecation. This example seems to underscore that pregnancy can serve as a wake-up call that one has needs, desires and limitations that preclude one from being the "perfect" mother or "perfect" therapist. This awareness can be helpful, not only for the therapist, but also for her patients; many of them either idealize the therapist or are engaged in a battle with their own perfectionistic superegos.

Working through one's countertransference does not always culminate in accepting and encouraging the patient's primitive material that involves the baby's health, deformities, the painful aspects of labor and so on. In fact, sometimes, subjecting oneself to it plays out an old masochistic-sadistic interaction for both patient and pregnant therapist. In this next example, Imber (1990) revealed how the elements of competition, denial of aggression fantasies of omnipotence, and reaction formation meld to form a sadistic-masochistic therapeutic interplay. Mrs. A. had been in treatment for one and a half years when Imber became pregnant and was one of the first to acknowledge her pregnancy.

> After enthusiastically congratulating me. . . . hoped that I had an easier delivery than she had had. She reminded me that she had had an emergency cesarian section at a small rural hospital. They were ill equipped to deal with her blue baby born with the umbilical cord wrapped around his neck. . . . her own recovery was slow and painful, I had heard the story before in context of an unsupportive husband. Hearing it in vivid detail while I was pregnant for the first time was a new and anxiety filled experience for me. At an earlier time I had felt sympathy for her and some anger at her neglectful husband. This time I felt personally threatened. Perhaps such a grueling, frightening experience awaited me 6 months down the road. If at this time in my life someone had tried to tell me such a story outside my consulting room, I might have felt free to protect myself by stopping them. Instead, I brushed away the impulse to do this and its implications. . . . Here, I believe was an interaction between personal neurotic need to deny weakness and a more objective response to the patient's dissociated aggression. I did suggest that she felt resentful at the idea that I might have an easier time of it than she had had. While there was, of course, truth to this, it was also in hindsight, meant to reassure myself that what she angrily and enviously wished on me, in her unconscious, would not come to pass. . . . What neither of us was willing to directly confront was how much buried envy and primitive sadism Mrs. A. had been expressing by making me sit through the recounting of her awful experience.
>
> Part of my defensive posture was to deny the significance of my anxiety as well as to feel sorry anew for Mrs. A. . . . It did not then occur to me that my response was a reaction formation much like Mrs. A.'s. While one could feel sympathy for her experience at the moment I was trying successfully to detach myself from my basic angry reaction. "I don't want to hear this."

I was avoiding her cruelty and my own wish to shut her up in order to escape from it. . . . What seems clear now is that my own competitiveness was stimulated by this experience, but was not at my disposal to use constructively. Because I needed to be blind to my aggression and competitive feelings I could not perceive the full extent of Mrs. A.'s. Among other factors contributing to my avoidance was an unconscious infantile sense I had that my good fortune really was at her expense. . . . I may have been playing out my masochistic need to be punished for having a baby.

(pp. 230–232)

Although on the surface it seems that curtailing the patient's diatribe against the therapist is in conflict with the task of becoming more maternal, allowing it to continue feeds the therapist's and patient's fantasy of striving to be an all-good mother (Imber, 1990). However, this initially unfolds with an analytic perspective; we almost always have other opportunities to explore it if the patient remains in therapy. What seems too toxic for both therapist and patient during the pregnancy may gain its rightful perspective after the baby and mother have successfully traversed the birthing process. Upon return from leave, the patient brought the therapist a gift. With exploration, the patient was able to acknowledge her abandonment anger and was able to understand her wish to make amends for her envy and resentment of the baby rival. For the patient, the therapist's pregnancy had parallels to the birth of the patient's sibling when the patient was just a toddler. Imber (1990) writes:

What permitted us to belatedly arrive at a more complete understanding of the reaction to my pregnancy was the diminution of my sense of vulnerability as well as Mrs. A's decreased sense that she needed to protect me from her anger.

(p. 233)

Another common reaction to intense anger and hostility is to allow and even encourage idealization of the therapist. Examples of this include a projection of the therapist as an ideal mother (e.g., "You will be the best mother and your baby will be the luckiest little child on the planet"). It is relatively easy to endorse these responses and not to question them, especially if the therapist is struggling with her own questions as to whether she will be a good mother. The danger of using this kind of personal reassurance is that it does not address the transferential elements of the patient's communication and can mask the patient's rage and sense of rejection (Pielack, 1989).

Therapist Reactions as Information About the Patient

In the beginning of this chapter, we noted that a contemporary perspective on countertransference entails the notion that those reactions of the therapist lying outside of the real relationship often provide the therapist with information about the patient's conscious and unconscious life. Yet, we focused predominantly on the therapist's reactions as a reflection of the therapist's psychology. We have embraced this perspective because we think the therapist's high level of awareness of her own conflicts and concerns provides the best context for examining her reactions as they bespeak of her patient's dynamics. However, if the therapist ceases analysis of the clinical material at this juncture, that is, if the therapist confines herself to exploring her reactions only to learn about herself, then valuable information about the patient will inevitably be lost.

Yet, how does the therapist disentangle those of her reactions that pertain to herself versus those that refer back to the patient? If we discard the framework of a binary classification, a fruitful approach is to assume that the vast majority of therapist reactions are complex: elements within them have roots both in the therapist's psychology and that of the patient. Consider the following vignette.

Vignette 4.11

A therapist in her third month of pregnancy found herself to be unbearably fatigued during her sessions with a particular male patient in individual therapy. She was mortified by her constant yawning, which she attempted in vain to suppress. She recognized that she felt tired in the presence of many of her patients. The exploration of her response yielded the awareness that her fatigue was in part due to the physical effects of her pregnancy and in part an expression of her annoyance that she had to work during a period when she would have preferred to attend to herself. Yet, with this patient, the fatigue was more pronounced. In trying to determine why this was, she noted that the patient expressed himself with a more impassive countenance than he had prior to his awareness of the pregnancy. He droned on with little attention to how the therapist was responding to him. In one session, the therapist's yawning was unremitting. She asked him if he noticed. He said he did but it didn't matter. He was feeling too empty to care about anything that she was doing. The therapist began to recognize that it was in fact an emptiness that she, too, had been feeling as he spoke—as if his treatment did not have any significance to either of them. His acknowledgment of his reaction, as well as the therapist's resonance with it, provided a basis for a very fruitful discussion of the patient's sense of life losing its vibrancy with his father's stroke, an event that at a very young age rather completely diverted his mother's attention from him. This patient, a sensitive man, was exquisitely attuned to the therapist's degree of preoccupation, and this shift was a stimulus evocative of the pain of an early childhood wound. The therapist saw the patient's disengaged style as itself a desperate communication to the therapist about a part of himself that was of critical importance to the treatment.

In this example, the patient acted in such a way that the therapist was led to experience a part of how the patient regarded himself. That is, the therapist felt, albeit partially and imperfectly, something akin to the feelings associated with the patient's view of himself as a discarded object. This experience provided the therapist with the affective basis to delve into new dimensions of the patient's difficulties.

Racker referred to this therapist's experience as a *concordant identification*[5] (Racker, 1972). In the example, the therapist was experiencing some part of the patient that he experienced as self. In structural terms, the therapist may have been identifying with the rejecting attitude of the superego toward the ego. In object relation terms, the therapist may have been identifying with an element of the patient's negative self-representation.

Concordant identifications are to be distinguished from *complementary identifications*, in which the patient treats the therapist as an internal (projected) object leading the therapist to identify with this object. In the next vignette, a complementary identification is at play in the pregnant therapist's treatment of a depressed elderly woman:

Vignette 4.12
Joan had been in treatment 3 years when the therapist announced her pregnancy. While Joan had been passive during the treatment, at this time, she assumed a heightened level of activity, relative to her own norm. She provided the therapist with a continuous and unsolicited stream of advice. The therapist interpreted the patient's activity as defensive: She was focusing on the therapist's condition rather than herself. However, the patient continued her barrage on the therapist. The therapist became increasingly impatient and would cut off Joan's inquiries into her health, recent medical findings concerning the baby, plans for the child's care, as soon as Joan would make a foray into this area. The therapist found herself dreading Joan's sessions and despite efforts to check herself, noticed that she was responding in a very rejecting way. She also felt that Joan was sensing her negative feelings. Joan's missing several sessions seemed to her to be a response to the therapist's behavior.

The therapist entered supervision specifically in relation to this case. The supervisor and therapist together were able to see that Joan's behavior was specifically designed to elicit the therapist's negative response. Continued exploration led the therapist to develop a hypothesis that Joan's solicitude was a reaction formation to her own hostility toward the therapist for abandoning her in favor of the child. Yet, as a disguise for her hostility, the patient's solicitousness did not entirely work: The therapist experienced the patient's officiousness as a hostile act. However, in this way, the patient accomplished another psychic aim. By responding to the therapist in such an off-putting way, she well-nigh guaranteed a negative reaction on the part of the therapist. She thereby found the means to mete out her own punishment for having had hostile feelings for the therapist.

The therapist's awareness, obtained through supervision, that she was acting out a role scripted by the patient, the role of the disapproving and rejecting object, enabled the therapist to emancipate herself from the role and achieve empathy with the patient. Oftentimes, complementary identifications interfere with concordant identifications (Racker, 1972). In this case, the therapist's own anger interfered with her empathy of the patient's anger over feeling displaced. The recognition of the complementary identification laid the basis for the formation of a concordant identification that would further the therapeutic relationship rather than jeopardize it.[6]

In Chapter 3, three thematic areas were delineated, areas of conflict that the therapist's pregnancy frequently stimulates in the patient. All of the diverse patient reactions we described can result in concordant or complementary identifications on the part of the therapist. An example was given of the emergence of concordant and complementary identifications in relation to the patient's perception of having been abandoned by the therapist. According to our scheme, this reaction lies in the first thematic area of symbiosis and separation. The second thematic area, that of envy and competition, also creates plentiful opportunities for diverse identifications. Patient envy in particular can be highly evocative of complementary identifications, because the wishes to destroy the object of envy, an inherence part of the envy experience itself (Klein, 1975), are likely to be extremely threatening to the therapist who will then be motivated to defend herself against the envy. The next vignette illustrates this dynamic:

Vignette 4.13

The therapist dreaded telling Tammy about her pregnancy because Tammy was at the end of her rope with a series of unsuccessful fertility treatments. She wondered if Tammy had suspected the pregnancy because Tammy had recently taken on a captious, biting tone with the therapist. The therapist felt that every comment was challenged and criticized. However, she found that Tammy was far less wrathful than she had expected her to be once the therapist shared her news. On reflection, she realized that she had made some self-disclosures, atypical for her, about some high-risk aspects of the pregnancy. In fact, she had exaggerated the risk. In effect, her communication to Tammy was, "I'm pregnant but not really and you should be kind to me because I (and my baby) have medical problems."

The therapist recognized that she had accommodated herself to Tammy's message in such a way that Tammy was able to submerge her emotional reactions much as she had in her early family life, a life in which Tammy experienced herself as getting little assistance from her parents in learning how to manage disappointments and deprivations. Tammy had contributed to the therapist's doing so by sending a clear message to the therapist about what might emerge in the therapy relationship that would be intolerable to her.

Hence, therapist and patient participate in an intricate piece of defensive choreography. In this case, the therapist's curiosity about the connection between her self-disclosure to her patient and her apprehension about the patient's reaction led her to abandon her complementary identification with a part of Tammy's internalized relationship world. In the place of this identification, she substituted an empathic awareness of how excruciatingly painful it was for Tammy to see the therapist obtain that for which Tammy yearned.

The third thematic area delineated, that of sexuality, jealousy and the Oedipal triangle, provides another host of occasions for concordant and complementary identifications, as in the following vignette.

Vignette 4.14

The therapist felt that she had made little progress with Jim, a patient she had been seeing for 13 months. In the sessions, he spoke in a detached way about various preoccupations, such as why he could not commit himself to any of his girlfriends. The therapist perceived herself as having no relationship with him at all. She felt she was regarded by him as little more than a sounding board. When the therapist had reached the sixth month of pregnancy, the patient had not commented on it at all. However, he had never commented on anything concerning the therapist previously. She apprised him of her pregnancy and upcoming leave. His reaction was totally unexpected. His initial comment, which the nonplussed therapist failed to explore, was, "It never occurred to me that you might be married."

Following the therapist's revelation, the relationship changed slowly but decidedly. The patient took on an attitude of tenderness toward the therapist. He inquired regularly about how the therapist was feeling. His speech became less ruminative. He would share, not his feelings, but various events in his life that he thought would interest the therapist. Sometimes he would talk about politics or other events in the news. The therapist recognized that there was a defensive component to many of his conversation excursions. However, she neglected to challenge him both because she had difficulty at this time challenging any of her patients and because his heightened awareness of her seemed to be progress.

The therapist began to doubt the comprehensiveness of her perspective on him when in one session he brought her a rose and she merely accepted it. She was embarrassed to admit to herself that there was some pleasure in being given the flower. She felt "an illicit" sense of triumph in having "won over" this unavailable male. She recognized that her embarrassment signaled the importance of her reviewing the case from the period prior to his awareness of the pregnancy to the present.

The therapist wondered if she perceived herself to be another in a long line of women the patient rejected/disregarded and ultimately discarded. For reasons she did not entirely understand, the pregnancy had increased his interest in her. She guessed that the patient's awareness of the likely presence of a husband led him to assume the role of sexual competitor. In accepting the flower, in not challenging his defensive verbiage, the therapist had allowed herself to be courted. Years later, in the treatment, she understood the patient's seductions as an effort to disguise more primitive longings to be nurtured and rage over the frustration of these longings by a mother who could only nurture when she was being charmed. At the same time, through the seductions, the patient could obtain some limited satisfactions.[7]

Thus, pregnant therapists are likely to establish concordant and complementary identifications in any or all of the three areas of conflict so commonly activated during this time. As in the examples just shown, an awareness of the nature of the identification is likely to enable the therapist to use it for maximum therapeutic benefit. The first step in the achievement of the awareness is the therapist's own curiosity about her reactions, not merely as they reflect her own issues and concerns, but as they bespeak of some possibly unidentified aspect of her patient's psychological life.

Recommendations for Addressing Therapist Reactions

Pregnancy is truly a time of emotional upheaval. Drastic changes in the endocrinological balance, alterations in the body image, reawakening of unresolved intrapsychic conflicts, and changing roles within the family, society and one's profession are the contextual backdrop for ongoing psychotherapy. In addition, this overwhelming, life-changing event creates the necessity for additional accommodation and alteration to the previously established therapeutic parameters; this intrusion is likely to be resented at some level by both the patient and therapist. With that in mind, we make eight recommendations.

1. **Accepting the tumultuous nature of this life change and acknowledging limitations**. As the pregnancy progresses, physiological and psychological changes conspire to require the therapist to limit her professional activities. Early morning and late-night therapy sessions and professional events often need to be curtailed. It may be wise to knowingly reserve these times for activities requiring little attention, energy and brain power.

   Pregnant therapists may find themselves less tolerant of certain kinds of patient problems; it may be uncomfortable working with antisocial and violent patients or with patients who have abortion-related issues (Nadelson et al., 1974). Likewise, it may be difficult for both a pregnant therapist and a woman with infertility problems to work together (see Chapter 5). The therapist's empathy for these problems may be limited and the patient's envy too great to work through these issues prior to delivery. Similarly, there may be some patients that are not able to tolerate working with a pregnant therapist (see Chapter 3). New patients may not wish to begin treatment with a noticeably pregnant therapist. Not all reasons are predominantly transferential.

2. **Balancing disclosure with privacy and anonymity.** The physical intrusion of the pregnancy into the therapeutic space does not permit the therapist to maintain complete anonymity, even if she desired that. However, it is not the only circumstance in the course of one's career that may impinge on the therapeutic frame. Pregnancy provides a provocative circumstance in which painful memories and distortions concerning mother–child relationships, dependency, sibling rivalry, sexuality and loss may emerge.

Discerning appropriate disclosures may be difficult. Consider the next vignette, which provides a typical example of a therapist's verbalizations on her struggle about what to reveal.

Vignette 4.15

There was much more disclosure. It was so personal. I usually do not self-disclose to patients. It felt foreign to me to be doing this. I did want to let patients know, but felt like I didn't want to impose my stuff on the session. I thought a lot about my approach of telling patients prior to the delivery or not. I debate, still now, about when to tell my clients. Not telling is consistent with my psychodynamic work. I felt like I needed to draw boundaries about how far I'd let the boundary go. In general, there was a pattern of: How do you feel? When are you due? Do you have other children? When patients asked: "Is your husband excited?" that was too far and I would say, "It sounds like you are really curious at this and I appreciate your excitement, but I want to keep focused on you."

Many therapists may enjoy revealing their status in their private lives and find themselves in the therapy setting being significantly more self-revealing than usual and desire to be even more so (Bashe, 1989; Fenster, 1983). Presenting too much information runs the risk of pure self-gratification. It changes the focus from the patient to the therapist and may mute or distort the unfolding transference (Lax, 1969). For others, in addition to feeling ambivalent about the upcoming changes in their personal lives, they may experience anxiety about altering the usual degree of disclosure and guilt that they may be transgressing the injunctions of anonymity and neutrality. A therapist who is too guilty, fearful, defensive, inhibited, or uncomfortable to recognize derivative material patients may leave little room for patients to express their "unacceptable" emotions. Yet, too little information about oneself may be unduly burdensome for the patient. The therapist will want to scrutinize her own inclinations with regard to sharing personal information. To some extent these disclosure preferences may be rooted in the therapist's cultural background. Evidence exists that cultures vary greatly in terms of the acceptability of self-disclosure (Wellencamp, 1995). Anonymity is maintained first and foremost to create an atmosphere of safety. The "breach" of anonymity required by the acknowledgment of the pregnancy does not preclude or inhibit the patient's reactions or exploration of them (Bassen, 1988; Greenberg, 1986). A few thoughts regarding disclosure are provided here.

3. **Consider the human response**. Most patients are both curious, which is most often intrapsychic and transferentially laden, as well as caring, which is the person-to-person human response. Certainly empathy is the most important element in the therapist's formulation of her response to the patient. At the same time, it is often difficult to find the appropriate and therapeutic balance between being appreciative of the patients' genuine caring while exploring their curiosities as projections of their fears and conflicts about pregnancy and the baby (Bassen, 1988). Many feel that self-disclosure is part of being human, and certainly in the moment it may feel less anxiety-provoking to provide a reality. Although the pregnancy might intensify the real relationship, it is often not necessary to disclose more than minimal facts. In general, the consistent maintenance of the usual stance enables the patients to recognize that despite the changes, the therapist can continue to function in her empathic and analyzing capacity as she had prior to her pregnancy. Bashe (1989) noted, "The patient can observe that the therapist's concern for the baby has not eclipsed her capacity to focus on the patient in the treatment room" (p. 19). Consider eliciting further thoughts from the patient first. It will allow time to consider how important the transferential elements are and give pause to formulate a response. In this vein, it is suggested for healthier adult patients that fantasies be explored before information is given (Fenster et al., 1986).

4. **Tailor disclosures while maintaining consistency**. With regard to the amount of personal disclosure, two seemingly contradictory guidelines may be helpful. The first is principally to hold a consistent disclosure posture toward patients. Revealing many details with one patient and very little to another may signal countertransference processes. When deciding about a specific revelation, consider whether the attenuation of anger or envy, desire for sympathy or avoidance of guilt underlies your motivation. The recognition of countertransference not only indicates a personal sensitivity, but also can guide us back to the patient's unarticulated and unacknowledged difficulties. Successful recognition and management of countertransference offers golden opportunities for therapeutic work.

The second guideline is to understand the importance in modifying elements of personal disclosure based on the goals of treatment, the patient's capacity to tolerate fantasy and reality, and their specific intrapsychic constellation of strengths, traumas and conflicts. What may be therapeutic for one patient may be counterproductive for another. For example, a patient might perceive silence in response to his or her accurate observation about the therapist's life events as an earlier parental prohibition that may have the effect of unnecessarily intensifying the transference rather than resolving it (Lax, 1969). Once again, cultural factors are likely to play a role in how the patient is likely to experience a self-disclosure by the therapist. For some cultures, a personal disclosure by an authority figure may be taken as a radical departure of an appropriate therapist role. For others, it may be well within the norm. Thus, the timing of announcements and the amount of detail given will fluctuate depending on each patient's needs (Abend, 1982). Recall the earlier example of the therapist who sent out birth announcements to all her patients. One potential problem with this act is that it disregards the uniqueness, problems and ways of managing anxiety inherent to each patient.

5. **When possible, disclose information in the therapy session rather than elsewhere**. In the office, rather than in the hall, many therapists experience more control over what they reveal. It feels more natural to explore the meaning of questions. During a brief telephone conversation, or an encounter in the hall, therapists report feeling more pressure to answer questions and find themselves divulging information they had not intended because they fear that patients will experience it as too depriving if it is withheld. Bassen (1988) reported that therapists she interviewed found that most patients did not feel a need to have their questions answered once this exploration took place. Therapists should also encourage office staff to refrain from divulging information about the therapist's status.

6. **Think through possible responses prior to sessions**. It is surprising how many therapists do not anticipate how to answer questions on the phone or think through the repercussions of positive reassurance. Even with careful thought, some feel the determination of what is best for the patient is considerably influenced by one's personal experience and bias rather than a more objective rationale (Abend, 1982). If giving factual information frequently serves the unconscious needs of the therapist, then the importance of consultation cannot be underestimated.

7. **Consider consultation or supervision.** Pregnancy is likely to occur relatively early in the career of the therapist. The pregnant therapist is likely to have a smaller reserve of professional experiences on which to draw when attempting to manage both transference and countertransference elements related to the intrusion of the pregnancy into the therapeutic space. The combination of neophyte status and accommodation to the frame required by altered physical state are likely to create therapeutic complications and precipitate a greater number of technical errors than might otherwise occur. Reading the literature is important. We reference more than 20 authors who have reported on their observations, and many have shared intimate aspects of their experiences and perceptions of their errors. However, the acquisition of information is often not sufficient to recognize one's own concerns and manage the alterations that may be optimal for therapy. Indeed, consultation can be valuable in reducing anxieties and recognizing countertransference (Ulman, 2001). Many senior colleagues have lived through the process. We encountered many who have openly talked of their experiences of pregnancy and expressed willingness to reach out to their younger counterparts.

They have wrestled with many of the same concerns, such as how and when to announce the pregnancy, and they have savvy advice regarding the political terrain concerning leave. In our interviews with a number of pregnant therapists, supportive colleagues were considered paramount to their sense of overall adjustment.

Regular supervision with a preceptor who has previous experience with pregnancy issues can aid in technical decisions, such as how and when to respond to questions, how and when to introduce the pregnancy, and how to determine a termination and return date. A sensitive supervisor may also be able to help the therapist sort out her priorities in her personal and professional life as they impact and alter her current therapeutic stance. Additionally, as Etchegoyen suggests, "Pregnancy challenges the analyst's ability to hold on to the psychoanalytic attitude" (Etchegoyen, 1993, p. 147). A supervisor can help identify blind spots created by unresolved conflicts and exacerbated by the therapist's altered state, identify transferences and offer information regarding parallel processes between patient and therapist (Fenster et al., 1986).

A number of the therapists that we spoke to were unable to recall many negative reactions from their patients and were even less able to recall instances where their own countertransference may have interfered with the therapy. Some therapists we interviewed indicated that patients were much more likely to express positive reactions than negative ones. Therapists who are not open to negative themes do not hear them when their patients "talk" about them.[8] Patients, too, sensing their therapists' vulnerabilities, cooperate in not openly acknowledging them.

In the best of circumstances, therapists have a great deal of difficulty acknowledging and are reluctant to speak openly with supervisors and colleagues about their doubts and blind spots and their impact on clinical work (Baum & Itzhaky, 2006; Bienen, 1990). The private status of the first trimester and the intimate nature of pregnancy exacerbate this difficulty. Even after this initial period of secrecy, it is surprising to us how many pregnant therapists are reluctant to consult a senior colleague or supervisor. Within our own institutions we have made offers to pregnant therapists who have not availed themselves of our expertise. We suspect that some of this reticence may have to do with the therapist's fear that her questions may expose some of her vulnerabilities, inadequacies, and even a sense of wrongdoing. Therapists in general acknowledge that once training has concluded, they are often inhibited to consult a senior colleague about their questions for fear that these colleagues who may have an ongoing role in providing referrals and references, may evaluate them negatively. As discussed earlier in the chapter, many therapists experience guilt that a personal life event has intruded into their work. This "disapproving attitude" is often projected onto supervisors and senior colleagues. Fearing negative judgment, the pregnant therapist avoids a potentially helpful individual, and sometimes precipitates the negative judgments they fear (Baum & Itzhaky, 2006). Even several therapists we interviewed and some who refused interviews expressed directly and indirectly their fears of our evaluation of their work. At a deeper level, these fears stem from a multiplicity of factors including historical societal attitudes of pregnancy as something to be hidden (Barbanel, 1980).

Fenster (1983) reported many pregnant psychotherapists she interviewed felt less open, more easily criticized, more distant, disapproved of, and uncomfortable with their supervisors fearing their envy. Although understandable, this is unfortunate because awareness of countertransference reactions during pregnancy can highlight and bring into focus certain significant dynamics within the treatment and can enable the therapist to use her experiences in the service of patient welfare (Bienen, 1990).

8. **Make time for personal psychotherapy.** Pregnancy is a time of vulnerability and loss of a previously established equilibrium (Ulman, 2001). The emergence of special feelings are likely to occur in every pregnant woman, particularly if this is her first pregnancy and child. These feelings, both psychodynamically and socially determined, need to be acknowledged and understood if the therapist is to use them advantageously in her therapeutic work. Although it is not possible to predict *a priori* which of her feelings will be the most difficult for a therapist to understand or to manage in the transference, a heightened awareness can help prevent future difficulties. If the therapist can negotiate the challenges of her changing self, the physiological and psychological changes that are occurring, the conflicts it has caused and the needs that it has created, she will be better able to hear her patients' themes and concerns and resist interchanges with the patient that emanate from her own emotional issues.

   The therapist's struggle to integrate her new self and status can reawaken old unresolved conflicts around identity, fears of damage, primitive anxieties about the body, sexuality, dependency and self-esteem. Irrational anxieties and fears with regard to this new experience of pregnancy can create havoc internally and interfere with her ability to do high-quality psychotherapy. To the extent that the pregnant woman is uncomfortable with her person or cannot contain her anxieties about her new role in her marriage and new role definition, she may find it important to enter or re-enter psychotherapy. Although the old psychoanalytic literature suggests that pregnant women, because of their self-focus, are not good candidates for psychotherapy, the more contemporary literature highlights the pregnant woman's heightened awareness of repressed fantasies and conflicts and increased attunement or sensitivity to others. In fact, pregnancy may upset the previous psychic equilibrium and provide the impetus and opportunity to work through earlier unresolved psychological issues such as ambivalent feelings toward and reconciliation with one's mother, issues of dependency, self-esteem, and competence (Deutsch, 1944, 1945). While therapy will not immunize a person from conflict and anxiety, it may help with understanding and perspective and reduce intense anxieties (Raphael-Leff, 2004). If a pregnant therapist intends only to enter or re-enter psychotherapy during this tumultuous time, we believe that it is important to choose a therapist who has some sensitivity and knowledge about the impact that pregnancy may have on the therapeutic environment.

Selecting a therapist who views pregnancy as a special opportunity in many therapeutic circumstances, not just a condition to be endured, may be growth promoting. At the same time, an enthusiastic view must be tempered with an appreciation for the negative effects that pregnancy may have on certain patients and a respect for the limits that it may place on the therapist's ability both physically and psychologically. Short-term psychotherapy that focuses on the therapist's internal upheaval as well as its countertransference manifestations in the therapy may be quite useful both personally and professionally. Separating out the countertransference that can be resolved from that which cannot is a very important function that a therapist may serve. For instance, as mentioned in the transference chapter, the pregnant therapist may not be able to tolerate working with patients who are considering abortion, or who threaten her safety (Nadelson et al., 1974). At the same time, a sensitive supervisor may be able to help a pregnant therapist work through her own fears of a patient's verbal expression of violent fantasies toward her fetus so that she may be able to appreciate and help her patients understand the many meanings of this fantasy.

Notes

1. While direct expressions of anger or the desire to harm the baby are not generally socially acceptable, they are often extremely salient in psychotherapy. However, it is our contention that societal norms, even in psychotherapy, are operative and more pronounced around pregnancy than toward other issues.
2. We acknowledge that we ignore many aspects of this incredibly rich example. There were also components of a real relationship that should not be forgotten. For instance, the patient's overt response was a caretaking one. The therapist's denial of her limitations did not permit her at the time to recognize the patient's caretaking efforts. These were interwoven with transferential components in that this patient had previously presented anger at her mother for being so sickly.
3. Sometimes, the therapist has apprehension about the patient's reaction to her pregnancy disclosure, particularly if this revelation is accompanied by the discovery of her sexual minority status. This topic is explored further in Chapter 7.
4. This therapist may have hampered the patient's ability to express herself freely and openly. However, in working with the patients who are more disturbed, "you don't mean that" could be a source of reality testing and comfort to the patient who feels that boundaries between thoughts and actions are blurred.
5. Concordant identification was one in which the therapist identifies "each part of his personality with the corresponding psychological part in the patient—his id with the patient's id, his ego with the ego, his superego with the superego" (Racker, 1972, p. 181).

6. It is also possible that Joan felt excited by the pregnancy—a breath of life into her depressive/vegetative state, but that the only way Joan could express her desire to share in this experience with the therapist was through a controlling and intrusive manner. It is not clear that Joan's behavior was necessarily defensive, or at least only defensive.

7. While we primarily presented this vignette to illustrate concordant and complementary identifications around the sexuality, jealousy and the Oedipal triangle, we also want to point out the way in which the pregnancy helped to make salient and perhaps even stimulate the transference and countertransference occurring in this dyadic relationship.

8. Also there are amnesic effects that occur in the postpregnancy time period, particularly for the many negative events that occur during pregnancy.

CHAPTER 5

Difficult Issues in Pregnancy and Parenthood

Many important issues in a therapist's life are not immediately apparent to their patients. Generally, therapists do not disclose them in treatment, except after careful consideration of whether such a revelation forwards the therapeutic process. Pregnancy for the female therapist does not allow for the event to remain unacknowledged, as was discussed in Chapter 2. Beyond "normal" pregnancy, difficult circumstances before, during and after the pregnancy also call for deliberation concerning the therapist's disclosure. In this chapter, we examine some of the problems with conception, reproductive technologies, miscarriage and loss, disruption of treatment during pregnancy, and ongoing infertility and childlessness, as they impact the therapeutic process.

Some of these circumstances may not be apparent to the patient and will be discussed in terms of indirect effects they may have on the therapist and her psychological and physical reactions and availability. Other events require time away from therapy. The latter are discussed in terms of the parameters of how, when and what to disclose about these events. All of these circumstances involve threats to the viability of a pregnancy and bringing it to fruition. Thus, we begin this discussion with a focus on the meaning of pregnancy within a broader bio-psycho-cultural context.

The Meaning and Context of Pregnancy and Parenthood

Having children is ensconced in the biological, sociological and cultural structures of generations before. Many cultures such as Hindus, ancient Greeks and Navajo have fertility gods or symbols that articulate a role of hope for conception (McDaniel, Doherty, & Hepworth, 2014). It is a biological imperative if the species is to continue beyond the current generation. The importance of pregnancy and motherhood is socially constructed and valued in all societies, traditional and contemporary (Sutherland, 1997). Even as twenty-first-century technology and feminism have conspired to give women more freedom and more choices, motherhood is a valued status in current gendered expectations for women (Ridgeway & Correll, 2004). The expectation to have and raise children is so significant that parenthood appears the norm and childlessness a deviation (Ulrich & Weatherall, 2000). There is a continuous distribution among women about the importance of motherhood in their own lives (McQuillan, Greil, Shreffler & Bedrous, 2015). In a recent survey by the Pew Center of unmarried, childless 18- to 29-year-old women, 74% indicate that they would like to have children (Wang & Taylor, 2011). This desire seems to increase with age; in a large national interview survey of women ages 25–45, only 12% of non-mothers desire to have no children (McQuillan, Greil, Shreffler & Bedrous, 2015).

To have a child is part of Erikson's (1968) developmental accomplishment of the task of generativity versus stagnation. The "reproductive story," as it is referred to by Jaffe and Diamond (2011b), is often unconscious and begins in early childhood. In the *Reproduction of Mothering*, Chodorow (1978) suggests that

> Motherhood begins internally in the conflictual, intense cauldron of childhood sexuality and object relations and is over determined, filled with . . . conscious and unconscious fantasy . . . and [is] foremost a gendered bodily, object-relational, and cultural experience for women.
>
> (pp. 4–8)

Many men and women feel a pressure and responsibility to one's culture, family and ancestors to produce, educate and raise children. Achieving parenthood confirms the couple's status as adults within their extended family. With this shift and redefinition in identity often comes a separation and individuation from one's own family of origin; they experience "greater authority, a confirmation of their sexual identity, and a fuller sense of themselves as equal to their own parents" (Jaffe & Diamond, 2011a, p. 34). Extended family, particularly grandparents in waiting, express a desire for renewed purpose and definition for their lives as their responsibilities to their own children lessen. Often articulated or unspoken is the narcissistic desire of continuing the family name or line.

As siblings and friends commence creating their own families, new kinds of activities are scheduled to accommodate the new generation. These events and activities are most fully enjoyed and utilized if the couple, too, is starting a family. The couple not pursuing or achieving parenthood has less in common in terms of life experience and activities with this new emerging identity of friends. In multigenerational social gatherings, childless couples can perceive well-meaning comments about their lack of children as negative (Sutherland, 1997).

Having a child allows for re-examination and reparation of one's own childhood hurts and conflicts as the procreated child's development corresponds to these painful time periods (Benedek, 1959). Earlier conflicts and events can be processed as they remember, rethink and redo from an adult perspective those stages in parallel to their child's development. A new appreciation for their parents' motives and behavior often enables a reconciliation if a rift has occurred.

Although the parent–child bond is unlike any that they have had, potential parents often harbor idealistic views and unrealistic fantasies of the anticipated relationship with the child. For example, they can and do feel excitement in anticipating and owning projected accomplishments. In mature and healthy adults, ongoing experiences modify the fantasies to be more realistic, as their own emotional abilities to love and nurture expand (Jaffe & Diamond, 2011a). Creating a child together can bring new excitement into the relationship. The shared creation provides an additional point of history together and can deepen the intimacy of the couple.

Awaiting Pregnancy

This section describes common demographic patterns associated with pregnancy and common dynamics when a sought pregnancy is unachieved.

Pregnancy Patterns

According to the Society for Reproductive Medicine (2012), a woman is most fertile in her twenties, with fertility gradually declining in the thirties. A 30-year-old healthy fertile woman trying to achieve pregnancy has a 20% chance of becoming pregnant each month, in contrast to a 40-year-old woman who has a 5% chance per cycle (American Society for Reproductive Medicine, 2012). Both egg quality and quantity decrease with age. For men, sperm quality decreases also with age, but this does not become a significant problem until men are in their sixties. For many therapist couples, education and its accompanying responsibilities have pushed them to postpone having a family after the optimal period. The more education a woman has attained, the greater delay in becoming pregnant (Yang & Morgan, 2003). The pressures and time-consuming nature of graduate training and its concomitant financial obligations press against the narrowing window of fertility. The medical advances in fertility and the sensational highlighting of older celebrity pregnancy have encouraged an optimistic view of the time line of fertility. In 2012, the *New York Times* (Dell'Antonia, June 12, 2012) reported that rates of pregnancy for women between 40 and 44 rose 65% over the last two decades. In fact, according to the CDC National Center for Health Statistics, pregnancy rates have decreased before the age of 24 and increased in the 30–44 range in the last two decades (Ventura, Curtin, Abma, & Hensaw, 2012).

The diligent use of birth control for decades leaves one with the underlying impression that cessation of protection will result in immediate pregnancy when training and financial obligations recede. If the desire for pregnancy is achieved within the anticipated time period and unfolds without a reproductive crisis (e.g., miscarriage or involuntary prolonged childlessness), the assumptions about having children and its accompanying characteristics often remain outside of consciousness. National Survey of Family Growth reports that infertility (as defined by 12 months of actively pursuing pregnancy) has steadily decreased over the last three decades. However, 25% of the married women in the 35–39 year range and 30% in the 40–44 year range still suffer from infertility, in comparison to 9% in the 30–34 year range (Chandra, Copen, & Stephen, 2013).

Imperiled Pregnancy

When the perceived timing for pregnancy does not result or other road blocks occur, the intrapsychic social and familial meaning of pregnancy versus infertility is catapulted into consciousness. A common complaint during this time is one of isolation from social and familial groups. Couples report loneliness both outside their duo and often even within the relationship as well (Jaffe & Diamond, 2011c). Couples express that life has come to a standstill; they feel unable to move forward, reluctant to relocate, change jobs, take on new clients, or even plan a vacation. Even professional women, despite their professional successes, are not immune from the helpless feelings of stagnation. As a McQuillan et al. (2008) survey suggests, educational level is not associated with the valued importance of motherhood. Couples feel that they are not easily able to transverse Erikson's (1968) developmental crisis of generativity versus stagnation. As the time passes, doubt in one's self occurs and family disappointments fuel personal inadequacies and shame.

As a therapist, she may become more preoccupied with her "infertile" state and is potentially reactive to clients with material around pregnancy and children. Emotions ranging from elation to despair may pull the therapist's attention away from her patients, as every little bodily sensation is interpreted in terms of whether or not she has achieved pregnancy status. As the months continue to pass without successful achievement of a pregnancy, the therapist may find herself acutely attuned to the pregnancy and maternal status of her patients. She may experience a lack of empathy or envy for patients who become pregnant while in treatment. In supervision, one therapist spoke about her feelings toward an impulsive crisis-oriented patient when the patient had revealed her latest crisis of accidentally becoming pregnant. The therapist said, "I have been planning for three months to become pregnant and she (referring to the patient) without a thought becomes pregnant. Where is there justice? I know I could be a better mother than she is." Likewise, a therapist in the position of wanting to become pregnant may find it especially painful when a pregnant patient considers terminating her pregnancy, as this next vignette reveals.

Vignette 5.1

I had been trying to become pregnant for several years. A patient who had missed her last two weekly psychotherapy sessions began the session on her return by stating that she had had an abortion the previous week. I was stunned. The patient expressed concern about how I might think negatively about her because she had had an abortion. At the time, I was aware of my anger toward her. As she was giving me the reasons that she couldn't take care of another child, I was thinking, "I'll adopt your baby. I can take care of your baby." I think I did ok with what I actually said to her, getting her to explore why she thought I would think negatively of her, but I was unable to take it further. I was upset but not for the reasons she thought. I wasn't against abortion, as she thought. I was upset by the irony of my wanting a pregnancy and her uninterest and rejection of it. I felt numb and detached from my feelings as I attempted to make meaning out of what she said. I thought afterward that other things may have been happening in the session as well, but could not focus on them.

Similarly, discussions by patients of burdens that their children place on them or intolerances of children and their development is often difficult for the therapist who worries she may never achieve pregnancy. One therapist who had great difficulty becoming pregnant remarked that she felt that she had been judgmental of her welfare patient with four children. This patient talked in therapy about how she could not wait until her children reached 18, so she would no longer be responsible for them. She was planning to tell them to leave her house. The therapist (now a mother) felt, in retrospect, that she had lacked empathy for this poor woman with limited personal resources; at this point in the discussion, she could better appreciate even with only one child the overwhelming experience that her patient must have felt as she struggled to manage four rambunctious children.

As a greater number of women are becoming pregnant in their thirties and forties, this experience of "infertility" can be temporary as the couple does become pregnant. There is a group of women who for some period of time are unable to conceive, but who eventually achieve pregnancy and a healthy baby, as discussed in Chapter 2. As age is often a pressing factor, the couple with little ambivalence about wanting a family will consider moving from the natural pursuit of pregnancy to a higher level of reproductive medical assistance depending upon their personal and religious beliefs. We will return to problems with reproductive technologies later in the chapter. In this next section we consider perinatal loss.

Loss of Pregnancy

Pregnancy is achieved when the fertilized egg implants in the uterus. Medical advances have allowed women to know if pregnancy has occurred earlier than in decades past. Blood tests administered in a doctor's office can detect the increase in hCG (human chorionic gonadotropin) about 6 to 8 days after ovulation (U.S. Department of Health and Human Services, 2010).[1] The earlier one knows of the achieved pregnancy, the sooner one can begin preparing and caring for the body. It is not possible to remain dispassionate, particularly if this has been long sought after. However, with the news comes the increased chance of disappointment. With sophisticated technological options for determining pregnancy, the awareness of a pregnancy loss is also more frequent for many couples who previously might not have known they were pregnant. Pregnancy loss can be further demarcated into miscarriage, genetic terminations and still-birth. Despite many similarities among the types of pregnancy loss, there are some differences that may impact both the therapist's psychological state and the therapeutic process.

Miscarriage Is Not Uncommon

Miscarriage is defined as the unintended termination of pregnancy prior to 20 weeks' gestation. Most spontaneous losses of pregnancy are due to chromosomal abnormalities (American Society of Reproductive Medicine, 2012). With each passing week, the chances of loss are reduced. The risk of miscarriage falls with advancing gestation between 6 and 10 weeks (Tong et al., 2008). The American Pregnancy Association (2016) indicates that overall miscarriage rate is 15% for women under 35 years. Age, however, is a significant factor in miscarriage. For women who are 35–45 years of age, the rate is 20–35%. For women over 45 years of age, the rate is 50%. These figures are probably underestimates because they are derived from when a pregnancy is confirmed in a doctor's office.

For decades, it has been thought that it is primarily the age of the female that matters in achieving a pregnancy; there are many instances where men who are 60 or 70 contribute to a healthy fetus with a much younger woman. However in the last decade, paternal age has been examined in more detail. Miscarriage risk increases by 43% when the partner is 35 years old and the risk increases to 90% when the male is 50 years old (Maconochie, Doyle, Prior, & Simmon, 2006; Slama et al., 2005).

Medically, miscarriage is generally viewed as a minor emergency.

> The medical model focuses on the event as a minor mishap which can be treated (ERPC, Evacuation of the Retained Products of Conception) and cured (try again in 1–3 months). There is no mention of a pregnancy, a baby, and any element of loss is ignored.
>
> (Moulder, 1994, p. 65)

It is not uncommon for the surgeon or obstetrician to discard early miscarriage remains in a hazardous waste receptacle. The medical approach conceptualizes the miscarriage as a medical condition actively treated and then followed up to avoid complications (e.g., infections). That approach detracts from and proba-bly trivializes the complexity of the psychological and social experience for the woman and her partner.

Emotional Response Following a Perinatal Loss

The intellectual awareness of high miscarriage rate and its fundamental func-tion does not dampen the immediate emotional experience for the pregnant woman. Zucker's (2014) description of her experience illuminates the potential intensity.

> This life-threatening, heart cracking experience eclipsed everything that had come before. It was a foggy mid-October afternoon muddled by spots of bewildering blood and foreboding cramping . . . how was I to know this when just hours earlier we had seen a strong heartbeat, and all had looked peaceful in utero?
>
> I attempted to take things slowly but still "go about my day" as my obstetrician recommended, but I abruptly felt overcome by terrorizing anxiety. . . . As I started to urinate something else happened. Something even now I have trouble writing about without feeling an urge, almost a compulsion, to scream aloud with sheer horror. My baby slid out. She dangled from me mere centimeters from the toilet-bowl water. My window-clad house should have shattered from the pitch of my prolonged primordial howl.
>
> (Zucker, 2014)

The response to pregnancy loss is highly individualized molded by cultural/political, familial and individual factors. Reactions can range from normal grief to longer-term symptoms of depression to relief. The incidence of grief is unknown. Most studies agree that no matter what the circumstances, most women experience sad feelings at least the first few days after the loss. If it is perceived as a loss, the grief can be intense and equivalent to the experience after any other significant loss (Brier, 2008). At one time it was thought that the experience of loss for the couple was proportionate to the age of the fetus. However, a large population study revealed that the grief reaction following a miscarriage can be as intense and severe as it is for a woman with a stillborn child or neonatal death (Robertson Blackmore et al., 2011).

Twenty to fifty percent of women experience significant depressive symptoms in the first month following a miscarriage (Slade, 1994), and anxiety also is common (Brier, 2004). Group data show grief as gradually declining over 6 months, although it is still elevated at 1 year (Robinson, 2011). The Robertson Blackmore et al. study (2011) found that those who experienced prior miscarriage were more likely to suffer from depressive and traumatic symptoms. These were often still present years later and not diminished by the later birth of a healthy child (Kinsey, Baptiste, Zhu, & Kjerulff, 2015). The greater the number of miscarriages an individual experiences, the more serious the psychiatric diagnoses the individual is likely to receive, and the more negative her current mood is likely to be (Toffol, Koponen, & Partonen, 2013). There is also little support for the protective effects of already having a family (Slade, 1994). Degree of investment in the pregnancy and concerns about infertility are generally related to increased depressed symptoms (Robinson, 2011).Research on this topic has focused on variables that predict intensity of distress and on "managing" the miscarriage. From a feminist perspective, this has the effect of reifying and pathologizing the emotional pain of loss and subtly reinforces a blaming of the victim (Cosgrove, 2004).

In many ways, the medical management of pregnancy has changed the experience for couples. Ultrasound technology and amniocentesis, which did not exist four decades ago, have allowed women to visualize their child at a very early gestational age. Some women begin to create an identity and thus a "personhood" for their anticipated child as soon as they learn that they are pregnant. Pictures and determination of sex may foster an early physiological and psychological bonding. Possible chromosomal abnormalities and other serious problems determined only by testing the amniotic fluid are masked and recede into the background as the visual creates hope and idealization of what this child could be. The same technology that can engage couples early in the pregnancy may make them more vulnerable to the loss. The question of "who" has been lost has evolved from the previous question of "what" has been lost (Sell-Smith & Lax, 2013).

The visual image and amazing medical advances conspire to help us believe in the certainty of healthy pregnancies and babies. DeFrain and colleagues articulated this most succinctly,

> Babies just do not die anymore. Or at least that's what most of us have come to believe . . . it's not a topic of conversation when it does happen, or it is talked about in hushed tones. . . . Couple our discomfort as a society with the fact that fewer babies die today because of medical nutritional, public health advances, and a perfect setting for a conspiracy of silence is constructed.
>
> (DeFrain, Martens, Stork, & Stork, 1990, p. 90)

The "scientisation of death" has placed the meaning and practices around the loss in the hands of professionals—doctors, coroners and undertakers—with the understanding that there is a "cause" (Frost, Bradley, Levitas, Smith, & Garcia, 2007). The problem with many miscarriages is that science has failed to prevent death and other than a general cause of fetus abnormalities or "hostile environment" for the growth, most women are not able to obtain more specificity. Thus, it is an "imperfectly scientised form of death" (Frost et al., 2007, p. 1006). If science has decreased infant mortality, then who is responsible for the loss? Many women look to their own behavior, wondering if they are responsible. Cosgrove summarizes this attitude:

> In light of the way in which the medical management of pregnancy has become normalized . . . it is not surprising that women who experience such a loss scrutinize their behavior during pregnancy and engage in self-recrimination and guilt over things such as sexual activity, what they should (or should not) have eaten, or the amount and intensity of exercise in which they should (or should not) have engaged.
>
> (2004, p. 113)

More than 40% of those surveyed felt that the loss was partly their fault and almost a quarter felt that others blamed them (Robinson, 2011).

Miscarriage, particularly if one of many, can create a loss of hope and agency, aspirations and bodily integrity. It is a disturbance in self-identity. As much of the culture still views motherhood as the primary female role, pregnancy loss not only represents an incomplete femininity, but a spoiled identity. Jones (2015), using a Kleinian framework suggests that

> the dead baby inside could be felt unconsciously as a horrible confirmation and concrete proof of the strength of one's inner destructiveness. . . . the dead foetus inside the mother's body can come to represent the damaged or destroyed maternal object in the psyche. It is not difficult to imagine how this kind of identification might cement or prolong depressed feelings where they could in other circumstances have been more transitory.
>
> (p. 442)

The miscarried baby comes to represent defective aspects of the self and of the internalized maternal representation.

Many couples are cautioned to wait until after 12 weeks to inform their closest relatives and friends. Thus, the early loss is often a private one, hidden from the public or even family. In Western cultures, funeral rituals for this unique loss are limited, particularly when there may be no physical object to bury and no public recognition (Sell-Smith & Lax, 2013). The loss, neither evident nor socially acknowledged, provides fodder for a complicated grief that is disenfranchised (McDaniel et al., 2014). This early loss is even more painful if aspiring parents perceive a lack of support by family and friends who do not appreciate the significance of the events. Potential social supports might be perceived as uncomfortable discussing the loss (Frost et al., 2007). Women with these losses expressed disappointment, hurt and frustration by the responses offered by friends, hospital staff and family. As Sell-Smith and Lax (2013) noted, "Terse adages may unintentionally hurt the woman who is struggling to find her own meaning of a devastating loss" (p. 5). Those never experiencing the situation are inclined to minimize the loss ("go back to work to take your mind off it") and "unbaby" the situation (Jones, 2015).

Many women experience their grief in isolation as they perceive their partners to lack the same level or type of grief besetting them (Franche & Bulow, 1999; Kong, Chung, Lai, & Lok, 2010, in Robinson, 2011). Stroebe and Schut (1999) articulate two types of orientations to the grieving process: loss and restoration. A loss orientation, more commonly found in women, focuses on affective expression of the lost interpersonal relationship, yearning for the deceased and a life together. A restoration orientation, more frequently seen in men, focuses on tasks to be done to rebuild life (e.g., making funeral arrangements) after a loss happens. Often some vacillation in the bereavement process occurs between these two orientations (Stroebe & Schut, 1999). Couples that remain in one orientation only can feel estranged from their partner if this is not recognized. Sell-Smith notes the difference between her and her husband's reactions to their losses.

> After our loss of Magdalene, I retreated far inside of myself, experiencing a depression like I had never felt before. I was unable to look outside of my grief, stuck in a loop of depression, anger, resentment and bitterness. I forced myself to go through the motions of everyday life, but with no emotional investment in what I was doing. I couldn't tolerate being around pregnant women, babies, happy people or anyone who didn't have this experience. I didn't think that other people deserved to be happy when I was struggling with misery. While I focused on what I had lost, my husband seemed to take a different approach. He was instrumental in contacting friends and family immediately following the loss, in scheduling my delivery and in making plans to cremate our daughter's small body. When I look back on the paperwork completed during my delivery and hospitalization, I see that my husband had signed many of the countless forms. He was planning for the future, looking forward to a vacation that we had planned before the pregnancy and helping our family adjust to a "new" daily life. I was initially baffled by what seemed to be a lack of emotional reactivity, only to learn later that we grieve in very different ways, one way not being privileged over another way.
>
> (Sell-Smith & Lax, 2013, p. 13)

DeFrain et al. (1990) note in their sample of parents suffering from stillbirth loss that men and women often responded differently to the loss, wives feeling husbands are insensitive and husbands thinking wives are going crazy.

Genetic Terminations

A couple may know that there is a possibility of a genetic defect when they are aware that they are carriers. In many cases, the woman does not have any risk, but encounters problems such as being exposed to Rubella during the pregnancy, and then must consider a pregnancy termination. Finally, as is the case with many therapists, because they are over 35, prenatal testing offers the opportunity to ascertain chromosomal abnormalities. The decision to terminate the pregnancy is based upon a host of cultural/religious/familial factors and is more difficult to resolve if there is greater ambivalence about the decision. The decision to end a pregnancy is an active one that must be made quickly when the natural course of pregnancy would not have ended in fetal death, which potentially makes it more stressful than other types of pregnancy losses.

If chorionic villus sampling is performed in the first trimester, a woman can terminate the pregnancy by dilation and curettage. If however, the decision is made after a genetic amniocentesis (in second trimester), a more difficult, more painful procedure of induction and labor must be performed. As with stillbirth, the couple should be given the opportunity to see or hold the fetus. Most women experiencing this kind of termination found it to be equal or more stressful than other trauma they had encountered (Robinson, 2011).

For those friends and family who know about the loss, the couple may struggle with whether to explain the decision or pretend a miscarriage has occurred. Honesty risks condemnation by those who may not approve. If the reason for loss is not shared, the couple may receive support, but suffers alone the guilt to end their child's life. Ambivalence and second-guessing whether they could have or should have continued the pregnancy and raised a disabled child is very common (Robinson, 2011). However, unlike other pregnancy losses, statistics suggest that a planned termination of a pregnancy does not increase a woman's risk of developing mental health problems (Munk-Olsen, Laursen, Pedersen, Lidegaard, & Mortensen, 2011). At the termination, the couple should decide whether they want to see the fetus. If they decide to see or hold the fetus, abnormalities may provide comfort that a good decision was made.[2]

Thinking through and articulating what to say to family and friends, including other children, may provide prelude and practice for thinking through if and what to share with patients. There is no correct answer, and much will depend upon the therapist's proclivity and comfort in personal disclosure, the patient's conscious and unconscious awareness of the pregnancy, and the anticipation of the capacity of the patient to tolerate the disclosure or ambiguity.

Stillbirths

Stillbirth is the death of a fetus after 20 weeks' gestation (or after reaching 14 ounces). It is much less common than a miscarriage, The Centre for Maternal and Child Enquiries reports that perinatal deaths (24 to 41 completed weeks gestation) affect 0.8% of all pregnancies in women over 35, and 1% of all pregnancies in women over 40 (Walker & Thornton, 2016). Stillbirth is more than 10 times the infant mortality rate[3] (Matthews, MacDorman & Thoma, 2015). Sometimes the mother notices the lack of fetal movement, but other times the fetus is alive at the beginning of labor and dies during the delivery process. Stillborn birth often occurs after prenatal genetic testing has been performed. Personal and professional contacts are aware of the pregnancy and all are anticipating a healthy baby. Half of stillbirths occur in uncomplicated pregnancies, so most women are unprepared for the "sudden" death as "anticipation and joy are replaced by despair" (Robinson, 2011, p. 572).

Technological sophistication has dramatically changed the experience, as it often allows for an earlier diagnosis, but women must then "endure the agony of carrying a baby who is dead for a week or even months" (Cosgrove, 2004, p. 115). Little has been known about this group of parents, as much of the research in the area has not differentiated early miscarriage from stillborn death. DeFrain and colleagues (1990), in a landmark study, received letters from 550 parents who had suffered stillbirth and were then able to obtain 304 completed questionnaires from that group. The investigators learned that recovery is a much slower process than was previously thought.

In this retrospective study of parents who had stillborn babies, slightly more than half saw or held the baby after it was born dead and all were "thankful" (DeFrain et al., 1990). DeFrain and colleagues opined that if the baby was without deformity, it may give parents hope that next baby will be alive and perfect. However, it is less clear when there is a deformity. The earlier medical practice of quickly removing the stillborn baby from the mother's presence was replaced with encouraging parents to look at the baby, hold him or her, or both in part because of this study. A Swedish study suggested that stillbirth mothers who reported not being with their babies as long as they wished, were at seven times the risk for later maternal depression (Surkan, Raadestad, Cnattingius, Steineck, & Dickman, 2008). Currently, the evidence that this procedure helps parents mourn is limited (Robinson, 2011). To the contrary, a later study (Hughes, Turton, Hoper, & Evans, 2002) found that mothers who held their stillborn babies had higher rates of depression (39%) compared to those who had just looked at their baby (21%). Both of these were higher than mothers who had no contact (6%). Women who held their babies also had higher rates of anxiety and PTSD, which persisted even at a 7-year follow-up (Turton et al., 2009). They often held vivid images of the dead baby, which continued to intrude into their everyday life.[4]

In the early days after the death, shock and denial are pervasive. An inclination is present to find cause and blame. Many blame the medical team; some blame God.[5] Parents search for the why of the event, and an autopsy may provide some information, although the rate of perinatal postmortem examination is less than 50% (Stillbirth Collaborative Research Network Writing Group, 2011). However, of those who request an autopsy, it is only helpful in about half the cases (Silver, 2007).

Intermittently, more than half of parents develop irrational thoughts related to the stillbirth—the baby was kidnapped, the doctor sold the baby, it is still inside the mother and so on (De Frain et al., 1990). Although some feel an initial guilt, as time passed, more and more acknowledged guilt. After few weeks, all of DeFrain's parents reported feeling some guilt that somehow they contributed to the death. The experience permanently changed all parents, and even after 8 years many reported not feeling a happiness that was felt prior to the event (DeFrain et al., 1990). DeFrain found that even many decades later, despite other positive aspects in their lives, including healthy children, they were still thinking about the lost stillborn.[6]

This may in part be due to lack of legitimatization by society of the stillborn as a real loss (Cacciatore, DeFrain, & Jones, 2008). The lack of research specifically about this group mirrors the social environment that denies this reality. Most people do not acknowledge the child who died at birth as a member of the family. Without a social recognition, there is an ambiguity to the event, a lack of established rituals of whether this was a lost child or an abnormality to be excised. The traumatic grief has no formal outlet for mourning. In the face of ambiguity, others lack a protocol to follow and shy away or offer clichés and quick fixes. Those who perceived family support during this period experienced lower levels of anxiety and depression (Cacciatore, Schnebly, & Froen, 2009).

Based on his sample, DeFrain et al. (1990) recommends that parents who attained an "optimism in the face of despair and encouragement to reach out to others for support" (p. 99) did much better. At the same time, he also encourages friends and family to give the parents some alone time to process the events as well. Ninety percent of his parents considered the baby as part of the family and named the baby. Two-thirds had a funeral, and most felt it was a good decision. Both of these acts mark the event and person, and decrease the ambiguity for the parents and their social circle. Most were aware of a support group available to them. However, of those who were aware of support group, only 21% participated. Most who attended support groups found comfort in participation. Both husbands and wives take about the same time to recover in terms of self-rated happiness, but husbands were perceived to recover sooner.

Managing Grief

"The death of a baby is a horrendous event that generates an endless cascade of profound and essentially impossible questions" (Cacciatore, DeFrain & Jones, 2008, p. 453). Couples experiencing a perinatal or infant loss search for understanding what they have endured. Some women are able to "recover" without a long period of grief, but others suffer a more complex and chronic bereavement. Jones (2015), in her review of the clinical and research literature, identifies three stages in the process of successfully managing the loss. The first is numbness, shock and denial. The second is pining and searching. The third is reorganization, recovery and creativity.

Jones' first two stages constitute the initial reactions to or defenses against the physical and psychological loss of part of the self. The first represents the affective response to the event—denial, dissociation. Some of the therapists we spoke with reported feeling not much of anything, and sometimes they perceived this as a signal that they "are over" the experience. This numbness can be short-lived, followed by an intense reaction such as Zucker (2014) expressed. Other therapists who experienced a loss felt a vacillation between numbness and intense sadness that lingered over months. Protracted numbness is often fostered by the larger cultural/familial expectations of the stigma, and women feel silenced to move on before they are emotionally ready. Therapists in that instance may return to their work, still in a state of shock, either thinking they are fine or believing they should be. It is only in retrospect that they often recognize that they were not fully available to their patients, as might be the case with any significant and sanctioned loss. Freeman (2005) articulates this point well:

> My memory of these months, during my hours with patients, is of a sense of relief from the relentless focus on myself. The days and weeks that preceded the miscarriages were most fraught with concern about my body. The in vitro fertilization cycle was a time filled with worry about my emotional state, in addition to an anxious awareness of changes in my body. At home, I felt intense, shifting moods, and I worried that my lability would distort my response to patients. I had the illusion that my office was a sanctuary from such emotional storms and believed that the effort of maintaining the status quo helped me feel most like myself during sessions. However, this self-control and dissociation held me apart from my experience, and consequently I felt less creative and spontaneous.
>
> (p. 51)

Jaffe and Diamond (2011c) encourage couples suffering from loss to identify and label those unconscious scripts that they adopted that outline how pregnancy and parenthood are "supposed" to unfold. Articulating the "reproductive story" helps couples become aware of the unconscious mandates that society, family and self placed upon them. Such a story gives form to the event and allows couples to decide upon its meaning to them.

In the category of Jones's pining and searching, we might place those who develop PTSD-like symptoms, where the body is still reacting often quite violently to the loss, but the conscious mind seems unaware. Sell-Smith describes this experience after her loss.

> My own experience of traumatic grief initially baffled me. My blood pressure spiked before my loss of Magdalene and remained elevated for several weeks after I gave birth. . . . the obstetric nurse . . . repeatedly stress[ed] . . . I need[ed] time to recover. I couldn't accept this as valid and remained convinced that part of my pregnancy remained. . . . My blood pressure eventually returned to normal. . . . My body had been reacting to a traumatic event in a normal, healthy way. My brain and body were overwhelmed and needed time to process what had happened. Cognitively I understood that my mind was experiencing a great deal of emotion, but I failed to recognize how overwhelmed the rest of my body was during this experience of traumatic grief.
>
> (Sell-Smith & Lax, 2013, p. 13)

The third step is most clearly articulated in Sell-Smith's autoethnography of her own attempt to make meaning "out of a messy situation":

> I suffered a miscarriage of a planned pregnancy, only to become pregnant again a few months later. The subsequent pregnancy was laden with anxiety

and constant worry that I would experience yet another loss. . . . events culminated in a stillborn delivery in the second trimester. . . . A few months later, I discovered that I was pregnant again, only to find out that I was carrying an ectopic pregnancy which would need to be terminated. I once again found myself feeling devastated, overwhelmed and in search of a way to understand what had happened and to heal myself. . . . I also found that looking at the literature in this manner gave me a new perspective when interacting with other women who have experienced pregnancy loss and with people who have not had this experience. The issue of perinatal and infant loss remains a painful and often avoided topic of discussion. From my own experience and from listening to the stories of other women in a pregnancy loss support group, I recognize the importance of discussing that which is often only spoken of in hushed tones. Giving voice to women who are often quieted is an important part of my grieving process and may be an important part of theirs.

(Sell-Smith & Lax, 2013, pp. 1–4)

Sell-Smith and Lax (2013) suggest the importance of giving personal meaning to the experience as an important step in coming to terms with the loss. In a study with women who had experienced early miscarriages, Frost et al. (2007) found that the meaning that the women created for their losses could be categorized into three approaches: pre-modern causation that utilized religion, nature and destiny (Judeo-Christian beliefs that loss is part of a grander scheme—God's way); modern explanations that highlighted medical and scientific knowledge (age, chromosomal abnormalities); and post-modern reasoning that challenges science as imperfect and acknowledge life's randomness.

Working Through the Loss

Social support is of critical importance (Swanson, 1999). Technology has provided an array of options to communicate to those around of the event, allowing family and other supports to learn of the event, but at the same time provide the necessary space for a more intimate or solitary processing. Sell-Smith offers her solution in an email sent to family and friends:

Hi everyone,
Sorry for the mass email. Just wanted to let you know that we received some very sad news today. At some point over the weekend, I lost the baby. We are pretty devastated, confused, and grief-stricken. This pregnancy had been anything but easy for me. Thanks for all of the support you've given us over the last few months.
—Julie

(Sell-Smith & Lax, 2013, p. 5)

In this case, Sell-Smith was clear about her emotional state as the result of the event. Because a range of responses can be felt, this articulation is particularly important. She left unspecified what she wished from her support system, although her clearly articulated emotional reaction provides some information about the appropriate response. While some social supports will have an intuitive understanding about how to respond to the message guided by knowledge of the couple, other caring and well-meaning friends and family without experience may not. If the couple expects a specific response, expressing that desire may result in others' responses that are more supportive and synchronous with what the couple feels they need.

No single way to work through the meaning of the loss exists. In her five stages of grief, Kübler-Ross (1969) suggests the importance of anger. Swanson (1999) has found support for the acknowledgment of anger as an important element in the process of healing. Using a brief counseling approach (accepting a loss, identifying what was lost, letting go and sharing the loss and going public), she found that the recognition and expression of anger is helpful in coming to terms with what was lost. Unresolved anger toward the self and/or others fuels depression, hopelessness and agency in the future (Cosgrove, 2004).

The meaning of loss is culturally and individually determined. That meaning will in turn influence the depth of the grief. The cultural context of whether the fetus or embryo is given personhood status influences how the woman and her family view the event. Given that the notion of personhood is largely culturally (politically, religiously, ethnically) and individually constructed, an approach to pregnancy loss that embraces a fluid interpretation of the loss may be the most compassionate framework for the salient aspects of the loss (Layne, 1996). A single, rigid definition of personhood does not allow for the variations that span society, religion and individual's psychology and circumstance.

As the meaning of the loss becomes clearer to the woman and her family, many men and women who experienced the loss espouse the benefits of memorializing the loss with a funeral or memorial service (Robinson, 2011). Many families "weav[e] babies lost in pregnancy into the fabric of the family" (Cote-Arsenault (2003, p. 23). In Sell-Smith and Lax 's (2013) online support group, many women wrote about the importance of holding on to memories that they had of their embryo, keeping evidence of the positive pregnancy tests and ultrasound pictures. If there were remains, many found ways to give permanent stature to them. Sell-Smith writes of having and sometimes wearing an urn locket with the cremated remains of her daughter.

Resolution is not the same as returning to a pre-loss functioning. A loss cannot be exchanged for a new life, erasing the memory of the loss. Many believe that grief is revisited throughout the lifetime. Sell-Smith describes her own movement from a quantitative dissertation on the topic to an ethnography, which involved the formation of an online pregnancy loss support group, an exemplar of a creative reorganization of the painful experience. In her personal reparative efforts to manage her loss and grief, she has tapped into a group that feels unacknowledged in their pain and loss.

Managing Psychotherapy After a Pregnancy Loss

Everyone grieves differently and in their own time frame. Many therapists perceive that something and someone important has been lost that needs weeks, months or even years to adequately mourn. However, not every therapist will feel that way. Many adjust well without digging into the strong affect-laden component of their experience (Reynolds, 2003). It is an individual determination of the ideal time to set aside before returning to practice.

Even if we need months, mostly likely we do not have the luxury to stay out of work or away from practice for the months that the grieving and resolution process may take. It is important for the therapist to be aware that a lull in the affective experience does not necessarily mean that the pain is over. Consultation, mentorship, personal psychotherapy or a specialized support group offers the opportunity to continue exploration and thus healing.

Returning to the Office

Only a handful of published reports include the effects of miscarriage on treatment.[7] When the miscarriage occurs in the first trimester, patients frequently have not been told of the pregnancy. The loss is a private one, often with little support from the outside world. Many therapists do not take much time off after this experience, and so re-enter the treatment situation with raw feelings and painful preoccupations. Even fortified with an awareness of this possibility, the therapist can be caught off guard.

One therapist with a miscarriage at 14 weeks found that she felt intensely for a male patient who reported that his wife had voluntarily terminated a pregnancy without his consent. She said that the intensity of her feelings at the time precluded her from considering the possible triangulation that this patient may have created between her patient, his wife and her. This patient was not apparently aware of his therapist's pregnancy, as the therapist felt his overt knowledge would likely have further complicated the treatment. The therapist is probably correct that exploration of this triangulation could have furthered this man's treatment. This exploration would not have required the therapist's personal revelation, a possibility discussed further in the next section of this chapter.

Patients discussing certain subjects, such as the burdens of childcare, laissez-faire attitudes toward abortion and unwanted pregnancies may bring into focus for the therapist her personal loss and become a cauldron of mixed feelings of anxiety, guilt, anger and resentment. In this next example, the therapist a decade beyond the loss reexamines a session with a contemporary frame of reference.

> The culmination of 2 years of infertility treatments resulted in an ectopic pregnancy. This coincided with a planned 3-week vacation over a major holiday. I returned to work recognizing that I still felt sad and unsettled about what further treatment I would pursue. I considered taking additional

time off, but the thought of having to call all my patients and cancel additional sessions seemed more than I could bear. I resolved to push forward, but felt no energy. I was overwhelmed by my patients' transferences to my scheduled holiday. That time period was very hazy. It was as if a fog had descended over me. I went through the motions of living, but retained few memories. I had no notion that I should have reasons to grieve, only to be grateful that it was diagnosed and my life was saved. Now more than two decades later I recognize that I was grieving a lost baby. My empathy for my patients was also compromised. Unable to manage my own private pain I hid behind a rigid analytic frame which prevented me from seeing the multiple relational dimensions occurring between my patients and me. I remember one session shortly after my return that was irritating to me. Now having a better perspective on my loss and I am able to recast the session in a different light. One patient had recently come back to therapy after she had a child, 4 months old at the time of the session. There was an issue with the babysitter not showing up. Instead of cancelling at the last minute, she brought the infant to the session. At that time I saw her actions as a break in the therapeutic frame and I was aware of my frustration. First she missed sessions for the delivery, then my vacation and now her baby was intruding into our work. There was a reality component of irresponsible adolescent babysitters, but was this payback for "my vacation"? I was annoyed that as we began our work again, the patient could not be fully present to our work. I felt a pressure "to progress" as she had previously complained of the slow pace of her progress. How could she focus on herself with the distraction of the baby wanting her? In retrospect, I was the one who could not focus, mired in my own grief and seeing her baby, my envy. Had I been more aware of my unadulterated envy bubbling under the surface and able to make use of it, I could have worked with the multiplicity of meanings in this act. On a surface level, the patient wanted to share this baby with me, seeking my admiration and approval for her accomplishment. At the same time she had also been competitive with me. She had a baby and I did not. This clearly marked a triumph over me, although she likely was not conscious of it as I had not openly acknowledged my loss. Her competitiveness and desire for approval paralleled those feelings she had expressed toward her mother. As we previously discussed her interactions with her mother, she had viewed the competitiveness as emanating solely from her mother. During the session the baby slept and did not interfere with the work we could have done. Years later, now that the pain of my loss has receded from focus, I recognize the missed opportunities.

The therapist is not incorrect in her assessment that the presence of the baby alters the traditional boundaries of the therapeutic dyad and could have been a distraction. Resistance for a more in-depth interaction with the therapist may have emanated predominantly from the patient for traditional neurotic reasons or for reasons having to do with the patient's unconscious awareness of the therapist's unavailability or pained state. However, as the therapist acknowledges, it is also a missed opportunity to explore a possible enactment. The patient has unacknowledged competitive strivings, flaunting a coveted ideal for both and at the same time desiring approval. The therapist in response is withholding admiration and has palpable envy. The example highlights how the therapist's task is complicated by her personal response to her loss and her countertransference specifically provoked by the patient's actions. The therapist cannot in that moment hold the patient's needs and preserve her personal task, and the event re-traumatizes her. At the time of the session, the therapist was unable to explore her own feelings in relation to the patient's actions, and thus could not offer containment or lead the way for the patient to discover her part in the enactment.

Lasky (1990), in a similar discussion about the management of the therapist's illness, suggests that emotional vulnerabilities of the therapist make it difficult to contain the material without interpreting the transference and placing the material completely on the patient, rather than seeing it as a product of the relationship between them. Time, support from colleagues and self-examination help augment this process. Freeman (2005) writes, "As I have felt able to be more in contact with my own experience, I have become more interested in analyzing myself and my patient's feelings about mothers, babies, and time" (pp. 66–67).

Lazar (1990) and Gerson (1996) wrote most poignantly and in-depth about their experiences. Lazar (1990) indicated that some of the most difficult reactions she experienced were her loss of anonymity, her anger, guilt and withdrawal. Both Lazar and Gerson had male patients for whom their negative reactions (their wish or relief at the occurrence of the miscarriage) toward male clients were extremely difficult to manage in the face of their recent loss. Gerson's (1996) description reveals her struggles:

> With some patients, however, my loss elicited. . . . rage, fear or disdain for me. Sympathy was replaced by pity and I became a sign of danger to them, a reminder of chaos or a carrier of badness. I found this reaction most difficult to work with at this time. In addition to the customary difficulties of negative transference remaining grounded required an enormous amount of psychological energy at a time when I felt depleted. Some of the attacks meshed with my own self-criticism. I felt less freedom, as did my patients to work with material that so obviously came from events from which I had no distance yet. My feelings were raw, and there was not a way to hide them.
> (p. 61)

When the therapist is likely to be most vulnerable and least able to handle intense interactions, the patients may be experiencing strong affects. Although some time off after the miscarriage is suggested, it is unlikely to be enough to enable the therapist to work through the loss. Thus, the therapist often returns to the therapy depleted and suffering deeply from her loss. Fears of patients' questions abound at a time when the therapist is least able to protect herself from intrusions into her personal life. Our recommendation is a reminder that setting boundaries can often be therapeutic and freeing for our patients, such as a simple statement like "That is something I do not want (or am not able) to discuss at this time." This type of response allows for the possibility that, with additional thought, the therapist might feel an answer may or may not be beneficial to the furthering of the therapeutic process. To the extent that the therapist is aware of her vulnerabilities, she may be able to guard against some of the most intense interactions by arranging her schedule so that she does not have difficult patients consecutively. Gerson noted that as she gained more distance from the event, she was able to utilize the event as an incredibly powerful focal point around which her patients could confront their central themes.

For many patients, the therapist's psychological unavailability and/or the unplanned missing of sessions present much difficulty. Fears of damage to the patient may lead to guilt or the denial of its significance. Cullington-Roberts (2004) provides her example of Mrs. X, whose mother had committed suicide and whose father had been idealized. She had a number of failed therapies where she "felt some glee at making them impotent; a reassurance to herself that they had nothing they could offer her of which she might feel envy" (p. 103). Initially, the patient was offered once a week therapy for 18 months by Cullington-Roberts. Instead of 18 months of therapy, they worked together for only 9 months, which was interrupted twice due to miscarriage, medical threats to the second pregnancy and then early termination. During these absences, the parental transferences were enacted as Mrs. X sought reassurance from the idealized male therapist who had originally referred her to Cullington-Roberts that her therapist had not died. Before a summer planned break, Mrs. X's

> anxiety increased about whether I would return, and her resentment grew at my taking a holiday on top of the earlier long absence, Mrs. X finally revealed her fantasy about my absence. She thought I had had cervical cancer, that I had had a hysterectomy. When I took up her wish and her anxiety about damaging me, she was very clear: she had not only been killing off any of my creativity in her mind, she had killed me.
>
> (p. 105)

Although this patient would have been difficult for any therapist (all her previous therapists had failed), the absences and early termination were particularly traumatic for a patient whose mother had committed suicide. As any therapist would, Cullington-Roberts struggled with her guilt and decision as to whether to continue the time-limited therapy as originally planned given these unexpected breaks. Cullington-Roberts (2004) writes that

> it is possible to sympathize with the patient and the immense impact on them but also reassure herself that what she has done is not a crime. Who

can help [the therapist] to recognize her omnipotent wishes to be perfect and her failure in that; to acknowledge damage to the patient without consuming guilt; to accept that . . . events being imperfectly under her control is part of life; and despite all, that these painful issues can be addressed— the impact from outside and the internal contribution—and is an essential part of the continuing work.

(p. 110)

It may seem that for those patients who have particular sensitivities concerning therapist availability and therapy in its nascent stages, the patients' best interests may be served by a referral to a therapist who is not likely to have limited availability. However, life circumstances are often not under our control, nor is our ability to predict who may need to absent themselves midway through treatment for personal reasons. Therapy unfolds imperfectly and is an acknowledgment of our humanness. From time to time, all therapies suffer from the strum and strife of ruptures in the treatment connection. It is then that the clinical acumen of the therapist is needed to repair the damage, and in the process the patient's ego is often fortified.

In the literature and in examples therapists presented to us, many of the therapists felt after the loss that they were responding in the usual manner, and relationally the interaction was "good enough." Yet in the years that followed, and after parenthood either was achieved or therapists were settled in their decision to be childless, many recognize that initially they were less present, less creative with their patients (e.g., Abbasi, 2014; Cullington-Roberts, 2004; Cosgrove, 2004; Freeman, 2005). When mired under a pall of loss, maintaining an authentic relational connection may be a daunting task. Yet, if patients remain in treatment, therapist and patient might work through this previous disengagement. In this next example, we see the way in which the therapist previously psychologically and physically unavailable is able to work with her own and the patient's reactions. Psychoanalyst Aisha Abbasi (2014) informed her patients of her impending and short notice absence for a number of weeks, which she explained was due to her secondary infertility and proposed treatment. The treatment was unsuccessful. She writes in retrospect of her reanalysis of her motivations for revealing her condition and treatment. (We will return to her example again when we discuss assisted reproductive technology):

So even as I thought that my telling my patients the reality of my situation would allow me to be as analytic as possible, I can see, looking back, that telling them was also based on my need to protect myself: by telling them I was inviting them to bring in all their feelings about what was going on with their analyst. At the same time, part of me was also asking them to temporarily suspend being the analytic patients . . . instead be reasonable adults who could understand my situation, and—at least for the next 6 months have associations that were tolerable to me in my somewhat fragile emotional state. . . . I asked my patients their thoughts and feelings about this new reality in my life. . . . My patients felt that these were useful analytic questions. . . . they responded . . . with rich and vivid associations. . . . Only months and years later was I also able to clearly understand how relieved I had been that I didn't have to deal with fantasies that I was leaving on a wonderful, spur of the moment vacation at a time when I was undergoing uncomfortable and sometimes painful procedures. . . . I did not have it in me to deal with certain reactions (e.g., rage).

(pp. 7–8)

Abbasi (2014) provides details for a case in which a female physician came for help with her emotions around infertility. Here is a short excerpt of their work together later in therapy after Abbasi's IVF procedure was unsuccessful.

[the patient] said hesitantly, "I think I'm gloating about my pregnancy and the fact that you could not conceive. It feels awful that I have such thoughts." I asked, "Awful in what way?" . . . she replied. . . . "It's hard for me to imagine . . . that you might be able to understand these feelings I'm having. I'm feeling glad that that I'm pregnant and you're not. That feels so mean, almost sadistic. I don't want to feel like that . . ." I said. . . "as though I couldn't possibly understand how deeply torn you feel about being so fond of me on the one hand and having thoughts of feeling glad about my loss and suffering on the other . . ." She replied, "I felt so angry at you over all those months when you were going through infertility treatments. I thought it was so unfair . . . you were going through the same problem that I was, except that you already had a child. I didn't even have one. . . . I really needed you and I needed your help with my feelings about what if you had your second child and I might not even have one." . . . [I added] "I would resent you and envy *you* as you resented and envied me."

(Abbasi, 2014, pp. 9–10)

In this remarkable example, where both therapist and patient are struggling with infertility, the therapist was initially hopeful that IVF would enable her to conceive as the patient struggled with infertility. Then later, when IVF has failed for the therapist, the patient becomes pregnant. The patient articulates the lack of the therapist's previous psychological availability. The therapist, despite her loss, is able to acknowledge and be attuned to her own competitive and envious reactions and contain those of her patient. With the therapist's help, the patient is able to acknowledge her anxieties, her gloating and the competitiveness in their relationship.

Principles of Personal Disclosures

In the preceding example, Abbasi informs the patient of the specifics of her personal circumstance. Given her circumstances, she felt that this information would allow patients the opportunity to associate and deal with these aspects of their analyst. It is only in retrospect that she recognizes the motivation of self-protection in this disclosure. It is not unusual for therapists to be able to identify some of their motivations, but be blind to others. Her example raises important questions, such as what to disclose and what could emerge in the therapy. In Gerson's (1996) edited volume on the impact of life circumstances and crises on therapists' work, therapists agree that one cannot remain completely anonymous; awareness of the transference-countertransference dialogue becomes the therapeutic gauge and tool. However, the optimal amount of disclosure remains controversial. Those who support minimal information to be given warn that more facts interfere with patients' fantasies and potentially manipulate them in service of the therapist's needs and limitations. Disclosures of bad news usually result in initial diffusion of patient attacks when there are alterations in the frame, such as missed sessions (Lasky, 1990). A reversal of roles can even occur where patients feel they need to take care of and listen to the therapist. Revelation of the therapist's loss potentially becomes traumatic for the patient, particularly if accompanied by the therapist's inability to contain her own trauma reactions to the loss.

In contrast to this position, Leibowitz (1996) and Gerson (1996) both argue that it is in the unwrapping of the patient's reactions to information about the therapist that becomes the most rewarding work. It is difficult to explore the reactions when one is in the throes of it. As we look back upon the event, we may find that we can gain a perspective in which we are more fully open to our imperfections as therapist, yet, a lamenting of our humanness remains (Gerson, 1996b). However, we see how Abbasi was able to utilize this material later in a productive manner.

Each therapist has her own vulnerabilities regarding and grieving the loss. She has her own level of comfort with disclosure and must judge patients' abilities to handle the disclosure and make use of it in therapy. We offer some thoughts and guiding principles in helping therapists make these decisions regarding disclosure.

Timing of the Loss

When the loss is early (before 12 to 14 weeks), the external physical evidence of the pregnancy is slight and procedures to deal with the loss are less invasive, thus requiring less time away from the office. As Freeman (2005) suggests,

> The problem of infertility has a particular impact on the therapist's capacity to be open and authentic because infertility is shrouded in secrecy . . . when the medical treatment did not "visibly" disrupt the therapeutic setting, there were external motivations not to speak of it.
>
> (p. 58)

The early loss does not require a specific disclosure, only acknowledgment of changes in frame (unexpectedly missing or changing sessions, phone or internet sessions). A simple message to the patient by phone or by email can be crafted. If the therapist wishes to reveal something more specific, a statement such as "I (had) have a medical issue, not life-threatening and is resolving (or is resolved)." Given the enormous psychic energy that most therapists experience after a failed pregnancy, the patient is attuned to the changes in the ways the therapist relates to him or her, even if the loss is not acknowledged. This relational change, we feel, should be acknowledged and considered if patients directly or indirectly refer to it (an acknowledgment that the therapist has been distracted if the patient notices or accuses).

As the pregnancy becomes more apparent before the loss and sessions are missed, some acknowledgment (and perhaps information) seems prudent. A call or email from the therapist or a designated professional should be instigated. Specifics of the problem are difficult to reveal on the phone, so that is best saved for when the therapist and patient are back in session. Some information regarding the unexpected absence (a medical emergency or a family emergency) should be communicated, as well as when the patient could expect to hear from the therapist ("you can expect a call in a week or two") and the emergency coverage that will be provided in the interim ("Dr. X will be covering for emergencies").

Evaluating How the Disclosure Will Have Specific Meaning to the Patient

We consider three relevant circumstances: the therapist's authenticity; the ways in which the therapist is perceived; and the special circumstance in which both patient and therapist are struggling with pregnancy and infertility and *therapist authenticity*. In some circumstances, focus on the therapist–patient relationship is secondary to the skills or techniques being taught. In instances such as these, the patient's awareness or interest in the therapist may not be central to the work being done, and thus the sharing of specific information about the therapist's state may not be crucial. In contrast, where the relational dynamics between the therapist and patient are the substance of therapy, the ongoing lack of authenticity hampers the therapy. Freeman (2005) shares the example of Ms. C, who had been in treatment for several years where she felt the patient's initial defensiveness was disruptive to their work.

> Neither parent provided a real connection with her, one that would have allowed C to know them or feel known herself. Consequently, she is hypervigilant to how others reveal or hide themselves . . . We were frequently in a battle over her desire to know more about me and her insistence that she could not modulate her own mood or contain her anxiety without gestures of support and signs of closeness with me. C is intelligent, talented, and competent. . . . however, she has veered between adequate self-care and

a capacity to work efficiently with others, and periods of schizoid withdrawal, somatic complaints, limited functioning.... C and I live in the same neighborhood, and she knew that I was also single. In retrospect, I minimized the meaning of both my physical presence near her and the many fantasies she had about my life. These fantasies gave her the sense that she knew me or had discovered things about me on her own . . . she noticed my wedding ring . . . C had an intense reaction. . . . she focused on her fear that a pregnancy would follow my marriage. Her insistence that I tell her if I was pregnant unfortunately matched my inability, at that moment, to deny that I was pregnant. I had already experienced one miscarriage, and, as the second pregnancy maintained itself, I became caught up with my own superstitions. I experienced her questions as a demand for me to negate my experience, something I was unwilling to do, even partially, because of my own fears. I acknowledged that she had guessed correctly (that I was indeed pregnant), even though I understood she did not need to know about my pregnancy. Her subsequent fury was expectable . . . she feared that a new family . . . would overshadow my concern for her. . . . She had believed that my life offered her the possibility of a model for living alone. And now she felt betrayed, envious, and destructive.

(p. 60)

At this point in treatment, the patient decompensated and resumed outpatient treatment with another therapist. She later resumed treatment with Freeman. During that time, she saw Freeman on the street holding hands with a child, which the patient thought was the therapist's. However, the child was much older than would have been the case if it was the therapist's baby. Her example continues:

I told her that I had had a miscarriage and also suggested that I thought she might have known this (because she had seen me during the year). I added that I believed she had not spoken of it because she had been afraid that she had hurt me and destroyed my pregnancy. I stated simply that her anger had not caused my miscarriage. . . . This moment was pivotal and difficult . . . to describe how different C's nodding, tearful response felt, and how unusual my commonplace explanation of my own experience sounded in the context of our recent history of intense confrontation. . . . there was directness and an intimacy to our connection, and I felt her relax in a profound way.

(p. 62)

Freeman acknowledged that her initial anxieties about the pregnancy led her to a less open exchange, which resulted in more awkward interactions with Ms. C. Freeman had worked through aspects of her loss when the patient resumed therapy. Her disclosure and change in authenticity enabled Ms. C to also shift in her defensiveness and ability to experience and express an intense and genuine emotional response. Authenticity was crucial for this patient to develop a sense of herself. As Freeman alludes, the "knowing" of the therapist's reality on multiple dimensions was likely also important to this patient's development.

THE PATIENT'S PERCEPTION OF THE THERAPIST

When the patient is confronted with the therapist's struggles, the patient is naturally prone to view the therapist as a vulnerable and flawed person. Zucker (2015) articulates,

> Would my patients be inhibited from freely discussing what might now, in the face of my fresh pain, seem like mundane details of their daily lives? I feared that they might want to protect me, comfort me, run from me or shield themselves from my anguish.
>
> (Zucker, 2015)

This inclination, then, might undermine the therapy. Zucker introduces Oliva, who did not return to therapy for a while, as learning of the therapist's loss at 16 weeks represented her biggest nightmare—"if it could happen to you, it means that it could happen to me." Fantasies of struggle, rage and destruction regularly exist between patient and therapist, particularly for patients whose sense of self and other is often merged; these patients now experience the "as if" nature of these struggles as dangerously close the realities of the loss. Despite the assurances that the patient has not caused any damage, she may still feel responsible, guilty and anxious about retribution.

PARALLEL EXPERIENCES FOR THERAPIST AND PATIENT

Sometimes, the patient and therapist are both undergoing transitions related to having a baby. Jaffe and Diamond (2011c) suggest that the therapist's disclosure of her status may be helpful when the patient is also experiencing infertility.

Our recommendation is for the therapist to remind herself that setting boundaries can often be therapeutic and freeing for our patients, with a simple statement like "that is something I do not want (or am not able) to discuss at this time." This type of response allows for the possibility that with additional thought the therapist might feel an answer may or may not be beneficial to the furthering of the therapeutic process. To the extent that the therapist is aware of her vulnerabilities, she may be able to guard against some of the most intense interactions by arranging her schedule so that she does not have difficult patients consecutively.

Assisted Reproductive Technology

Assisted reproductive technology (ART) refers to a constellation of fertility treatments in which eggs and/or sperm are handled outside of the body. Examples include intracytoplasmic sperm injection, in vitro fertilization, and surrogacy, which enable couples to have offspring that could not occur naturally. In vitro fertilization (IVF) is the most common ART procedure.[8] Procedures involve surgically extracting eggs from a woman's ovaries, combining them with sperm in the laboratory (either the father's or a donor's) and transferring them to the woman's body or donating them to another female through the cervix. ART is inextricably linked to the diagnosis of infertility, both of which create stresses and potentially long-lasting effects in the lives of therapists. We will briefly discuss issues of infertility, then ART, followed by an examination of clinical issues that arise during the process.

Infertility

A diagnosis of infertility is given if a woman is not able to achieve pregnancy after 1 year of unprotected sex.[9] Approximately 6% of women of childbearing age are diagnosed with infertility and approximately 12% of women in the 15–44 age experience difficulties achieving pregnancy and birth (impaired fecundity) (www.cdc.gov/reproductivehealth/infertility, updated December 19, 2016). As discussed earlier in the chapter, these percentages increase with age for both males and females. Options include pursuit of a more specific diagnosis and fertility treatment, adoption or no action. As couples become more intentional about achieving pregnancy, intercourse transitions from pleasure and intimacy to an act that is more mandated.

Infertility creates stress, and stress affects infertility (Loftus & Namaste, 2011; Lynch, Sundaram, Maisog, Seeney, & Lewis, 2014). Couples describe infertility as the single most stressful experience in their lives (Hajela, Prasad, Kumaran, & Kumar, 2016). Just 20 years ago, the label of infertility was as devastating as a diagnosis of AIDS or cancer (Domar, Zuttermeister, & Friedman, 1993). A diagnosis of infertility may affect individual identity and self-worth, the couple's relationship and one's place in the familial/social group.

A diagnosis of infertility precipitates psychological anguish and hopelessness (Cousineau & Domar, 2007). It is experienced as a loss of control, which may alter the perceived capacity for self-regulation (Beebe, Jaffe, & Lachmann, 1992). Many have likened it to a trauma, and there is increased risk of post-traumatic symptoms (Daugirdaite, van den Akker, & Purewal, 2015; Deka & Sarma, 2010; Klock, 2011). There is self-blame, desperation, grief and depression (Clay, 2006). Self-esteem can suffer, as infertility challenges identity (Loftus & Namaste, 2011). Therapists report a questioning of their competence during this time. Freeman (2005) writes,

> during this period of infertility I had become plagued by a sense of insecurity I felt I had outgrown earlier. My past internal dialogue had been dominated by feelings of inadequacy and questions about my behavior. This dialogue created an awkward self-consciousness that was familiar and

uncomfortable . . . that I had lost access to my secure, satisfied self and was instead stuck with a more anxious critical self.

(pp. 52–54)

For the individual, the stresses of infertility and its meaning may reawaken old losses, narcissistic vulnerabilities and perceptions of defectiveness. Intertwined with our own dynamics, dysfunctional aspects of our character may be exacerbated (Mann, 2014).

Couples may experience challenges in their relational equilibrium. Earlier studies suggested that prolonged infertility could lead to relationship discord. However, more recent work has suggested that results are highly varied, and that almost a third of couples report that the experience enhanced their relationship (Pasch & Sullivan, 2017; Peterson Pirritano Block & Schmidt, 2011). Even unsuccessful infertility treatments do not have to have a negative impact on the relationship (Reporaki et al., 2007).

Identity and relational struggles are exacerbated by cultural and social norms (Deka & Sarma, 2010; Klock, 2011; Ranjbar, Akhondi, Borimnejad, Ghaffari, & Behboodi-Moghadam, 2015). Freeman (2005) reminds us that "our society often seems to equate childlessness with negative characteristics, including selfishness, immaturity or. . . . being cold or withholding . . . or not nurturing" (p. 54). In ethnicities and cultures ascribing to more patriarchal values, women with infertility problems experience a sense of failing to meet obligation of marriage and expanding family (Klock, 2011; Ranjbar et al. 2007; Sutherland, 1997). Many women struggling with infertility protect themselves by choosing not to talk about their infertile state. Familial and cultural shame and guilt abound (Allison, 2011). Depending upon the culture, there are various degrees of attitudinal and perceived stigmatization toward the infertile woman and couple. Thus women unable to naturally conceive retreat from social circles in silence, feeling stigmatized by their "friends" and family (Allison, 2011; Sternke & Abrahamson, 2015). Patients too often have transference reactions that mirror that of society (Leibowitz, 1996).

The pursuit of parenting taken to the next level is a process of acknowledging the probabilities as they present (e.g., the probability of achieving a natural pregnancy if over 40) and making decisions about a course of action as couples fit their personal characteristics and attitudes into what is known. Many a therapist in this situation has described the series of disappointments and psychological adjustments needed to decide upon a course of action and to change that path as new information about her personal situation becomes available.

The pressures of time and the difficulties of making decisions when nothing can be said with certainty cost enormous psychic energy in the therapist's personal and professional life. Freeman (2005) remarks on the importance of maintaining a cautious balanced view

of the meaning of each microscopic development. This hyperawareness [of] more external changes in her body creates room for fantasies and magical thinking that link subtle physical sensations with the desire to make meaning, create hope or counter superstitions. This sensitivity—physical, emotional, and cognitive is both a distracting and an isolating experience. It is difficult to admit to oneself the range and intensity of fantasies and the intricate way in which they are linked with subtle or imagined physical experiences.

(p. 51)

In Vitro Fertilization Treatment

There have been remarkable technological improvements in assisted reproductive procedures that have increased the success of producing a full-term, healthy infant. A stressful, technologically sophisticated procedure requiring precise timing, in vitro fertilization can be physically demanding, very costly[10] and emotionally draining, often involving immediate and difficult decisions.

Success Rates

In 2014, 173,198 cycles were started with the intent to transfer at least one embryo, which resulted in 57,323 live births (www.cdc.gov/art/reports/2014/national-summary.html, reviewed December 19, 2016). Although this one-third statistic is very hopeful, the percentage of cycles that result in normal weight, full-term singletons is correlated closely with age.[11] There are several steps in the process, which are focal points for increased anxiety. Successful completion of a step increases the likelihood of achieving a healthy baby, but is still very much age dependent. For example, if one or more embryos are viable, then for those under 35 years the probability of a healthy term baby is 30%, and for those aged 43–44 it is 5%. Less than half the transfers result in a pregnancy (implantation), with increasing age resulting in a lower percentage of implantation. There is a rapid decline around 40 years of age in the use of one's own eggs. The use of a donor egg remarkably increases the likelihood that a pregnancy will result in a full-term, normal weight infant. The use of donor sperm or donor eggs offers an alternative hope for building a family but may complicate the family dynamics, regardless of whether the donor is anonymous or a family member. Statistics do not predict an individual course and outcome. Treatment may aid in quickly achieving pregnancy or may result in unsuccessful attempts and failure to become biological parents. Such unpredictability contributes to the stress of the experience.

Physical and Emotional Demands

Multiple tests are used to pinpoint fertility problems. These often require exact day timing so that all other events in life are subject to cancellation. These tests may also be uncomfortable, although generally physical recovery time is minimal. A woman's cycle is recreated as multiple medications are introduced prior to the procedures and throughout the pregnancy to stimulate multiple ovary production and follicle growth, induce ovulation, prevent premature ovulation, and create a more favorable uterine environment. The most common side effects of these medications are depression, mood swings, breast tenderness, vomiting, dizziness and headaches. (http://americanpregnancy.org/infertility/ infertility-medications/). Frequent blood tests are used to monitor the effects of medications and further specify the timing. The use of the term "side effects" minimizes the emotional turmoil that many report. Women undergoing fertility treatments are more prone to high levels of anxiety (Yakupova et al., 2015). Almost 40% of the women and 15% of the men meet criteria for major depressive disorder (Holley et al., 2015). Therapists report intense and quickly shifting mood swings (Abbasi, 2014; Freeman, 2005). For those who have confidence in their ability to contain strong affects for both themselves and their patients, this may create a great deal of anxiety around managing even their own moods; the psychic cost may be a less creative, less spontaneous presence in the sessions.

What is surprising to many is that some women who become mothers after prolonged infertility treatments remain depressed and anxious (Oshlansky & Sereika, 2005). They and many around them find these feelings confusing, given the enormous resources that they devoted to achieving what would be deemed by all to be a successful outcome. They are less likely to articulate their emotions because of their shame and confusion about their reactions. This silence fuels their isolation and may deepen their depression.

Couple Functioning

Couples often make difficult decisions as medical tests reveal new information. Some decisions, such as when and whether to proceed with treatment, require the garnering of new information, multiple consultations and lengthy couple deliberations. These may be considered over months and even years. Other decisions, such as choosing an egg donor, how many embryos to transfer and whether to reduce the number of embryos implanted in IVF,[12] require more immediate attention. Beliefs about life and birth, religion and one's social and cultural anchors influence and often create conflicts for the couple. ART procedures and the choices that come with these decisions highlight differences in couples' beliefs and ethical systems and priorities for having a biological family. The couple's compatibility in decision-making processes eases the stress or exacerbates it. Strategies for coping with the unknown and the degree of needing and wanting control become salient. Whether failure to achieve the agreed-upon goals is temporary or permanent, how the couple manages disappointments and lack of success is prominent. If members of a couple have similar coping strategies about fertility treatments, they experience it as a less stressful time (Pasch & Sullivan, 2017). To the extent women are more involved and want to talk about it, and to the extent their partner is in synchrony with that, it is a more positive event. Use of avoidant coping strategies produces greater stress and has a negative impact on relationship (Peterson et al., 2009).

How the couple responds to the intrusion of a medical team into the most intimate aspects of their life together becomes an important variable. This group of specialists "appears to have omnipotent powers to give or withhold a baby and promotes intense transferential feelings of dependency, infantilization and vulnerability" (Allison & Doria-Medina, 1999, p. 163). If couples have similar ideas about perceived levels of control over the treatment, there is also less relational discord. Some infertility clinics have support groups for couples, but many do not.

Handling Treatment Concerns Arising From ART

Many of the issues arising in the psychological treatment settings have been covered earlier in the chapter. There are three aspects inherent to infertility treatments that may affect a therapist's work: the amount of time required; the inability to predict in advance when procedures and monitoring need to occur; and the psychological energy invested and consumed in each step of the treatment, making less interest and energy available for patients and their therapy.

First, infertility treatment is time-consuming. Educating oneself about the treatment and choices, medical consultations, treatments and monitoring may take enormous amounts of time, particularly if infertility specialists are not nearby. A full-time job or practice may be difficult to maintain if infertility treatments are initially unsuccessful and require additional cycles.

Second, the timing of the infertility treatment cannot be precisely determined months or even weeks in advance. Short-notice cancellations are very likely, particularly if therapists engage in more than one cycle of treatment. The therapist has to be able to cancel other activities, often with less than 24 hours' notice. Problems are likely to occur in jobs that have little flexibility. In practice, patients who have little flexibility (either for psychological, familial or vocational reasons) will have difficulty rescheduling cancellations with short notice. Patients with severe abandonment issues and a propensity to act out will have difficulty tolerating the sudden disappearance of their therapists. Some of these issues can be ameliorated if patients are adequately prepared for the impending abruptness of cancellations that may occur. As the therapist begins to prepare for infertility treatments, they may consider referring new patients who present with these difficulties to another practitioner. However, student therapists might not be given the latitude to make such decisions.

Third, achieving parenthood through this route requires an enormous individual investment. Each step is monitored such that success creates hope, and failure introduces disappointment, grief and despair. Therapists, like all participants in ART, are keenly aware that despite extraordinary efforts, they might in the end encounter failure. In short, they are on tenterhooks. With a slew of medications supporting the pregnancy function, the experience is an emotional roller coaster. Minute bodily sensations intensify the emotional state and are potentially distracting from the therapy work at hand. To see patients under these circumstances is quite difficult. Some therapists report that the opportunity to work is a relief and distraction from the intensity of the emotional experience. Freeman (2005) writes, "My memory of these months, during my hours with patients, is of a sense of relief from the relentless focus on myself" (p. 51). As Freeman implies and others more directly report, the ability to dissociate their personal experience from what happens in the therapy hour works as an effective immediate coping strategy (Zackson, 2012). Under the circumstances, the therapist might be able to offer no other response. We must recognize that we are not perfectly available and attuned to our patients at all points in our lives and in their therapy. Both Freeman (2005) and Abbasi (2014) have suggested it is often only in retrospect that therapists recognize their lack of presence and their patients' sensitivities to it. If patients persist in spite of these therapist lapses, the opportunity to work with their accruing reactions presents itself more directly. We will come back to this point after the next section.

What Should We Disclose?

The first factor in disclosure is a consideration of the therapist's personal circumstances. For each therapist, there is an initial calculation of time periods that will be needed for infertility treatment to occur. For example, blood draws are often required in the mornings, so therapists should plan temporarily to move patients' sessions so that travel, waiting time and procedure can be accomplished. If some of the procedures necessitate travel to another state or town, this needs to be considered in disclosure and session arrangement. Anticipated time away may figure in the decision on whether and how much to disclose to patients as well. Abbasi (2014) delineates her rationale for disclosing to patients prior to treatment:

> I would be in a state of great emotional upheaval, pumped up with high doses of hormones, and undergoing a variety of medical and surgical procedures. The thought of having to announce to my patients, without any explanation that I needed to cancel a batch of upcoming sessions (for visits to the local treatment centre), followed by another announcement that in a couple of days I would be leaving for 2 weeks—and repeating this abrupt routine twice over a four to six month period—seemed grotesque to me and unfair to my patients.
>
> (p. 7)

Abbasi writes later that she recognizes that dealing with her patients' anger at a time when she felt so vulnerable unconsciously influenced her disclosure decision. We feel that regardless of the primary motivation for disclosure, a lengthy and abrupt absence without explanation is too burdensome, even for relatively healthy patients. A sudden illness or accident may amount to the same lengthy interruption as infertility treatments. However, the possible intrusion of time can be predicted in the case of infertility treatments, whereas it could not in sudden illness or accident. Such a change in boundaries and frame without prior acknowledgment, if possible, is disrespectful to our patients' time and commitment.

The second factor in disclosure is the setting in which the therapist works. Working for organizations in which there is frequent patient turnover may be more an issue of coverage for the functions in which the therapist participates, rather than preparing patients for anticipated absences. At the other end of the spectrum is private practice, where emergency coverage can be anticipated and obtained, but one therapist cannot easily stand in another's stead. What population is treated within the setting is also a critical concern. For example, therapists who treat children might consider discussing the matter with the parents rather than the child. For patients at the lower end of the ego functioning spectrum, knowledge of the therapist's effort in having a child might be overly stimulating and regression-promoting.

The third factor is frequency of therapy. A therapist should consider the pros and cons of disclosure for each of their patients, given their histories and psychopathology. If patients are seen once monthly or less frequently, it may be possible that a particular patient does not miss any sessions. In this case, a disclosure may be more burdensome to the patient than a single abruptly cancelled session. The more frequently a patient is seen, the more likely that person's treatment will be interrupted by infertility treatments. Abbasi's patients were in analysis and some preparation seemed essential.

What a therapist discloses will be more dependent upon the therapist's orientation and preferences. As we previously discussed in the lost pregnancy section, one may decide to reveal only general information (e.g., "I need to attend to a personal medical situation. It is not life-threatening, but is important. I don't exactly know when it would happen, but when it does I will be out of the office on short notice for approximately . . . days."). Many patients are familiar with the therapist's lack of transparency and will either talk about their reactions or not. This particular scenario as presented offers only the first cycle of treatment. If one is planning on several cycles, if the initial ones are unsuccessful, then revealing the scope of absence should be considered.

Abbasi (2014) offers more specific disclosure in her announcement:

> I decided to inform my patients that I was struggling with secondary infertility and was about to begin a series of treatments that would over the next 6 months periodically require me to cancel—on short notice—appointments scheduled for the following ten to fourteen days . . . if they had questions . . . how we dealt with them might reveal dilemmas and complex choices for us

to negotiate . . . and whether boundaries were being crossed or too much reality introduced . . . how we dealt with them would ultimately deepen our work together.

(p. 6)

We particularly liked her introduction to the potential consequences of her revelation, including the possibility of further questions, personal issues that it might highlight and the issues of boundaries. Of course, the disclosure is likely to usher in new patterns of patient and therapist reactions. For example, some patients might feel a need to lessen their introduction of material about their own children, lest it arouse the therapist's negative feelings.

Revisiting the Impact of the Therapist's Infertility With Patients at a Later Time

Most patients, even those with considerable psychopathology, can at least briefly function as caring individuals when a therapist experiences a crisis. In our discussions with therapists undergoing infertility treatments, they report that most patients express empathy and mute their irritations at the disrupted schedule. As previously discussed, therapists undergoing these procedures do not feel psychologically able to deal with the many negative feelings that patients harbor. At some juncture, the situation is resolved either in successfully having a healthy baby or in accepting and working through the failure and loss. It is only then that many therapists are less distracted by these other desires, less vulnerable and more energized in their work. For patients who have remained in treatment throughout the process, therapists are ready to more fully and deeply explore the hidden emotions and their patients feel freer to reveal how they felt. Abbasi eloquently describes this experience:

> as I stabilised emotionally, that patients began to talk about the envy they had felt regarding the possibility that I might conceive a baby; their fear that I would be preoccupied with the baby if I had one; the anger that I was already preoccupied with the trying to have a baby. . . . and finally their ultimate pleasure and satisfaction that I had failed in what I was trying to accomplish. . . . I can understand only in retrospect that it was truly not possible for me, during the period when I was trying so hard—and wanted so much—to conceive a second child, to talk with my patients about their wish for me to not have a child, their rage that I wanted to have a child . . . while maintaining the same degree of neutrality, genuine curiosity and compassion I generally had. Discussing their glee about my trials and suffering might have felt impossible then.

(pp. 19–21)

This, of course, is only possible when patients continue or return to therapy after the fertility "crisis" abates.

Recommendations

We offer three broad recommendations for therapists confronted with difficult situations in relation to the task of attempting to build a family.

1. We have described a number of difficult circumstances that a therapist may face, such as pregnancy loss, pregnancy complications, stillbirth, infertility difficulties and the use of assisted reproductive technology. We have left death of an infant or young child for others to examine. One or more of these are not uncommon occurrences among therapists. Yet very few have shared their experiences in writing. Most therapists express some anxieties about some of these possibilities, but many suffer in silence with their occurrence. The frequency of these events ensures the presence of many supervisors and colleagues who could help those therapists who are struggling with these issues. We recommend that therapists take advantage of such resources, although unearthing them might be daunting. An advantage of disclosing one's status to colleagues is that others might self-identify as having undergone such challenges.
2. The therapist should be aware that these events, despite their private character, might infuse and influence the therapy situation. The therapist must be ready to tackle complex decisions in relation to self-disclosure and do so by recognizing the multiple dimensions that should inform this decision such as the timing and extent of the disclosure. Decisions should also take into account such factors as the age and psychopathology of the patient and his or her life situation with respect to parenting.
3. Therapists should keep in mind that while in the midst of one of these crises, they might be too vulnerable themselves to help their patients deal with the intrusion of the event (e.g., therapist's distraction, absence, inflexibility) into the therapeutic situation and the patients' more negative emotions surrounding it. Obtaining special resources (e.g., supervisory input) or time off might be helpful to all.

Notes

1. Some drugstore urine tests boast of equality of results, although they are less accurate.
2. Seeing and holding the fetus may result in increased risks for depression, anxiety and PTSD symptoms, as will be presented in the section that follows.
3. Eight percent of infants die within the first year of life. Many worry about sudden infant death syndrome (SIDS), but actually this accounts for only 7% of all infant deaths (Matthews, MacDorman, & Thoma, 2015).
4. Reynolds (2003) suggests that parents who have suffered this loss be informed of the option to hold and see their dead infant, and that those professionals involved in the process help parents assess the risks and benefits of these options.
5. Cacciatore, Froen, and Killian (2013) also found a significant number of women blame themselves, although not all.
6. Bennett (2005) refers to the loss as a traumatic grief that does not dissipate even with subsequent pregnancy.

7. See Barbanel, 1980; Cosgrove, 2004; Freeman, 2005; Gerson, 1996; Lazar, 1990; Leon, 1992; Zucker, 2014, 2015.

8. More information can be found on the Reproductive Health Infertility section of the CDC website (www.cdc.gov/reproductivehealth/Infertility/index.htm, last updated April 16, 2016).

9. When women do not have predictable menstrual cycles, are over 35, or have other high-risk factors, they may be encouraged to consider their options sooner than one year (www.cdc.gov/reproductivehealth/infertility, updated December 19, 2016).

10. In 2014, *Forbes* reported that the average "fresh" IVF cycle costs $12,000, before medications, which typically run another $3,000 to $5,000. (https://www.forbes.com/sites/learnvest/2014/02/06/the-cost-of-ivf-4-things-i-learned-while-battling-infertility/#3050a27124dd, February 6, 2014). However, this seems like an underestimate. A large-scale study (Katz et al., 2011) found the median cost for IVF and IVF-donor egg groups were $24,373 and $38,015 for IVF and IVF-donor egg groups, respectively. Cost of successful outcomes (delivery or ongoing pregnancy by 18 months) averaged $61,377 for IVF. Most insurance does not cover these procedures, but may cover a portion of some of the medications.

11. For example, the percentage of cycles resulting in a full-term, normal weight, single birth for under age 35 is 23%, 38–40 is 13%, 43–33 is 3% (www.cdc.gov/art/reports/2014/national-summary.html, reviewed December 19, 2016).

12. ART has dramatically increased the number of multiple births that occur. Multiple births increase medical risks and complications to both the mother and infant prior to birth. They also are more likely to result in premature births and increase maternal depression after birth. Implanting several embryos, as is common practice, can result in no pregnancy, but it also can result in several fetuses (www.acog.org/Resources-And-Publications/Committee-Opinions/Committee-on-Ethics/Multifetal-Pregnancy-Reduction).

CHAPTER 6

Therapist as Father

The transition to parenthood is an important transformation for a male therapist as well as for a female therapist. Fatherhood is deeply rooted in biology and the structures of society and culture, belief and custom. Although the historian's data source and point of view to some extent determines the emphasis of the descriptive role, throughout history "Father" has claimed a number of significant roles—as a companion, care provider, spouses' protector, model moral guide, teacher and breadwinner (LaRossa, 1997). Sociocultural forces have drastically changed the relative importance of each of these roles over the past few hundred years (Brooks & Gilbert, 1995; Demos, 1994).

The role of the father today has its roots in the religious ideology of ancient Greek and Roman times, during which he had the responsibility and capacity to control all non-religious aspects of the lives of his wives, children, concubines and slaves (Rotundo, 1985). The "patriarchal father" in the imperial Western world had an enormous influence. As parents and children worked the land together, his role was an intricate and tethered part of domestic and work life, as a caregiver, a companion, a model, a moral teacher, overseer, educator, benefactor and guidance counselor. He *was* the primary parent, psychologically and physically present in his children's lives, and this was particularly true when it came to sons (Pleck & Pleck, 1997).

According to social commentator Blankenhorn (1995), men's shrinking involvement in the home was set in motion with industrialization, when factory work led to the physical separation of work and home. The father assumed the primary role of economic provider (Lovett, 2007). The writings of the time also emphasized the child's development of conscience and self-government rather than simple submission; the childrearing literature placed increasing emphasis on persuasion and coaxing and less on coercion, and mothers were assumed more capable of obtaining obedience through love and understanding. Thus, a new ideology developed in which the chief responsibilities for raising the young were allocated to the mother, as she became the primary parent (Demos, 1994). Thus, as the mother's importance in childrearing expanded, the father's role was marginalized. He became a more part-time figure in his children's lives as his role as teacher, moral overseer and companion waned and his role as provider and protector became central. His best attributes of ambition and aggressiveness were often viewed as at odds with domestic life, and he was frequently viewed as incompetent as a caregiver on the home front, a rival to his children for attention from the overburdened mother.

In the twentieth century, principally after the Great Depression, a central function of the father was as a "pal" or chum in addition to breadwinning and moral guardianship roles (LaRossa, 1997). Although infant care (and particularly care of the sick infant) was the province of mothers, many childrearing manuals and books were aimed at "parents" working together, giving fathers an increased role. Letters written to the Children's Bureau, founded in 1912 to protect children, indicated that there were fathers (albeit a small proportion) who took a more significant and warmer role in caring for small children than has generally been acknowledged (LaRossa, 1997).

In the 1960s, the "Participant Dad" became the ideal as the demand for his physical and psychological presence in the family dramatically increased. Although breadwinning remains a key role for the father in most segments of society, this "nurturant" father was (and is) expected to be more actively involved with his children, particularly in focusing on the fun activities and displaying warmth, affection and chumminess (Demos, 1994; Lamb, 1986, 2010; Pleck & Pleck, 1997). Indeed, in large subcultures of today's society, fathers are expected to be available when their children and spouse need them.

In our pluralistic society, the confluence of the women's movement, the gay fathers' movement, and the single fathers' rights movement have emphasized that a variety of concepts of the "ideal" father can co-occur; variations on these ideals occur as each subculture, ethnic group and class define and redefine their spoken and unspoken norms around appropriate fatherly behavior. As such, these "ideals" are built on shifting family and cultural demands and expectations. Such shifts create tension and loyalty conflicts for men in relationship to their families, work and the larger society. The "successful" father is defined in terms of his child's development and the demands of his sociocultural and familial context (Franklin & Davis, 2000; Lamb, 1997a).

The literature has begun to reflect a burgeoning appreciation of the positive influence that an active father can have on his children's development, as well as the tensions and issues experienced by the new father (Raeburn, 2014). However, much less has been written about the development of a paternal identity (Cath, Gurwitt, & Ross, 1994; Diamond, 1995; Lamb, 2010a, 2010b; Osherson, 1986, 1992, 1999; Ross, 1994). Our own experience in reviewing the therapist's pregnancy and parenthood literature parallels this general trend. Prior to our previous edition of this volume, nearly nothing had been written about the male therapist's entrance into parenthood and its impact on the therapeutic interaction. Unlike our female therapists, who often worried a great deal about many of these issues, the male therapists, more frequently than not, felt as if they had been caught off guard with their patients' curiosities and their surprise at the emerging issues.

Over the past 20 years, we conducted a semi-structured interview with 16 male therapists whose wives had been pregnant within 2 years from when we interviewed them. Some were interviewed during the third trimester of pregnancy and again a month after they returned to work, and some were done entirely retrospectively. Therapists were asked general questions about their personal reactions and reactions of their patients at each trimester and when they returned to work. Additionally we obtained written or oral vignettes and experiences from approximately 20 other male therapists (Fallon & Brabender, 2004; Fallon, Famadoor, & Brabender, 2009). Notably, the theoretical orientations of these therapists were varied.

Based on our discussions with these male therapists and reading of the scant literature, we present their observations and struggles with the hope that male therapists, their female colleagues and their collective supervisors will give some of these issues consideration prior to their occurrence in therapy. Additionally, this chapter can be utilized by the pregnant therapist in understanding her spouse's response to the pregnancy. Our focus in this chapter is on (a) the development of an identity as a father; (b) a discussion of the impact that their wife's pregnancy can have on the therapeutic hour; (c) a review of some of the tensions experienced by the father-in-waiting and father of the young child; and (d) a final consideration of the some of the technical dilemmas in the therapy.

Developing an Identity as a Father

Although becoming a father is an important life cycle event, many of the male therapists we interviewed often neither consciously contemplated nor incorporated into their professional identities their budding fatherhood. As Osherson (1999) noted, unlike career achievement, fatherhood is generally not rehearsed or practiced as a child and does not become a central part of identity until fatherhood status is actually achieved. The development of this identity, certainly for a therapist, is aided by an appreciation for the central role that a father plays in the development of his child. Osherson (1999) eloquently described this role in the following poignant passage:

> Fathers play a vital role in the child's normal drama around separation from mother; they safeguard and nurture their child's healthy self-respect, and they are the guardians and custodians of their children's healthy aggression and mastery . . . The father beckons to the child at many different ages. For the baby who only has eyes for mother and is disconsolate when she leaves the room, for the toddler who wants to explore the world beyond mother's lap yet timidly wonders if safety lies only in her arms, for the school-aged child taking the school bus for the first time wondering if it's better to stay home with mommy, for the normal teenager tottering on the edge of adult

sexuality and power—for all of these children, father's attention and interest are a bridge away from the comfort of mother toward the comfort and challenge of the larger world.

(p. 216)

The father acquaints the infant, and later the child, with an exciting and larger outer world, promoting differentiation and individuation, while the mother provides a safe haven from which to explore (Gunsberg, 1994). Although this viewpoint originates from the psychoanalytic and developmental theoretical stance, an explosion of research since the 1980s supports the important contributions that fathers make throughout their children's development (Coley, 2001; Eberwein, 2017; Lamb, 1997b; Ross, 1994; Silverstein & Auerbach, 1999; Raeburn, 2014).[1]

Until recently, it was felt that the father's relationship with his child became important only later in infancy. However, newer research suggests that expectant fathers' mental status and involvement with their wives' preparations for the child significantly impacts infant well-being (Alio, 2010; Shah, 2010). Infants are capable of forming early significant attachments to their fathers, even if the father does not take significant responsibility for caretaking activities (Bretherton, 2010; Yogman, 1994).

Fathers also provide a unique and qualitatively different way of interacting with infants than mothers do. For instance, with regard to differences in playing with the infant, mothers tend to play in a more conventional manner (e.g., games and toys), and fathers tend to do so in a more unpredictable, idiosyncratic, and physically stimulating fashion (Lamb, 2010b). Whereas mothers are generally more rhythmic and containing, fathers engage in staccato bursts of both physical and social stimulation with their children (Yogman, 1994). Fathers hold their infants as part of play, whereas mothers hold their infants more for care giving activities and to restrain from them from unsafe activities. Fathers' play with their infants also differs with regard to the gender of the infant; they are much more active with their male than female children, even at 1 year of age, whereas mothers are equally active (Gunsberg, 1994). Similarly the synchrony of emotions with their infants is much more intense, particularly with their sons (Feldman, 2003). Thus, differences in infant–parental interactions provide the child with exposure to different and complementary cognitive and emotional organizations of the world.

By preschool, children with highly involved fathers are characterized by increased cognitive competence, increased empathy, less gender role stereotyping, and a more internal locus of control (Pleck, 1997). Surprisingly, a child's language development is more closely related to the father's language skills than the mother's (Leech, Salo, Rowe, & Cabrera, 2013; Pancsofar & Vernon-Feagans, 2010).

A father's presence and influence is particularly salient as the child steps into the outside world. A father's "destabilizing" and activating interactions with his child enhance transition to school, decrease behavioral problems, and increase popularity with teachers and peers (Paquette, 2004; Parke, 2002; Sarkadi, Kristiansson, Oberklaid, & Bremberg, 2008). In adolescence, positive and greater paternal engagement is associated with good self-control, high self-esteem, intelligence, life skills, and social competence (Coley, 2001; Koestner, Franz, & Weinberger, 1990; Pleck, 1997; Russell, 1986). For girls, it is associated with less risky sexual behavior (DelPriore & Hill, 2013; Tither & Ellis, 2008). Overall, a father's consistent and active engagement is associated with an array of positive outcomes including cognitive, social, emotional and behavioral (see Sarkadi, Kristiansson, Oberklaid, & Bremberg's 2008 review of 24 studies).

High paternal involvement also has indirect positive effects for infants and children. Research suggests that the husband's support of his wife lessens the degree of maternal distress prenatally and during labor (Cummings & Reilly, 1997). By supporting the mother after the birth, a more effective mother–infant relationship occurs, which facilitates positive adjustment by children (Yogman, 1994). In addition, a father's capacity to reduce or resolve conflict with his wife enables better child adjustment (Pollack, 1995).

The weight of the research suggests that the father's involvement in the development of his child offers something complementary and healthy to the mother's role. In addition, many personal rewards accrue for the father, which include delight, a sense of renewal and the opportunity to be creative (Yogman, 1994). Pruett put it this way:

> What makes tending babies so powerful, moving, even healing is that it often allows men to attend to a gender-blind childlikeness in themselves. The abiding wish for intimacy, the capacity for unambivalent love, hope, and forgiveness, and the rewards of vulnerability and dependency are what make children so wonderfully human. . . . In physically attending to his child, a man is reaching back into himself, into his own experience for something he cannot necessarily remember, in which he may have lost faith and trust, and for which he probably has no role models from his own childhood—an abiding wish nurturing male presence. Here his baby has a very important impact. What his child actually provides is unforbidden access to the childlike (not childish) part of the father's unfinished incomplete, pre-gendered/role self.
>
> (Pruett, 1987, pp. 230–231)

The Impact of the Emerging Pregnancy

While having a baby happens at the same time for a couple, men and women don the parental cloak in different ways and meanings to the event. The emerging reality of pregnancy and parenthood for each parent may vary. In this section, we review his tasks, personal feelings, experiences and transferences as they evolve by trimester. According to Campbell (1989), all men progress through three phases of pregnancy that correspond only very loosely to the prenatal trimesters: the announcement, the moratorium (an emotional withdrawal) and the redefinition of themselves and their roles. We discuss the impact of pregnancy on the therapy and male therapist by trimester beginning prior to conception and ending with ongoing fatherhood issues, as most of the therapists we interviewed related their experiences through the trimester time lens.

Achieving Pregnancy

The transition to becoming a father is an important but stressful one, often accompanied by personal upheaval and disorganization. If the pregnancy is planned, several months prior to the impregnation, an intense internal and external reworking of old relationships in relation to the self unfolds (Osofsky & Culp, 1993). The previously established equilibrium surrounding conflicts of sexual identity, career and marital choices is again challenged, although perhaps less obviously than for the mother to be. Still, it is a stressful developmental crisis (Chandler, 1998). The preparation for pregnancy and the newborn commences and renews a renegotiation of previous and present relationships with parents, siblings and spouse. A process of self-resynthesis continues throughout the pregnancy and well after childbirth (Gurwitt, 1994, 1995). One therapist told us that he thought a great deal about his father during his wife's pregnancy:

> I wondered if I was beginning to hear things differently from my patients. I think that as a therapist there may have been shifts in my identification in subtle ways. In general, I felt I was now listening to the other side of the generational divide.

Most men at this stage begin to set goals for themselves as fathers, often based upon their own childhood recollections, choosing to compensate for their fathers' deficiencies or to emulate them. These goals are often modified as observations of families around them and emerging interactions with their own children restructure the realities of being a father (Lamb, 2010).

When pregnancy is finally achieved, although excitement and a sense of accomplishment are present, most fathers-to-be feel some ambivalence about their new status and it seems to take longer to work through this ambivalence than it does for their female counterparts (Cohen, 1993; Ellsbury, 1987). They acknowledge anxieties about finances, their capabilities in their role as father and the loss of the freedom that came with the childless portion of their life (Campbell, 1989). Their anxieties concerning their new life often silently dominate their thoughts. As Fainman articulated it, "There is no obvious biological sign of pregnancy that others can respond to, which will denote their status, like a pregnant 'bump or bulge.' The male's bump is invisible, certainly physically and for many preferably dynamically too" (p. 27).

First Trimester

In the first trimester, as with female therapists, most male therapists we interviewed did not feel that the pregnancy changed how they conducted therapy. The exceptions occurred when male therapists worked closely with their wives in a practice or hospital setting. For example, one group therapist whose wife was his co-therapist was acutely aware of his wife's needs and felt the need to be protective of her, which he felt put him in conflict with the needs of the group. Male therapists reported that they were in general much more aware of themes related to birthing and being parents. Whether patients were picking up on unconscious aspects of the therapists' behavior or whether the therapists were more sensitive to these ever-present themes remains unclear. One therapist conducting a group put it this way:

> The group did not find out about the pregnancy. . . . The group made the co-therapist more like a spouse and asked us more questions regarding how we were as moms and dads or sometimes what we would have done as parents if we were in a certain situation . . . my co-therapist was a vibrant woman of 65. This was a new development for a group that had been together for half a year.

Described as a "whirlwind or unreal experience," this term is marked by psychological disequilibrium, and our male therapists reported concerns about the viability of the pregnancy and fears of losing the baby and/or spouse. Guy et al. (1986) wrote about his anger toward an unmarried patient having an abortion when he was concerned with a possible miscarriage of his own child. He also spoke about his secret guilt and feelings of betrayal for conceiving in response to a depressed female patient who was grieving the loss of early menopause.

Our therapists reported awareness of certain pregnancy-related themes that appeared in their patients' issues and meanderings, but most shied away from any kind of exploration. In retrospect, they speculated that they felt that they were not prepared to be questioned about their personal status and felt uncertain in separating their own issues from their patients. In our supervision of male therapists, we have come to believe that further exploration is likely to lead to a patient's more personal exploration rather than a questioning of the therapist's status.

An interesting phenomenon occurs with many men in this trimester and again in the third trimester: they develop physical symptoms that mimic their wives' symptoms, such as appetite loss, nausea, vomiting, emotional lability and other aches and body pains (Mason & Elwood, 1995). Known as Couvade syndrome, or sympathetic pregnancy, this phenomenon occurs in many cultures and there are some studies that suggest that up to 87% of men report at least one of these symptoms during their wife's pregnancy (Klein, 1991; Devi & Chanu, 2015). This response is said to be partly in response to identification with his wife, but also partly arising from his own internal state. As Gurwitt (1994) stated, "the experience of powerful magical forces being at work. . . . The couvade phenomenon in its many forms would be an attempt to ward off the powerful internal and external forces to which all members of the society are subject" (Gurwitt, 1994, p. 298). Feinman (2002) detailed possible psychological etiology for this syndrome, which included identification with the expectant mother, identification with the father of his childhood, identification with the fetus, reawakening of the Oedipal strivings, rivalry toward the fetus, intensification of dependency, parturition envy, and sexuality and gender issues. Recently, some have attributed these symptoms to increased prolactin and cortisol levels in men during their wives' pregnancies. However, the data suggests that the increases occur in the third trimester rather than the first, and will be discussed in more detail in a later section (Feldman, Gordon, Schneiderman, Weisman, & Zagoory-Sharon, 2010; Storey, Walsh, Quinton, & Wynne-Edwards, 2000).

With one exception, none of our interviewees announced his wife's pregnancy during this trimester, although in a few instances when the therapist missed a session at the last minute, support staff revealed the status of the therapist without the therapist's permission. Interestingly, this was less likely to happen with female therapists who guarded their status more closely so that support staff generally did not know during this trimester and therefore could not spill the beans. The single exception demonstrates how one's status as a prospective parent can be disclosed in unanticipated ways: one therapist revealed to a patient that his wife was pregnant after the patient, a grandmother, questioned him about his status of being married and having children.

Second Trimester

During the second trimester, the expectant father may remain somewhat ambivalent and feel emotionally detached from the pregnancy (Levant, 1995). This can be a stressful period in the couple's relationship, because his wife's relief from nausea, fatigue, and emotional lability of the first trimester, coupled with her experience of fetal growth, has moved her toward an acceptance of the pregnancy and a productive, exciting period. Thus, the couple's levels of connection to the pregnancy and acceptance of their new status as parents are not synchronous and can lead to conflict in the relationship. Frequently fathers resolve their ambivalence relating to the baby once they experience fetal movement. How easily this happens depends on each person's prior sense of self, family of origin relationships and current social supports (Campbell, 1989).

Usually, fetal movement ushers in awe in achievement from both prospective parents and a more secure connection to this new nuclear family. At the same time, many men see the child as a rival for attention and support that conjures up memories of an envied sibling. Envy of the mother's ability to bear a child is also a typical part of the affective picture (Gurwitt, 1994).

These personal feelings may find their way into the therapeutic interaction. Ambivalence, guilt, envy and so on can often affect the way the therapist responds to the events in a patient's life. For example, one male therapist who expressed considerable ambivalence about his wife's pregnancy reported that one of his patients wanted to become pregnant and he found himself withdrawing and pulling back from her because he did not want to get "too involved." He recognized that he felt similarly toward his wife and her pregnancy. Another therapist reported:

> My wife had a healthy pregnancy, but I was much more aware of my potential to be hurt . . . more conscious of where I sat. I often positioned myself near the door. There was a heightened awareness of the vulnerability of my family.

During this trimester, conflicts about revealing versus not revealing the pregnancy emerged. None of the male therapists we interviewed (unlike their female counterparts) announced the pregnancy to their patients. Occasionally, patients would discover that their therapist's wife was pregnant from other sources. It was at these points that male therapists were desirous of some collegial or supervisory input.

Yet, almost without exception, each therapist was acutely aware that his wife's pregnancy had changed the way he was personally feeling. They were sensitive to the fact that it certainly influenced the material that they heard and perhaps on what and the way that they focused on this material. Most felt conflicted: a desire to reveal and an internal admonition not to reveal personal information. (We focus more on the question about whether and how to reveal the pregnancy in the next section of this chapter.) Toward the end of this trimester, most of the male therapists that we interviewed considered how much time would be sequestered for the new family unit. While there was some acting out on the part of the patients, most therapists felt that because there was little direct disclosure, it could not be attributed to their wives' pregnancies.

Third Trimester

In the third trimester, the reality of impending fatherhood sets in. Our male therapists were personally more excited, and at the same time fraught with anticipatory anxieties. Each had his own way of dealing with anxieties. For example, some read, others surfed the internet to allay their fears of envisioned tragedies, and still others used denial. Fewer marital differences are apparent as the father-to-be has developmentally accepted his role. Couvade symptoms again emerge or intensify (Feldman et al., 2010; Johansson, Edwardsson, & Hildingsson, 2015). Recent studies have suggested that, similar to women, men have an increase in their levels of prolactin and oxytocin (Feldman et al., 2010;

Storey et al., 2010). These hormones have been linked to increases in maternal caregiver behaviors.

Unlike female counterparts who more readily spoke with co-workers and supervisors, male therapists were more solitary and silent in their concerns. One male therapist who never articulated any concerns during his wife's pregnancy, when probed a year later, said the following:

> My wife was set to deliver as I was finishing my training. I did not yet have a job. I was so worried. My wife was not working and a new baby was coming. How would I support them? I could not concentrate and could not sleep. My wife ended up having to console me. "It will be ok she said." A real reversal of roles.

In therapy, three technical points should be considered: whether and how much time to take off from work; whether to announce a hiatus before the birth or after; and how much to reveal about this major life event. The first issue is often dictated by personal circumstances and the professional setting in which one practices. Although all the male therapists we interviewed intended to be at the birth, a striking difference along gender lines about the time expected to be away from their practices and jobs was evident. Although some planned for a longer paternal leave, male therapists expected to take 1 day to 1 week off on the average. A number of them felt conflicted about taking this time. Some in outpatient practice expressed the increased financial pressures; days with the family meant days unpaid. Others working for organizations expressed guilt about leaving work responsibilities to colleagues during the additional days after the birth. Many felt a countervailing pressure from their wives or other children to remain with their families. This difference is interesting in light of US-mandated law, which allows for unpaid parental leave, available equally to mothers and fathers.[2] About 40% of the men who are aware of paternity leave opt not to take it (Martin, 2013). California and New Jersey are the only states that have paid paternity leave (Reuters, 2011).

Because none of the therapists we interviewed had announced the event prior to this trimester (although some patients had discovered it), most felt some uncertainty about whether and how to reveal the pregnancy. Many acknowledged seeking supervision or consultation for these issues. Of those who did not, a number expressed regret over not doing so. An optimal candidate to provide supervision, fathers observed, is a therapist who has had the experience of becoming a father and is therefore likely to be most sensitive to relevant issues. The therapist in the following vignette articulated many of the questions expressed by our therapists:

Vignette 6.1
When I told my patients that my wife was expecting, they all expressed joy. I said "thank you" and tried to move on to the agenda that I had for the

session. Even if they wanted to talk further, I shifted to the agenda. If they asked other questions it was hard for me to figure out what to do, whether to dwell on it, whether I would lose my sense of competence . . . They did want to spend more time on it. . . . part of me wanted to talk about it, but would I be depriving them of what they needed to talk about . . . when I talked to my supervisor. I wanted to shift the focus because I was uncomfortable. I wanted to talk about it because it was a novel experience . . . but I was not sure if there were rules about it in doing therapy . . . would I be crossing boundaries . . . also a fear of losing control in the role as a therapist.

Although this therapist broached the topic in supervision, he felt that in a parallel process the supervisor, like he, focused his attention on the therapy agenda. Another male therapist had the following experience in supervision:

Vignette 6.2

My wife and I decided that I would take a week off from my practice, beginning when my wife went into labor. So, for some patients I would be missing one session. For some, I may not miss at all. How could I announce that I would be away when I did not know the dates? In our prenatal classes, they told us to prepare a bag ahead of time and that it could happen rather quickly. Should I treat it like an illness and just cancel at the last minute? Or should I tell my clients ahead of time, but then would I need to tell them why? They would wonder and question me. I also had the other problem of who would call them if I was unavailable and would I have the presence of mind to remember to do this? I talked to my supervisor about this. He was very clear. This was my issue and not my patient's. To paraphrase, what I heard him say was that my vision was clouded by my own excitement and sense of accomplishment and I should talk more about that in my own therapy. If I was only planning to miss a maximum of one session per patient, I should call when it happens and cancel with the simple explanation that I needed to cancel for personal reasons. When I return, I should explore their feelings about my missing a session. I was completely deflated, but dutifully complied with my supervisor's advice. I still wonder about that.

Disclosure of the pregnancy is a concern to many of the male therapists we interviewed. About two-thirds of the therapists felt that their patients never knew that they had become fathers. Most who did inform their patients of their newfound status did so at the time of the missed session. Some others said that they needed to cancel for personal reasons.

If patients learned about the pregnancy from other sources and inquired about it, the acknowledgment by the therapist was usually followed by a perfunctory "congratulations" with little discussion. Most of the therapists revealed their discomfort discussing the topic and so were relieved when discourse about it waned. In general, unlike their female counterparts, male therapists were not asked very much information about the baby and they did not feel pressed to reveal personal information. One therapist whose group found out about the pregnancy through other sources acknowledged that he "was disappointed that the group members had little reaction and wished that group members had shown more envy or jealousy." A few therapists regretted that they had not taken more initiative in exploring issues related to the pregnancy and their new status when they felt it was present.

The expressed patients' reactions to their therapists becoming fathers were very different in quality and in intensity than females' experiences. Although it is possible that patients were truly unaware of their therapists' major life transition, it is also likely that at least some therapists were not aware of derivative material that existed, and patients sensed that their therapists did not wish to discuss this personal information.

Disclose or Not Disclose the Pregnancy, and When?

Although most expectant fathers with whom we spoke revealed little information about their new status, a legitimate question is whether a strategy of revelation moves the therapy forward. The optimal approach is probably situation specific. Some relevant factors to consider are setting and the nature of the therapeutic relationship; the amount of time that the new father will be away from his patients; the potential sense of betrayal that a patient may experience by discovering this information at a later date; the therapist's level of comfort with the personal revelation; and the ongoing impact that this new status will have on the therapeutic relationship. Each of these five factors is discussed briefly.

Setting is one of the most significant factors. In some settings, such as the psychiatric hospital, therapeutic connection is brief, with patient turnover every few days. Patients come to expect that hospital staff will precipitously disappear for emergency coverage, vacations, conferences, and other hospital duties. In this whirlwind of pebbled and inconsistent treatment and providers, the particular impact of this event on patients may be minimal. For settings that involve longer-term treatment and therapists' commitment to specific patients, the nature of the therapeutic relationship becomes more significant. The possible effects that the upcoming absence has on each patient is another important consideration. One might decide to disclose to one patient, but not another (Fainman, 2002).

Most therapists were more comfortable revealing the particulars with patients who were in a more supportive treatment, with the worry that revelation in a more dynamically oriented treatment was originating from the therapists' own preoccupations. As one therapist put it, "For my patients in psychodynamic therapy, I felt like it was their therapy. To say anything when they did not bring it up either directly or derivatively would have made it my therapy." This, of course, is the traditional analytic stance with regard to personal disclosure, and implies that such divulgences would be countertransference. Yet, even when countertransference motives are present, insights can be culled. In one example, a therapist revealed to a grandmother patient about the upcoming birth. While he recognized that his initial revelation in part was based upon his own feelings of isolation, this enabled this female patient to begin to talk about her experiences with both her children and grandchildren, because she felt that now that he was going to be a father, he understood her dilemmas.

We would contend that therapists' judicious personal revelations can sometimes lead to good modeling and growth promoting experiences in patients (Yalom & Leszcz, 2005). Here is an example of the way in which disclosure of the pregnancy augmented the therapeutic process.

Vignette 6.3

One of the more special opportunities during the time I was expecting my first child occurred with Trish, a 43-year-old woman who had devoted 20 years to caring for children with physical handicaps. She came into treatment after an inpatient stay for a serious suicide attempt. She had been a recovering alcoholic for about 7 years and had just lost her sister to a drug overdose. Her sister had been instrumental in her recovery.

At the time my wife and I were expecting our first child, I had already seen Trish in once a week supportive-expressive individual psychotherapy for 4 years. Trish had also been in group therapy with my wife during several stays in the inpatient service. She knew that my wife and I were married because it was common knowledge around the hospital. Trish at this time had weathered several bouts of serious suicidal despairs. Her anger at being abandoned by her sister had reached a fevered pitch in acting-out behavior with others. We talked about her angry outbursts as her attempts to convey to others the righteous indignation she felt about being abandoned and misunderstood. She showed a gentler side to me in the transference, which took on a mildly eroticized but generally positive tone. Others saw her as the quintessential Borderline, and despite her anger at me in the treatment (for not seeing her side of the story, for hospitalizing her once when she had a slip and became unwittingly suicidal) we had a relationship characterized by mutual respect. I remember being literally trepidatious that she would experience my wife's pregnancy as an abandonment, especially because she had never married and her serious depressions and alcoholism had cost her a career in public service with children. I was already mourning the loss of our generally peaceful trusting relationship. Although my orientation is interpersonal in nature, and I readily disclose my subjective reactions to patients in the service of working our way out of sticky issues related to core maladaptive patterns of interaction, I rarely disclose other personal information to patients. My belief is that treatment with Trish took a turn for the better when I started to share more personal information about the expected baby. I decided to begin seeing Trish twice a week shortly before the baby was born feeling that this would provide her with a measure of support around the time of the baby's birth. Trish began to encourage me to bring in pictures of my child after the birth. Instead of railing at me for abandoning her when I took off around the time of the birth and for not bringing in any pictures of the baby after the birth, Trish grew more serious about exploring the issue of abandonment in a productive manner. She began to express her anger directly at me in sessions especially about hospitalizing her when she had become suicidal and "abandoning" her to staff who did not understand her. Her sense was that she was able to trust me more because I had "loosened up" by being more human with her (accepting a gift for the baby and sharing my feelings about the birth). Trish grew less explosive during these months after the birth showing a firm assertiveness. She was more peaceful. I eventually placed a picture of my daughter in my hospital office, which Trish correctly ascertained was an indication of greater trust. I had, in fact, been plagued by the fantasy that if I brought a picture in she would eventually abduct my child in a fatal attraction retribution for my rejecting her. I feel strongly that this was a turning point in the treatment. Three years after my daughter's birth Trish feels hopeful again, she does volunteer work with children, and feels a sense of trust with not only me but several people in her life. She has encouraged me to share stories about my daughter's development, which usually produces a moment where she can share her expertise in child development and education. She says it makes her feel that she can really give me something back for the help she has received. We have moved to working on her guilt and gratitude in this regard. I could not have predicted that my daughter's birth would have deepened the treatment in these ways.

In this vignette, rich with transference/countertransference interplay, the therapist uses disclosure and the birth of his child as a stepping-stone to explore productively the presumably long-standing issue of loss. This particular disclosure may have been especially meaningful to her; perhaps her therapist trusting her with information about his baby was reparative to her self-esteem in light of her previous failure in her former vocation. Part of the initial repair may have been the therapist's acknowledgment (to himself) of the fantasy of the patient's envy (abduction of his child). This potency of the fantasy, a projective identification, was deactivated and metabolized for the patient by placing a picture of the child in plain view, a recognition that this was only a fantasy and that the patient could be trusted. This vignette provides an example of how the woven tapestry of the personal circumstances of the therapist, his ensuing disclosure, and the details of this particular patient's background enable particularly meaningful therapeutic work to be accomplished.

How long a therapist may not be available around the birth and thereafter may compel the therapist to provide more specific information. For instance, if the therapist will be curtailing availability after the birth, he may want to acknowledge the event at least a month prior to its occurrence in order to work through the patients' possible feelings of rejection. If the therapist intends to take less than a week off, which may mean that a number of his patients will never perceive any break in treatment, then it may behoove the therapist to consider other factors that may obviate his imparting information. For instance, if this is the first child, will the new father be too preoccupied, tired, or excited to devote a reasonable amount of energy to his patients? What are the realistic probabilities of a complication that would necessitate additional time off (e.g., a wife's cesarean section may require the father to care for another older child longer than anticipated)?

If longer than one week will be missed, we recommend that the therapist give anywhere from 2 weeks' to 2 months' notice to the patient. The longer the hiatus and/or the more patients who are more anxiously dependent, may require some warning, exploration, and reassurance that adequate coverage will be available and that the therapist will return. If the therapist is planning to miss only one session or less (as most of the male therapists that we interviewed did) and there are no other extenuating circumstances, we do not believe that the therapist is required to announce the event. Unfortunately, extenuating circumstances cannot always be predicted. If the therapist is unable to return when planned, some information provided to patients allows them to utilize the healthiest parts of their ego to muster understanding. Whether and what the therapist reveals depends upon the nature of the patient's issues and the therapist's level of comfort with the personal revelation.

In discussions with many senior colleagues, considerable disagreement prevailed concerning the disclosing of information regarding fatherhood and information about the baby. Many of our colleagues are of the opinion that for a number of patients, not being told this information at the time of the birth, and discovering it later on their own, leads to a sense of betrayal and erosion of trust that far outweigh the therapist's fears of unnecessarily contaminating the treatment with personal information. For example, one female patient (a therapist herself) learned from a mutual colleague several months after the event that her male therapist had become a father. On this discovery, she expressed that she felt a sense of betrayal by her lack of awareness. She, too, was a member of the same professional community and felt humiliated by not knowing this when other colleagues did. Their relationship had a certain tenuous balance in terms of power and equity. The lack of disclosure made salient the inequity in their relationship and exacerbated her premorbid sense of intense shame. This was coupled with the fact that she recently had painstakingly shared many "dark secrets." For her to share and remain in therapy, she had to believe that they had a certain kind of mutuality; this lack of disclosure, she felt, was a disregard for the relationship and her needs. Despite continued attempts by the therapist to explore her sense of humiliation and betrayal, the previous level of trust could not be salvaged and the patient discontinued therapy. This example highlights not only issues of betrayal, but also the importance of taking self-esteem and personality factors into account when considering a pregnancy announcement. For other patients, this humiliation, sense of betrayal and lack of trust often could be worked through. The therapist must weigh the risks of betrayal against the complications that personal disclosures create in the treatment, and recognize that non-disclosure might not always be in the best interests of the client (Henretty & Levitt, 2010).

In this next example, the patient confronted the therapist with her knowledge and the therapist was able to use therapeutically the material that ensued.

Vignette 6.4

While I was expecting my daughter, I told all my patients, with the exception of one, that I was expecting a child and that I would be taking my regular August vacation (my daughter was expected then), but might have to vary it a bit based on when she arrived. The one patient I did not tell about the pregnancy was Rebecca, an attractive, youthful professional woman in her late fifties who had just undergone a radical hysterectomy. Rebecca had also been in a childless, loveless marriage with a man many years her senior. A long-suffering self-involved woman, Rebecca had made good progress in three times weekly psychoanalytic psychotherapy. I rationalized not telling Rebecca about the expected baby, feeling it would add insult to injury, especially because she herself would be away the 2 weeks following my scheduled vacation. Furthermore, she had never asked me personal questions throughout the course of therapy. I had clearly underestimated Rebecca. Four weeks after my daughter was born, she asked me "So has your second child been born?" She had evidently known that my wife was expecting because she surmised that the woman who shared the suite with me was my wife and she had not seen her return to her office because of the maternity leave. I answered her question honestly, saying that it was my first child, and we began to explore the significant meaning of my not sharing this news with her. She felt I had underestimated her progress in the treatment and was treating her like the fragile, highly constricted, and isolated woman that had begun treatment with me many years earlier. We entered a new phase of treatment where she was able to chide me in a good-natured way about my limitations and I was able to acknowledge the changes she had made. Although I still find that I share little personal information with her, I do disclose considerably more countertransference material in the here-and-now of our therapy interactions than I did prior to the birth of my daughter. Not surprisingly, over the years since my daughter was born, Rebecca reconnected with several nieces and nephews with whom she had lost touch and now frequently takes trips out of state to visit them.

Although the therapist did not initially reveal information about the birth of his child, when the patient brought it up, he was able to acknowledge the countertransferential elements of his behavior and avoid an irredeemable betrayal. The discussion fostered growth for both the patient and therapist.

The male therapists we interviewed were more tentative in revealing information about their new status than their female counterparts. In accordance with this trend, Simone, McCarthy, and Skay (1998) found that for female therapists, with experience, self-disclosure increases but eventually plateaus as they move to an intermediate level of experience. For male therapists moving from intermediate to high levels of experience, self-disclosure diminished. These gender differences in self-disclosure might be, in part, a psychology shaped by generations of cultural norms as to appropriate role behavior. However, other factors could affect this lack of disclosure as well: too much interest in family life may be seen as a feminine characteristic; or perhaps they may perceive that concern about their personal life will be viewed by others as being uncommitted to their profession (Pleck, 1993). With regard to the latter reason, often male "contexts" do not give them permission to give this event its due. This is supported by observations that women receive more personal gifts and gifts for the baby than men do. Fewer men sought senior colleagues or supervision than their pregnant female colleagues. Those who did often did not find it helpful, as one of the earlier examples illustrates. It also may be that they felt less comfortable talking with senior colleagues to gain some insight, and so were less able to work through these unspoken values.

Another possibility as to why our male therapists did not reveal information about their newfound status may have to do with their social roles as protectors. One insightful therapist articulated his reluctance to clarify his unexpected absence from the clinic in this way:

> I don't want my patients to know that I have a new baby. I am seeing a lot of disturbed, dangerous individuals. I feel this need to protect my new family. When I think it through, I know it does not make sense.

In another example of unanalyzed disclosure, a therapist revealed to a male patient recently out of prison about his wife's pregnancy. The patient began to talk about his own lost years with his daughter while he was in prison and thwarted attempts to reconnect with her. The patient moved from weekly therapy to monthly med checks when the therapist's wife delivered. The therapist, distracted and tired by his new responsibilities, was relieved that the patient spontaneously wanted to make this change. The patient did not directly mention the therapist's baby again. Had the therapist been more attuned to this change as related to his newfound status, he might have attempted to address this with the patient. However, in retrospect the therapist recognized the unanalyzed pain that the patient felt when the therapist had the opportunity that the patient would never get again. This became apparent at the time of final termination, when the last words of the patient to therapist were words of advice that he (the therapist) "better not mess up this opportunity."

We recommend that each therapist examine his own motives for revealing information or neglecting to do so. We feel fairly secure in recommending that in cases where the therapy is impacted in an ongoing way, that the question should be not whether the newfound status is disclosed but how much to reveal. For instance, when the therapist sees patients in his home or home office, where evidence of the situation is potentially impinging on the treatment (e.g., sounds of the baby crying, the storing of child gear in view), the new reality ought to be acknowledged and addressed in treatment. Even when patients do not openly articulate their reactions, derivative material will often allow the therapist to open the discussion.

Whatever the therapist decides to do, he must make his wishes known to the other professionals involved in his patients' care (e.g., co-therapists, trainees, covering therapists, social and case workers, professional unit staff, and administrative support). In the context of co-therapy, the therapist must also collaborate with the co-therapist in determining how to facilitate the processing of any shared information. Otherwise, the prospective or new father might be left unprepared to handle patients' responses to information revealed by his colleagues, such as the therapist in the next vignette who was co-leading an LGBT support group.

Vignette 6.5

Without advance notification to the group, I missed a session after the baby was born. When I came back to group, the co-facilitator asked me in the group without warning if I wanted to tell the group why I was gone. I did reveal that my wife had a baby. But I felt "out-ed" because the group suddenly became aware of the fact that I was not only a new dad, but also, a heterosexual man. I ended up disclosing more than I usually do, like the name and sex of the baby. The discussion then moved to the topic of my sexual preferences in the third person. "I guess that means he's straight." They seemed to almost settle on my being straight and then someone said, "I guess he could be bisexual." There was more discussion, and they eventually agreed that they did not have enough information. Finally after 10 or 15 minutes, one member asked if I was straight. I said, "I guess I can come out now as a straight person." I felt vulnerable and exposed. Although there was some closure to the issue, I still wondered how this may affect the group. The subject was quickly changed by one member for the rest of the group session.

When such disclosures are made, the therapist can feel ambushed and unprepared, creating considerable tension between the new father and other professionals. McNary and Dies (1993), in their study of co-therapists' tensions, found instances of pregnancy disclosure by the non-pregnant therapist to create considerable tension. In the previous example, the therapist recognized the parallel between the exposure of his sexuality and the group members' similar experiences. Had the therapist not felt so vulnerable and been better prepared for this potentiality, he might have used his awareness of his vulnerability to pursue the parallel process that his group members may have felt about their sexuality being exposed.

There is a notable decline in marital satisfaction for men, with its peak occurring between 6 and 18 months postpartum (Osofsky & Culp, 1993), although a meta-analysis of 97 studies suggests the decline is not as steep as it is for mothers (Twenge, Campbell, & Foster, 2003). For fathers, this decline is likely to be particularly great if the pregnancy was unplanned (Lawrence, Nylen, & Cobb, 2007). With higher levels of perceived stress, this dissatisfaction increases as well (Chandler, 1998). Such dissatisfaction is potentially likely to affect the infant's care, in that research has shown that the father's level of support to his wife affects her adjustment and the care she provides for the infant (Osofsky & Culp, 1993). Hence, the father's importance in his child's development occurs not only directly through his relationship and attachment to the infant, but also indirectly through the support and protection of the baby's mother (Gurwitt, 1994).

Health status also declines over the first 8 months of fatherhood (Bartlett, 2013; Ferketich & Mercer, 1989). Although fathers obtain more sleep at night than mothers, they accrue less sleep overall and report fatigue commensurate with that of their wives (Gay, Lee, & Lee, 2004). Health and self-care issues are likely to exacerbate any already existing psychological anxieties and marital discord. Most male therapists feel the impact of this life-changing event on their work. Similar to his female counterpart, the male therapist is able now to experience many of the parenting struggles that his patients report; evoke transferences that might not otherwise manifest themselves; and enjoy the increased credibility in dealing with children and their families. At the same time he, like his wife, is faced with establishing a work–home balance that involves identity issues, increasing the efficacy of his parenting skills, fostering the nurturant aspects of his personality and striking a time management equilibrium between childcare, professional activities and personal development.

New Knowledge, Empathy, Credibility, Transferences and Countertransferences

One of the significant benefits of this life experience from a therapeutic standpoint is that having a child provides a new forum for the acquisition of knowledge and the gaining of hands-on experience. One child therapist exclaimed, "At least 50% of the knowledge that I have of child development comes from my own experience. It's like on the job training." Most reported an increased capacity to empathize with parents and their struggles around childrearing; they expressed their appreciation for the complexities of the parent–child interaction. One male therapist put it this way: "I look at children differently now. I am more balanced now in that I don't empathize solely with the child. I can empathize with the pain parents feel when things don't go well." This statement also highlights their recognition that this life transformation had altered their previous attunement balance. How this process unfolds might be more idiosyncratic to the therapist–patient dyad. For some it was a personal identification (i.e., "I see certain problems with my adolescent clients and my first thought is that I hope that my child does not turn out to be an alcoholic or drug addict"). Others were aware of their increased affinity to the child and their protective responses. One therapist working with a deprived young female child told us that he bought his patient a present, something that he had never done with any other patient. Although he never gave it to his patient, with supervision, he recognized in this act his wish to protect this child as well as his own daughter from the effects of emotional deprivation.

In contrast, some therapists worried that they might be too supportive of parents because of their own newfound identification as a parent. A therapist put it this way:

> It takes me out of the position of being neutral and brings up a lot of comparison stuff like "I will never do that to my child" or "How would I manage that hyperactive child if he were my son?"

Another therapist who had an adolescent daughter said, "Every time I sit with an angry mother whose anguish and anger are tethered in her verbalizations, I am reminded of my own reactions to my sometimes self-absorbed and often exasperating daughter."

The therapist's newfound life change elevates expertise as someone capable of understanding and providing reasonable solutions to parental dilemmas, both subjectively and objectively. One male therapist observed:

> The pregnancy has given me more credibility with parents because now I will have kids too. They say things like, "Now you will know." I don't even have the child yet. It is like not having a child actually means you know about what it is like or how to raise a child, but patients seem to think so.

This last statement highlights the transferential elements of the therapist's newfound status.

The male therapists we interviewed described many interesting patterns of transferences and countertransferences. They commonly expressed uneasiness in knowing how to manage them, which highlights the void in mentoring during this process. Frequently, these reactions were similar to those articulated by their female counterparts (see Chapters 3 and 4). We discuss a few of the more interesting examples to stimulate further thought and curiosity about how the reader might handle them should they occur. As is true of their female compeers, some male therapists noticed differences in male and female patient responses and concomitant differences in their own responses to each gender. One therapist commented, "My male patients have been more congratulatory and macho. They were usually brief. My female patients seem more maternal, wanting to know more about my wife and the baby's health." Likewise, some male therapists felt more discomfort talking about it with their female patients. It seems that there can be different origins to this discomfort; at least for some, it seems to be similar to the female therapist discomfort involving the more erotic transferences and countertransferences in the therapeutic relationship. One male therapist acknowledged being aware of actively hiding information about his newfound status with female patients, one of whom later overheard a clinic staff discussion. This discovery, he noted, coincided with this patient having less interest and energy for therapy. This change in her made him aware of some unaddressed erotic aspects to the relationship, both transferential and countertransferential.

Another fairly common transference among both child and adult patients is their envy of the new baby and their wish to replace the baby. Next is an interesting vignette illustrating these reactions.

Vignette 6.6
I had a picture of my wife and new son on my desk. One grade-school child who came from a chaotic family and had just been separated from his physically abusing father asked about the picture and the name of my son. I told him. Three months later in therapy, he asked to be called by P., the name of my son. When I commented that that was the name of my son, he denied the link and explained he wanted that name because it was the name of a rock star of a popular group. He went through a phase when he wrote this name as his name on all his school papers. During some of the sessions, he would beat a BoBo doll that he had given his name, K. He would berate the doll and call it a loser. He would also at the end of the session drop to the floor pretending to cry and google like a baby. When I would say that perhaps he wanted me to be his dad, he would not acknowledge it. One day after I said it, he referred to himself in the third person, and took my hand and his mother's placing them in his chest saying "P. wants Mommy and Daddy." I brought it up at the next session, but he continued to deny it. Eventually, he was able to leave the sessions without this behavior. His use of P. as his name has decreased, although he uses it occasionally when something upsetting has happened at home or in school.

Children act rather than verbalize this transferential wish of having the therapist as their parent, a wish that is common for many patients. A new baby in the therapist's life brings this wish into sharper focus. The therapist reported that he felt his own personal situation had made him more sensitive to this child's needs and he was able to handle his tantrums at the end of the session with less annoyance and more empathy. In this instance, the therapist provided a positive male role for this child. Although the child was never able to acknowledge his wishes in words, the articulation of them by the therapist seemed to contain the child and so was important. Although maintaining a picture of the family on one's desk is an individual matter, in this instance, the therapist was able to allow it to be used by the child in the enactment of his wishes.

The direct or indirect expression of patients' envy is also a common response to the pregnancy. It can also cause considerable discomfort and guilt in the therapist, as is evidenced by this next example.

Vignette 6.7

One middle-aged single man that I was treating in therapy for anxiety and depression went to the emergency room the day that I missed our session for the birth of my child. My secretary had called to cancel the session. I never found out what she said to him. I heard that he left the emergency room AMA and had been somewhat belligerent during his stay. When the patient and I met a week later, the first thing that he said to me was, "I guess congratulations are in order." I felt a pressing need to explain my absence at the same time I felt vulnerable. He quickly moved on to another topic. During the session when we talked about his ER visit, he said, "They made me feel like an incorrigible child." I again felt a pressing need to apologize, but didn't. I was relieved when he changed the topic and began to talk about his brother's children with some envy.

During supervision, the therapist recognized the importance of his patient's response and his own discomfort, but had not made the connection between the secretary's phone call and his patient's description in the ER ("an incorrigible child") until it was pointed out to him. The patient's background included being physically and emotionally abused by his father. We suspect that the unexpected missed visit elicited the patient's feeling of being abandoned by his therapist "mother," perhaps in his mind because he was "an incorrigible child," and he went to the ER to fill the void. In the ER, by way of projective identification, he reenacted the beating by his father. It is possible that this patient sensed the therapist's anxiety around this issue and moved to more derivative material in discussing envy of his brother's children. Trying to help this patient make the connection between his behavior in the ER and its relationship to the therapist's cancellation may have helped the patient begin to explore the manner in which he recreates these old traumas. This example also highlights the importance of preparing those covering for the therapist's absence and how unanalyzed parts of the therapeutic dyad may come to be acted out in the more extended therapeutic setting (e.g., the hospital ER).

Here is a good example of the way in which an astute therapist was able to work with the material that became salient during his wife's pregnancy.

Vignette 6.8

One of the more difficult scenarios during the time I was expecting my first child occurred during the treatment of a gay student in his late twenties whom I had been seeing in a three-times-a-week interpersonally oriented psychoanalytic treatment. Chip suffered from severe separation panic at the end of sessions and especially around weekends and vacations. He felt that he could not hold me in his mind when I was not physically present and that I was his only hope for salvation. He led a socially isolated life and severely underestimated his robust intellect, academic achievements, and charm. He felt extremely unaffirmed and neglected by his father and felt alternately abused or smothered by a mother who had been seriously abused as a child.

Reluctantly, I shared the news of the pregnancy with him earlier than my other patients, perhaps knowing that we would be going into a particularly difficult phase of treatment. He had suffered bouts of fairly serious depressions with some psychotic features, for which he had been medicated. During my wife's pregnancy, these depressive episodes were characterized by paranoid thoughts that I wanted him out of therapy. He would often self-mutilate while at home, cutting himself delicately on his abdomen, with the magical hope that I would know he was doing this and would drive out to his apartment to rescue him. Efforts to discuss the seriousness of his behavior, medication and hospitalization were met with the replay that I could not cope with his envy, ostensibly, of my full life. Fortunately, enough time remained before the birth actually occurred to explore his wish to be inside of me and to be held by me. I had mistakenly thought that his envy was related to my having a life partner. What he really wanted was to be my child held in a protective cocoon. When I was finally able to set myself at ease about his safety, I turned my attention to fully immersing myself into the concrete way he felt that being in my office and my physical presence held him. Interestingly, he was the first patient I told that I was expecting a second child, this time having completed his education and embarked on a career, but still feels unloved and not held. He no longer mutilates himself and accepts measures such as medication and extra support from the verbal holding that the psychotherapy provides him. He finds the idea of my having a boy less threatening, for reasons we have yet to understand.

This therapist recognized the serious impact that the hiatus in treatment may have on this seriously disturbed patient and gives sufficient notice. He is able to utilize this personal event to help his patient develop strategies to hold the therapy and therapist in his mind when his therapist may not be physically present. Here, too, the therapist learns and acknowledges that the stimulus of the pregnancy enabled him to recognize that his patient's desire to be held in a protective cocoon was more central to his intrapsychic structure than his envy of the therapist's life situation.

Male therapists with whom we spoke expressed interest in understanding these transferences and countertransferences and at the same time, were often reluctant both in the session and with colleagues to explore the material. Their sense of vulnerability, intensified by new parenthood, was often particularly disturbing to them. Yet, as with their female counterparts, exploration of the patients' projections of the therapist's transformation offers a wealth of opportunities for the patient as well as personal growth for the therapist.

Recalibration of the Professional Personal Balance

The Importance of the Breadwinner Role

For the therapist, marriage and the birth of the first child often coincides with the initial phases of his career, as many wait until their education is completed before starting a family. A man's identity is still tied to the breadwinning role, despite the large proportion of women in the workforce and a movement toward egalitarian values at home (Antil & Cotton, 1988; Hiller & Philliber, 1986; Lamb, 1986). Many of the male therapists we interviewed were acutely aware of the pressure that this value creates. Here is one therapist's remembrance of how pressure as provider impacted the therapeutic hour.

> **Vignette 6.9**
> When I had my first child, I was just out of school and desperate to make a life for my new family. Many family and close friends questioned, how are you going to manage, as I wanted a practice, not to work at a job. I previously had not had to ask for payment, always being generous with my time and in treating indigent patients for little or nothing. Now I needed money, and I had to ask patients to pay at the end of the hour for my services. I felt like a vulture. It really affected my sense of myself as a humanitarian. The success of my practice became the exaggerated barometer of my self-esteem. It was absolutely awful in those years. Now with the coming of my third child, I feel so differently. I feel financially stable. I know what my abilities are and what my deficiencies are. I feel comfortable asking for payment because I feel worth it and have accepted that I cannot be as gracious as I would like because I have a family to support.

Statistics suggest that there is a significant decline in the proportion of income that men actually provide to their families due to the influx of women into the workforce. In a household survey, the Pew Research Project found that wives whose income exceeded their husbands' income increased from 4% in 1970 to 22% in 2007.[3] However, while men are willing to share the provider role, there is still resistance to accept their wives' role as co-provider (Deutsch & Saxon, 1998; Zuo, 1997). Social pressures on heterosexual men to be the primary breadwinner still remain. The majority feels it is important to make more money than their wives (Hiller & Philliber, 1986). In contrast, gay men demonstrate greater role flexibility on this dimension, and if anything, prioritize childcare over other activities (Stacey, 2004).

A cultural assumption exists that women, but not men, will decrease their involvement in work outside the home to take care of the additional demands required by this new family life (Silverstein & Auerbach, 1999). In conformity with this assumption, men—including male psychotherapists—are reluctant to take advantage of the official family leave policies when they work for hospitals or agencies, for fear that they will be perceived as uncommitted to their job or unmasculine (Hochchild, 1997; Pleck, 1993). Most fathers (and the male therapists we interviewed were no exception) do not take formal paternity leave. In fact, as we have noted earlier, many of the therapists we interviewed did not miss sessions with many of their clients and most did not miss more than a week. This is in sharp contrast to the female therapists who took considerably more time. Thus, despite changing cultural values and the infusion of feminist thinking into the culture, both men and women in general believe that bread-winning is still an important component in men's family role and a critical component of their gender identity (Crowley, 1998; Zuo, 1997)[4]

Expectations for Life at Home

At the same time that heterosexual men are expected to fulfill the breadwin-ning role, there is both an internal pull and external pull to become more involved at home. Internally, men derive considerable psychological satisfac-tion from their families, for many perhaps even more than their work (Pleck & Lang, 1979). Men acknowledge that they want to be part of life at home (Pru-ett, 1987). When asked, most will spontaneously articulate desires to nurture their offspring (Cohen, 1993). Externally, babies take time. With large numbers of women entering the workforce, they can no longer take sole responsibility for household and childcare duties. Societal norms depict the good father as a nurturing parental figure who actively involves himself in a more expressive and intimate way with his children than his own father did (LaRossa, 1988; Pleck, 1995, 1997; Rotundo, 1985). The good provider role is expected to be nurturing and to share in the household duties (Bernard, 1981). The belief in co-parenting is most prominent in the upper-middle classes, which is an important departure from the past (Pleck & Pleck, 1997). In 1976, even Spock, in his "bible" on childrearing, reversed his 1946 position from suggesting that it did not make financial sense for mothers to go to work and pay other people to do a poorer job in raising children to maintaining that both parents have an equal right to a career if they so desire and an equal obligation to share in childcare. However, the practice of co-parenting has been quite common for lower-class couples where both spouses worked different shifts. Each parent would take full responsibility for the household when not at work (Russell, 2011).

If the "new" breadwinner-nurturer did not himself have such a father, how could he be expected to become one? There is some evidence that new fathers have "fragmented models" of ideal behavior, selecting behaviors that incorpo-

from a variety of others, especially peers, rather than modeling after a single individual (Pleck, 1997). It is also likely that positive caregiving experiences earlier in life foster higher parental involvement. Highly involved fathers can be spotted even earlier than childbirth from their enthusiasm and daydreaming of fatherhood (e.g., reading books on childcare before and during the pregnancy, attending the birth, daydreaming about being a parent, excitement about quickening, taking days off from work immediately after the birth). Personality characteristics such as sensitivity, perceptiveness, openness to experience, accepting obligations and commitments, and viewing fatherhood as an enriching experience all positively contribute to a higher level of involvement on the part of the father (Pleck, 1997).

Given that society expects on some level that both parents have rights and obligations to home and career life, the birth of the first child is likely to create a crisis in terms of role expectations for the couple and will require a renegotiation of allocation of responsibilities. Although each couple may create a unique arrangement, research suggests that there are a number of trends in terms of expectations and actions that each partner brings to the relationship. We feel that the male therapist, operating in a whirlpool of personal uncertainty, competing responsibilities, and high affect will benefit from an increased awareness of these trends. Such knowledge may facilitate a higher level of home life satisfaction. Thus, we are presenting a summary of the findings.

According to a report from the Pew Research Center (Parker & Livingston, 2016), 66% of all families with children under 18 are dual-income families, whereas 4% have only the mother employed and 28% only the father employed. This report further indicates that since 1965, fathers have more than doubled the amount of housework they do, and tripled the time they spend with their children. However, when couples maintain a traditional household (with either the mother remaining at home full-time to care for the children or a shared view that the mother's employment is not representing a significant part in the family support function), both mothers and fathers expect that fathers will be less likely to participate in home activities (Wilkie, 1993). When mothers do contribute a significant portion of financial support to the household, most couples expect that childcare should be shared. There is, however, considerably less agreement on whether and how housework should be shared. In addition to this lack of agreement, there is evidence that spouses misperceive their partners' expectations fairly often (40% of the time), with one study suggesting that husbands are more able to accurately articulate what their spouses expect of them than wives can (Hiller & Philliber, 1986; Pew Research Trends, 2015). Whether the men are more perceptive or the women are more effective in communicating their expectations is unclear. In any case, these differences in expectations and misjudgments of the others' perceptions can affect marital satisfaction. The ability to recognize these differences and misperceptions and to negotiate a mutually satisfying agreement is critically important to the ultimate happiness of the family unit.

How Do Expectations Translate Into Behavior?

Overall, after childbirth, there is a definite shift to traditional marital patterns, even if this was not the case before birth; men work as much or more outside the home, while women reduce their efforts in the labor force and increase their childcare and housework efforts (Moss, Bolland, Foxman, & Owen, 1987). However, women who delay marriage and childbearing until their thirties (often due to their pursuit of education) are much more likely to stay in the workforce and continue to show a major commitment to career (Goldin, 2006); many female psychotherapists would fall into this category. Fathers, in general, spend much less time with children than mothers do, particularly if mothers are not employed outside the home (Walker, 2015). Hochchild's data of 25 years ago suggested that fathers spent an average of 12 minutes per day with their children. Based on a 2008 survey, this number has increased substantially, averaging 3 hours per workday in interaction with their children (Aumann, Galinsky, & Matos, 2011). There are different kinds of parent–child interactions, and the level of the father's involvement varies depending on the type and whether the mother is employed. For instance, when the mother is unemployed, the father spends approximately 20% to 25% as much time as the mother directly interacting with the child: if the mother is employed, this is increased to about one-third the time. In this latter case, fathers do not spend more time with their children, but rather the proportions increase because the mothers are doing less. In terms of accessibility or availability, the father is available only about a third as much as the mother if she is unemployed, but two-thirds as much if she is employed. When it comes to taking ultimate (administrative) responsibility for the child's welfare, fathers are generally not involved regardless of whether the mother is employed (Pleck, 1997). For the single wage earner, the level of paternal involvement is much more dependent on the personality of the father, whereas for dual earner families, involvement is more a function of structural factors (Lamb, 2010a). One additional fact: the father's emotional support of the mother should not be underestimated as having a significant impact on child development, although it is not generally counted in any of these measures of paternal involvement (Lamb, 1986, 1997a).

In general, participation in household tasks and childcare is determined more by ideology rather than time availability, with those males who hold a more traditional ideology being less involved with childcare tasks (Deutsch, Lussier, & Servis, 1993; Perry-Jenkins, Seery, & Crouter, 1992; Pleck, 1997). Nonetheless, as time progresses in terms of age of parents, length of marriage, and number and ages of children, women do increasingly more household tasks, such as cooking, cleaning, and shopping relative to their husbands (Lachance-Grzela & Bouchard, 2010). From a gender construction perspective, men's avoidance of household work is an effort to protect masculine identity (Erickson, 2005). Consistent with this perspective is Arrighi and Maume's (2000) finding that the greater the challenges men experience at work, the fewer the hours they devote to household tasks. Although the number of hours that women work outside the home has no impact, as males' income and hours worked increases, there is less likelihood that he will participate in these more stereotypically feminine tasks (Antil & Cotton, 1988). When fathers are asked, their reality and ideal preferences are discrepant; many fathers express a desire to work less and spend more time with their children (Moss et al., 1987). They are happier when they are doing a little more work at home with both childcare and some of the stereo-typically masculine household chores (e.g., repairing, mowing the lawn).

Although most couples agree that childcare and household chores should be shared, a majority of fathers say they participate equally in only half the iden-tified childcare tasks and about one-third of the household tasks, even by their own admission. There is a significant disjuncture between wives' and husbands' perceptions of how much each participates in childcare and household duties. In both household and childcare tasks, husbands and wives see themselves partic-ipating more than their spouses see them contributing. The percentage of wives who view their husbands as doing or sharing these tasks is even lower than the percentages of husbands who see themselves completing them (Miller & Phil-liber, 1986). Husbands are especially more likely to see tasks as shared, whereas wives see themselves with major responsibility, particularly because they are frequently in a position of having to delegate tasks (Russell, 2011). Thus, for most couples, even those with dual earning arrangements, these activities con-tinue to follow traditional patterns in spite of spouses' expectations for greater equality in their relationship (Pew Trends, 2013).

Some evidence exists, however, that change is underway. A survey of the Families and Work Institute revealed that those dads who are currently in their twenties spend more time with their offspring than older fathers do.

Interestingly, the gender of the first child may influence how men and women negotiate their responsibilities in the parental subsystem. In dual income fam-ilies, couples who reported that they shared childcare were found more likely to have a male firstborn, compatible work arrangements, and similar levels of income than were couples in which the wife takes primary responsibility for the children. They also reported feeling that their relationship was egalitarian and that the division of labor in the household was satisfactory (Fish, New, & Van Cleave, 1992). There could be many reasons for this: perhaps fathers are more comfortable being physically intimate with a son than a daughter and so it allows for the development of an unprecedented interaction.

Obstacles in the Development of the Nurturing Self

Forty percent of fathers claim that they would like to spend more time with their children (Lamb, 1986). Presumably, at least some of this complaint has more to do with self-imposed limits or perceived incompetence. With greater childcare comes less freedom to move in one's social and work environment. Also, either parent could experience many of the tasks associated with childcare as monotonous and less stimulating than other possible involvements. More time at home could mean less opportunity to engage in the kinds of activities outside the home that bring social approbation and other kinds of external rewards. This same ambivalence, also reflected at a societal level as the push for a nurturing good provider, is potentially sabotaged by a number of obstacles: the dearth of social supports to achieve a self-perceived competence; the hostility and negative stereotypes that men receive from relatives, friends and employers; and spouses' discouragement as a result of their ambivalence about sharing the nurturing domain.

Self Obstacles

A man's traditional role has been to interface with the greater society and family. Consistent with this, his network is designed to supply him with information about how the system works rather than the personal contacts that are characteristic of his female counterparts (Lamb, 1986, 1997b). Thus, men's networks provide them with inadequate encouragement and a paucity of resources relevant to childcare. In actuality, evidence is lacking for the notion that first-time mothers have more skill and competence with their children than do fathers. Many fathers are not aware that first-time mothers are just as bungling and intimidated as they are. The societal expectation that women know what they are doing prevents them from withdrawing (as their male partners may do) and forces them to feign a competence until they actually acquire the skills they lack. In a sometimes subtle interpersonal dance, fathers who lack confidence in their parenting abilities defer to and concede responsibility to mothers. Mothers agree to assume responsibility, not only because they view it as their role, but also because their partners do not seem to be especially competent care providers, exhibiting such behaviors as clumsiness and hesitancy. Lamb (2010) suggests that those fathers who experience themselves as competent are more likely to spend time with their children because they find it rewarding; in contrast, situations that instigate feelings of ineptitude are likely to be avoided.

Obstacles Created by Family and Friends

Involved fathers may encounter hostility from acquaintances, relatives and friends. Pruett (1987), in his study of fathers who are primary caregivers, found that they experience a sense of isolation from friends and family when they declare their atypical childrearing plans. As they engage in childcare, they are likely to encounter negative attitudes (Pleck, 1997). One author (VB) remembers the shock that her husband encountered from her child's classmates' mothers when he volunteered to be the homeroom parent. This was a task that was implicitly perceived as women's work. Likewise, fathers and their children are often not invited to be members of playgroups when mothers organize those groups. At work, coworkers and supervisors are sources of disapproval because fathers are more likely to miss work or be later than non-fathers, presumably due to childcare difficulties. Few fathers avail themselves of the full leave available to them, in part because the law is not in line with the unspoken attitudes of men's involvement in childcare (Hochschild, 1997). Not availing themselves of family leave policies results in less opportunity for contact and achievement of comfort and competency as a father.

Obstacles From the Workplace

The job setting is often a major obstacle to father's involvement. Frequently, the workplace provides little accommodation for men to be active forces in their children's lives. According to a study of the Families and Work Institute (Aumann, Galinsky, and Matos, 2011), 16% say they could not keep their jobs if they worked fewer than the number of hours they currently work, and 14% indicate that they must work long hours to keep up with the demands of their job. This same study uncovered the fact that for fathers, the boundary between home and the workplace is blurred due to technology. Whereas in 2002, 32% of fathers were contacted at home by a work associate, only 6 years later, the percentage had climbed to 48%.

Spousal Obstacles: Maternal Gatekeeping

Mothers, too, play a role in fathers' degree of involvement in childcare. Recent research has identified the phenomenon of maternal *gatekeeping*, which refers to maternal attitudes that encourage or inhibit father's involvement in childcare (Fagan & Barnett, 2003). Maternal gatekeeping is a determinant of paternal involvement, and according to some research, is mediated by the mother's perception of the competence of the father (Fagan & Barnett, 2003). Yet, additional evidence suggests that whether a mother sees a father as competent is rooted in certain of her personality characteristics. The more perfectionistic the mother and the poorer her psychological functioning, the less likely she is to see her husband as a competent parent (Schoppe-Sullivan, Altenburger, Lee, Bower, & Dush, 2015).

In addition to personality characteristics, painful emotional reactions in the mother might also strengthen maternal gatekeeping. In Pruett's study (1987) of men who were primary care givers, most of the women struggled with unwelcome envy of their husband's competence and shared intimacies with their children although they felt deeply that their spouses' involvement was vital. Mothers reported that when they saw their husbands and babies responding to each other, they felt competitive feelings, fearing the irrational that sharing the nurturing domain diminishes the mother's status, relationships and sense of self. As to why, Pruett offered this comment:

> Women do not want to give up their preeminence in this vital area, for the nurturing domain is that psychological place in which our children are

cared for, protected, and helped to grow into their own unique selves. Both noisy and silent, sustaining and frustrating, depleting and fulfilling, sensual and abstinent, it is confusing but never trivial in purpose or company.

(p. 241)

Russell (2011) talks about the natural hurt either parent feels when the young child refuses his or her attention while demanding the other's. She underscores, however, that the family derives rich benefits when there are two equally available and competent caregivers.

Maternal gatekeeping has not been studied in couples where one of the parents is a mental health professional. Presumably, when the father is a mental health professional, he would bring an understanding to both the child's and the mother's inner world through which he would establish his competence, in the eyes of the mother. When the mother is a mental health professional, one would anticipate that she might look beyond the mundane tasks of parenting to discern the father's capacity to appreciate the inner life of the child. It would seem, then, that the phenomenon of maternal gatekeeping would be beneficially investigated in terms of the background each party brings to the parenting enterprise.

Tensions Between Work and Home

According to a Pew Research Center investigation, productive work time for men (job, plus childcare, plus household duties) is approximately 58 hours a week (Parker & Wang, 2013). In this same study, 50% of fathers said juggling home and work is difficult. Although this survey encompasses men from many professions, managed care and other economic influences are likely to have increased the male therapist's time at the office. The upshot of these combined influences is that the new father-therapist is typically exhausted. One therapist said,

Initially I was very tired because I was up a lot. I tended to be a little less crisp because of fatigue. There were times when I would have rather been home. This feeling lasted over 3 months. The fatigue lasted over a year.

This, in combination with assaults to personal competence, mixed messages from society in terms of role identification and ambivalent messages about wives' expectations, is likely to result in tensions between the couple and tensions around loyalties to home and to work. Employers and patients become annoyed and angry when childcare interferes with the daily work schedule. In some treatment environments (e.g., outpatient clinics), the nature of the responsibilities precludes others from covering. There is a loss of income for the organization, which leads to an intensification of pressures on the male therapist. Of course, private practice does not allow for paid leave of any type. Spouses become frustrated and angry when they feel deprived of emotional and practical support. Divided loyalties are bound to create stress and tension for the new father. Financial pressures can be an added burden. Although the new baby is exciting, home life is also likely to be chaotic and lead the new parents with desires and guilt over wishes to retreat to work where things are more stable and less chaotic (Hochschild, 1997). The father often has more of an opportunity to realize these wishes. It is here where patients can often gratify the therapist's own desires in terms of self-esteem and competence. In the following vignette, the therapist had some recognition of his own potential desires for illicit gratification in this therapeutic relationship.

Vignette 6.10
I had to be careful with my female clients, particularly those who had loving feelings toward me. Things were chaotic at home; I felt my worst in terms of competence there as well. I often needed to remind myself that I could only do things if they were for the good of the client. So I had to not do things for me. I needed to keep the client in mind and not act on my own needs. At times I felt like, this is really nice here, and at home it felt like I heard, "you are not available" all the time. It was a very confusing time for me.

Although this therapist appeared to be particularly aware of his circumstance, the combination of sleep deprivation, a loss of control and lack of freedom, constant assaults to self-esteem, and the perceived loss of a partner who seems too busy with the new baby could lead to the therapist's inability to keep the patients' issues in the foreground.

Perhaps the most common struggle for the male therapist as a new father and relatively young professional is the balance between who needs what, the most, and when. Balsam (1974) referred to this as "divided loyalties." Osherson (1992) gave us a good example of the internal division that men can experience.

Often I'll be working here at the office thinking about how I'd rather be with my kids. I'll hurry to finish a brief to get some work to my secretary so I can be home on time so I can see them. . . . Then I'll be at home, playing with my kids and I'll be thinking about the work I ought to be doing, or how I'd rather be at the office.

(p. 213)

This issue takes on an infinite number of iterations with concerns for patients and family, requiring one to prioritize. Patients become keenly interested in who is being offered more gratification at any given moment. Although female therapists balancing home and work might face this issue more frequently, male therapists do not escape it, as we can see in the next vignette.

Vignette 6.11
There was one patient in crisis who I was concerned about. I made a post-birth appointment with her the next day. She said to me, "How are you

going to do this? You are being ridiculous. You are not going to be able to see me that quickly." I assured her that I would be available. The next morning I realized that it was as she had predicted. I had to call her and say, "I can't make it. You were right." I felt guilt about not being available enough and wanted to keep going with my practice. It was partly that I was concerned for her, but I was in the mode of building a practice and with my wife not working, and with a new baby at home, I felt more pressure to produce financially.

Re-establishing Balance Between Work and Home

Combining work and family roles for fathers creates as much or more stress than it does for the new mother. Fathers who are more involved with childcare report that they feel the lack of time to pursue their careers and that their family responsibilities interfere with their work. However, they also feel less strain in their family role as compared with those fathers less involved at home (Pleck, 1997). It appears that higher paternal involvement extracts some costs to fathers immediately, in that the more available fathers are more likely to feel distressed about their non-traditional role, suffering more decline in self-esteem. However, these disturbances do not reduce satisfaction with parenthood and do not longitudinally negatively impact careers. In fact, although fathers with high levels of involvement in childrearing appear to suffer from an initial disequilibrium, in the long run they appear to have a modest positive impact on career success (Pleck, 1997).

It is our impression that male therapists have a greater appreciation for the importance of their role as a father than many of their peers and are generally fairly involved at home. They often socialize with other therapists who embrace these same values. Thus, their peer group supports their greater empathy for the plight of their wives, and their decisions to spend time at home. How fathers and children engage might be as important than the amount of time they spend together. Equally important is how fathers, mothers, children, and other important people in their lives perceive and evaluate the father-child relationship (Lamb, 1997).

Recommendations

Since the last edition a few more papers have been written from the perspective of the new dad therapist. While research about the importance of fathers in child development has been growing it still lags behind maternal research (Raeburn, 2014). As fathers are increasingly obtaining their due in the parental and developmental literature, awareness is increasing of the importance of this milestone in the personal and professional life of the male therapist. Our own interviews of the expectant male therapists suggest that becoming a father is a multidimensional event that does affect the male therapist's work. Moreover, the male therapist's reactions seem to change in fairly predictable ways as the birth approaches and following the birth. Post birth, fathering entails a balance between the urge to achieve independently and the equally pressing need to be connected to meaningful others. As Pollack suggests,

> It is a balance between men's often less than complete experience of nurturing caretaking from their own fathers, in the past, and their opportunity for achieving a different model of fathering for the next generation—and through this struggle to change, achieving a personal, psychological transformation for themselves.
>
> (1995, p. 330)

In light of these observations, we make the following recommendation:

1. Fathers should expect the achievement of the balance between professional and personal development to be challenging. Along with writers such as Levant (1995), we suggest that male therapists take steps to develop an emotional self-awareness, which in turn, will aid them in their ability to understand their own reactions, communicate their wishes and needs to their families, and maintain a healthy personal professional balance.
2. Fathers should recognize that social norms are changing rapidly, particularly in terms of how mothers' and fathers' roles are perceived. Knowing that part of the stress of being both a new parent and a therapist derives from cultural pressures is likely to lessen such stress.
3. Even though the workplace might define the father's new status as a parent as irrelevant to his or her work, this profound change in status is likely to imbue his interactions with patients, and he should strive to recognize.

Notes

1. Silverstein and Auerbach (1999) made a convincing case that neither mothers nor fathers provide genetically unique or essential contributions to child development. Rather, parenting involves a variety of caregiving functions that are fulfilled according to the specific bioecological context in which the family exists. Research on mothers and fathers during the newborn period suggests that neither are natural parents and there are few significant differences in parenting behaviors between them. Mothers tend to appear more competent as a group, because after a year's time, they have spent much more time with their infants and have become more familiar with their biological rhythms and needs, etc. (Lamb, 1997b). When fathers have assumed the primary caretaking role, they are as sensitive and competent as mothers (Pruett, 1987; Russell, 1986).
2. Papua New Guinea is the only country in the world that does not permit paternity leave. (Addati, Cassirer, & Gilchrist, 2014). "U.S. behind most of world in parental leave policy: Study; Papua New Guinea, Swaziland & U.S. lag". *NY Daily News.* 24 December 2011.

3. Fry, R., and Cohn, D. (2010). *Women, men and the new economics of marriage.* PewResearch Center: Social and Demographic Trends. Retrieved from www.pewsocial trends.org/2010/01/19/women-men-and-the-new-economics-of-marriage/

4. Zuo, J. (1997). The effect of men's breadwinner status on their changing gender beliefs. *Sex Roles, 37*(9), 799–816.

CHAPTER 7

Non-traditional Family Structures: Adoptive, Single and LGBT

Like much of the literature on families, the scholarly corpus on expectant families emphasizes the traditional family constituted of a mother, father and biological children. The one respect in which the literature is inconsistent with this social scheme is that whereas the traditional family is predicated on traditional roles (mother, homemaker and caregiver; father, provider), the expectant parent/therapist literature, which focuses primarily on women, assumes that the woman is working during and often following her pregnancy. Rarely, however, does the literature extend to the alternate family structures that have been increasingly common since the 1950s, so much so that from the perspective of prevalence, the non-traditional family can be accurately regarded as the new traditional family (Livingston, 2014). In this chapter, we cover only a subset of structures. We focus specifically on adoptive, single parent, and LGBT families. Various family structures such as blended or parent-cohabitation families are not covered. However, our intent is to create a stimulus for other writers and researchers to pick up the mantle *en route* to the development of a literature that includes families of all types. Certainly, if one is a therapist and an expectant parent, regardless of what that family structure is or will be following the arrival of the child, assistance in anticipating one's own likely reactions and those of clients as well as guidelines for solutions to common problems is useful. It is also the case that to varying extents, the family structure determines some of the particular issues that are likely to present. In this chapter, we provide multiple illustrations of this point. Therefore, most of the existing literature will have relevance but limited relevance to the therapist/expectant parent whose family departs from the traditional structure.

Being in a non-traditional family has implications for expectant parents. Despite the decreasing presence of traditional families on the societal landscape, the traditional family continues to be seen as both normative and desirable. Alternative types of families are subjected to devaluation, often in disguised form, and sometimes, outright discrimination. The expectant parent might begin to encounter negative reactions or the absence of positive reactions as he or she approaches the arrival of the child. For example, colleagues at work might respond differently to the arrival of an adoptive versus biological child. Although others' lack of enthusiasm is likely to be hurtful, any distress can be lessened by the realization that such responses, rather than being personal, are part of a larger sociocultural picture. On the other side of the ledger are various strengths that non-traditional families bring to the enterprise of raising a child. For example, families with individuals who have encountered prejudice prior to a child's arrival are particularly able to help that child develop coping skills in relation to others' intolerance. As we will see, each type of family has a distinctive strength profile, the awareness of which can enable the expectant parent to put it to best use. In the sections that follow, we characterize both the challenges faced and the opportunities enjoyed by adoptive, single and LBGT families.

Adoptive Families

One relatively common means of building a family is through adoption. In 2012, for example, 119,514 children were adopted in the United States (Child Welfare Information Gateway, 2016). Although adoption often follows attempts to conceive a child biologically, a variety of other roads can lead to an adoption. For example, adoptions are very common among same-gender couples (Goldberg, 2010). Single individuals who have not found a partner are increasingly motivated to adopt a child. As well, some individuals adopt children in response to disasters such as the Haitian earthquake of 2010, which led to the adoption of approximately 1,500 children in the United States.[1] A strong tie between foster parent and foster child might lead to an adoption.

Therapists who adopt a child might be tempted to see this life transition as irrelevant to their professional work. Several factors might discourage the therapist from realizing its importance to his or her professional life. First, the female therapist does provide a changed physical profile to those around her. The baby is quite literally not in the room. During the expectancy period—as the parent is making a near approach—nothing extraordinary appears to others (a circumstance she shares with both adoptive and biological fathers-to-be). Second, whereas during pregnancy, others in the workplace are requested or mandated to make accommodations for the pregnant therapist, the expectant adoptive parent generally requires no particular assistance or consideration from others. Of course, once the child arrives or once the parent departs to retrieve the child, the parent's transition does affect her workplace presence. Third, as the adoptive parent looks at the literature, he or she is likely to find next to nothing suggesting that the field does not define it as a matter of professional importance.

We suggest that the adoption is a matter of great consequence for the prospective parent's professional life. Even though an adoption is not visible in the way that a pregnancy is, it is nonetheless a public event. Whether the therapist chooses to announce the adoption to the patient, its public character makes the information easily accessible. For patients in inpatient, day hospital, and residential treatment centers, the likelihood of overhearing staff talking about such an event is great. Once a single patient learns of this transition, it is likely to be known throughout the treatment community. However, the child's arrival into the family often entails some disruption of the treatment. The perceived disruption might be even greater if the therapist does not give the patient sufficient advance notice. Most importantly, perhaps, given that the monumental character of adoption necessarily transforms all adopting individuals, including therapists, the treatment that therapists conduct during adoption passages must be affected.

Distinctive Aspects of Adoption

Adoptions differ greatly from one another (Brabender & Fallon, 2013). Variation among adoptive families is created by the locus of the adoption (e.g., domestic versus international), the broker of the adoption (e.g., private agency vs. public agency vs. private attorney vs. informal arrangement), the relationship between the adoptive and biological parents (i.e., closed vs. degrees of openness), the prior relationship between the child and adoptive parents (relative vs. non-relative), and the sameness or difference between the child and parents on a number of identity facets such as race, ethnicity, sexual orientation, ableness and the age of the child at the time of adoption (Pavao, 2007). The relational status of the parent is also relevant (e.g., single, cohabiting, married in a heterosexual relationship, married in a same-sex relationship, married in a blended family). All of these factors in isolation and combination with one another potentially affect the adoptive parent's experience and his or her behavior within both home and professional settings.

Despite variation, the process of adoption differs from that of biological parenting in several broad ways, each of which we describe in the following sections.

The Logistical, Sociopolitical and Affective Uncertainty of Adoption

Building a family through adoption is often a less certain process than the more customary route of conception, pregnancy and birth of one's own biological child.

LOGISTICAL UNCERTAINTY

Perhaps the most fundamental uncertainty that can persist through the adoption process is whether the adoption will be completed. Certainly, biological births carry risk. However, oftentimes, prospective parents take on the risks of biological parenting (if an identified child is yet to be born), the potential that the biological parent will at some point be unwilling to forfeit parental rights and the possibility that some external entity (e.g., a governmental unit) will fail to approve the adoption. This particular source of uncertainty might continue even after the child is brought home. In international adoptions, uncertainty exists over whether adoptions will remain open in that country. For example, one of the authors had been awaiting a child for a period of a year when the country closed its doors to adoptions. Such a development requires that the parents submit an application to an alternative country, a very lengthy and again, unpredictable process. The entity providing adoption services might also raise questions in the minds of pre-adoptive parents. For example, Roy, Schumm and Britt (2014) describe the case of one couple that had to switch from one agency to another, thereby lengthening the waiting time. A lengthy waiting period occurred with the second agency also. Finally, they were told by the second agency that the route that would likely be most successful for them was to first become foster parents with a hope to adopt a child they fostered. Such a circuitous process cannot but engender doubt as to whether parents have chosen the best routes to pursue adoption.

When the adoption will occur is another major source of uncertainty for most adopting parents. Although for biological parents, some question might be present as to when their baby will be born, the indefiniteness spans only a few weeks and at the very most a few months. As this first vignette illustrates, for adoptive parents, the period of uncertainty is potentially much longer. Particularly in an international adoption, once a child is assigned, innumerable factors can create delay in the adoptive parents' assumption of custody.

Vignette 7.1

After one of the authors (VB) and her husband were assigned a baby, they proceeded through a successful evaluation in a Central American country 3 months later, at which time they were able to spend 1 week with their new daughter-to-be. They were sent back to the United States with the understanding that they would be able to return in 2 months and bring their daughter to her new home. However, delays were innumerable. For example, late in the process, it was discovered that the stamp on a document was unclear. Government offices were closed for an extended holiday period, preventing the author and her husband from remedying this problem. Because of the accumulation of such difficulties, they were unsuccessful in receiving authorization to obtain custody until an additional 4 months had passed—crucial months in the life of a very young child.

For many families, the wait on assignment of a child is much longer than they expected or were led to believe. Furthermore, in the face of delay, the anxiety is easily aroused in adoptive parents that some obstacle has arisen that will derail the adoption altogether. Compounding the problem of delay is the fluid character of the timetable. Often, pre-adoptive parents need to transition into parenthood with stunning promptness, a pattern that Weir (2003) describes as leapfrogging.

One difference between biological expectancy (i.e., pregnancy) and adoptive expectancy is the locus of the factors creating uncertainty as to whether the longed-for child will enter the family. In the case of pregnancy, the factors are primarily internal. The impediments to a successful delivery (particularly in the case of professional women who generally do not face external challenges to their nutritional needs and are guaranteed reasonably competent medical treatment) primarily exist within their physical selves. Even when there are external factors, the pregnant therapist typically has some measure of choice and control. In the case of adoption, the emergence of external impediments is not unusual.

Added to the uncertainty about the reality of the adoption is the fact that both before and after the adoption, adoptive parents are subjected to an intensive screening process (Brabender, Swartz, Winzinger, & Fallon, 2013; Kirk, 1981). Rather than being a minimal screen, the evaluation is most often comprehensive and invasive. It is likely to include the excavation of the prospective parents' early family history including troublesome events (e.g., "Did your parents ever use corporal punishment?"). In a sense, therapists who are seeking to adopt might find these questions and the answers to them especially worrisome because they are likely to understand the implications of particular responses. Through the information they submit and their presentation during interviews, pre-adoptive parents, in some cases, must establish not mere adequacy but also, superiority to other prospective parents in the pool. Rosenberg (1992) expressed it well:

> Because the supply of available healthy young children is far below the demand, adopting parents find themselves in a competitive arena. If they compete through an agency, they need to prove their desirability according to the agency's values and increasingly, according to birth parents' preferences. They must face the reality that if they do not agree with the values and practices of others, they may not receive a child.
>
> (p. 169)

Rosenberg also made the point that adopting parents, on receiving approval, obtain a validation that is inaccessible to biological parents.

After a child is placed in the home, a caseworker visits the home periodically to ensure that the match between child and parents is a good one. The constant scrutiny of adoptive parents (which of course contrasts strikingly with its total absence in the cases of biological parents) undermines the parents' sense of entitlement to the assumption of a full parental role vis-à-vis the child. On the other hand, at times, it can serve as a source of support.

Sociopolitical Uncertainty

The institution of adoption is constantly in flux. However, in more recent decades, change has occurred at a particularly stunning rate. As Pertman (2011,

p. 168) writes, "so many changes are taking place that they're dizzying even for active participants, and it's hard to think through all the implications of the tumult." Here, Pertman is referring to bewildering array of decisions with which today's pre-adoptive parents are confronted, such as when to discontinue fertility treatments, what type of adoption to pursue (e.g., international versus domestic) and whether to participate in the increasingly common phenomenon of an open adoption (i.e., an adoption in which, to varying degrees, birth parents continue to obtain knowledge about, and involvement with their child's life). As pre-adoptive parents are negotiating these decisions, they know that broader socio-political factors will affect their own adoption story. For example, new legislation at the state or federal level can facilitate or hinder an adoption process. In international adoption, the economic and political realities within the host country will be critical in whether a prospective parent's efforts reach fruition. A couple might await news of an election in a foreign country to obtain indication of whether the adoption policy in that country is likely to change.

AFFECTIVE UNCERTAINTY

Another type of uncertainty is affective, and concerns the bonding itself. Adoption, often following a protracted period of attempting to conceive a biological child, includes the frustrations of unsuccessful fertility treatment. When parents discontinue their efforts to conceive a child, what ensues is understandable grief over the loss of the dream of having a biological child (Brabender et al., 2013; T. Fallon, 2013). As Rosenberg (1992) wrote:

> With time, they cannot help but fall into a state of despair. Realistic hope is now abandoned. Instead, there is pain, depression, and helplessness. They recognize that they have failed to fulfill what was an essential function of their lives.
>
> (p. 53)

The adoption process sometimes begins while the pre-adoptive parents are still actively grieving. Part of the work they need to do is realizing that even though adoption is an excellent way to build a child, it does not replace the sense of loss over not being able to have one's own biological child—a loss that can remain throughout a person's life (Pavao, 2007). Still, if pre-adoptive parents have sufficiently addressed their sense of loss, then, their apprehension about adoption as a means of becoming a parent will combine with feelings of exuberance and excitement. Also, following protracted fertility efforts and the ultimate disappointment, prospective parents experience an urgency to complete the adoption process (Swartz, Brabender, Fallon, & Shorey, 2012), a reaction that can discourage them from taking advantage of supports available to them, such as participation in a pre-adoption exploration group (Pavao, 2007). Yet, these negative reactions typically exist alongside feelings of exuberance and excitement (Brabender & Fallon, 2013).

Pre-adoptive parents worry about their capacity to bond with their adoptive child, and the child's ability to attach to them. Qualitative investigation by Swartz, Brabender, Fallon and Shorey (2012) and Wingzinger, Fallon and Brabender (2016) revealed that before the actual adoption takes place, adoptive mothers contemplate the bonding process deeply and educate themselves on the attachment literature. They ponder how their bond with their adoptive child might be similar to or different from bonding with a biological child. Whether those around them will see their bond with their adoptive child as genuine and robust also stirs up anxiety. These anxieties are likely to be particularly intense for mental health practitioners who tend to be highly aware of attachment and its implications for later development.

All of these uncertainties that adoptive parents face carry psychological consequences, two of which have particular influence on the therapist's work. The logistical uncertainties leave adoptive parents in a state of perplexity over their degree of progress toward their goal of adoption. Accompanying this felt lack of control over the process is a range of negative emotions such as apprehension, anger and exasperation, all blended into a most troublesome medley. To mute these uncomfortable feelings, adopting parents might engage in various behaviors designed to provide a sense (often illusory) of mastery over the situation (Grotevant & Kohler, 1999). For example, in the 2007 movie *Juno*, we see Vanessa Loring, the pre-adoptive mother, exhibiting an obsessive preoccupation with the details of the baby's eventual room. It seemed to be at once an assertion that the adoption would occur and a denial of her myriad anxieties about the dependability of the birth mother, Juno, with whom she and her husband had developed a plan.

A second consequence is that the pre-adoptive parent encounters a host of difficulties in planning his or her professional life. Psychotherapists Civin and Lombardi (1996) described how they had been prepared by their adoption agency that they would be able to pick up their baby, born in November, in February at the earliest. However, in December, they received a call from the same agency informing them that they would need to be in the South American country the next day to retrieve their daughter-to-be. Civin and Lombardi wrote,

> We booked the airplane flight and launched our own flight into mania. We had two days to buy everything we ever might need as parents, pack, and deal with our professional obligations, both to our students and our patients.

(p. 89)

Under these circumstances, not atypical for adoption, the psychotherapists were forced to notify their patients of the separation and the reason for it by phone and in some instances via answering machine.

When pre-adoptive parents experience affective uncertainty—doubting, for example, whether they will love their adoptive child the way they might have loved a biological child—they are likely to feel self-critical in relation to this reaction. Being angry over roadblocks to adoption is likely to be quite acceptable to pre-adoptive parents while doubt over the decision to adopt far less so. Those of our reactions that are objectionable to us, we attempt to suppress. If they find expression, it is usually through indirect means, enabling us to ignore their presence. The therapist who is also a pre-adoptive parent is likely to enter therapy sessions with this emotional complexity. Certain responses of the client might be threatening because they bring to the surface those very elements the therapist seeks to keep out of awareness. For example, a client talking about relationship ambivalence might be subtly encouraged to explore only the positive pole of the ambivalence, or push the client toward a premature resolution. Alternatively, the therapist might shift from an exploratory stance, or encourage the patient to shift to a topic that circumvents the therapist's sensitivities.

The Invisibility of Adoption

Another distinction between the pre-adoption period and pregnancy is that whereas the latter is unmistakably and progressively visible (Stuart, 1997), the former is not. The adoptive child does not enter the sessions in the same physical way that the child of a pregnant therapist does. This visual absence does not mean that the adoptive child is absent from the treatment: the patient might detect subtle changes in the therapist. Anxiety, excitement, preoccupation and joy might be among the feelings and cognitive states sensed by the patient. The therapist might also take travel and maternity leaves. However, all of these changes do not lead the patient to draw the inevitable conclusion that the therapist is adopting a baby in the same way that a patient can see that the therapist is pregnant. The pre-adoptive therapist must, typically, make a more active declaration.

Strengths of Adoptive Families

Although adoptive parents face challenges not present for biological parents and greater stress (Rijk, Hoksbergen, ter Laak, van Dijkum, & Robbroeckx, 2006), they also possess strengths that can be mobilized in pursuing parenting tasks (Brabender & Fallon, 2013). The intensive screening and waiting period through which adoptive parents proceed ensures that overall, they are likely to bring sound psychological characteristics to the parenting enterprise. Adoptive parents tend to show a higher level of relational stability (Rijk et al., 2006) and marital satisfaction (Leve, Scaramella, & Fagot, 2001) than other parenting couples, including those in a traditional marriage. Once the child enters the home, adoptive parents show a smaller decrease in marital satisfaction relative to biological parents' experience (Ceballo, Lansford, Abbey, & Stewart, 2004).

These features do not necessarily distinguish them from the population of mental health professionals who are new parents, but do distinguish them from the population at large. As new parents, adoptive parents tend to be committed to a high level of equal sharing in childcare. For example, Holditch, Sandelowski and Harris (1999) observed 21 heterosexual couples and 49 biological parent couples. They found that the discrepancy in time the mothers and fathers spent with their children was significantly less for the adoptive than the biological parents. This characteristic of adoptive parenting is not only a benefit for the child but also, for the mother in that the father's participation is likely to reduce her stress, which benefits her professional life as well as her personal life.

Therapist Reactions

The distinctive features of adoption affect the therapist's work in both the pre-adoption and post-adoption periods. In the vignettes that follow, the interplay between therapist and patient responses is seen. The next one examines those therapist reactions tied to the vicissitudes of the adoption process.

Vignette 7.2

Margaret, a therapist who had been assigned a child from an Eastern European country, was scheduled to appear in the country in 2 months with her husband to obtain custody and emigrate the child. Margaret and her husband chose to pursue adoption after several years of fertility treatment that did result in a pregnancy. However, Margaret miscarried the fetus at 5 months. She and her husband had been in an adoption waiting pool for 2 years.

Margaret had recently spoken to another person being served by the same agency who had made the trip only to discover that the abandonment decree of the child had been revoked. Apparently a cousin of the child had appeared to claim her. Although Margaret had some joyful and hopeful moments in the weeks leading up to the trip, her experience was dominated by fearfulness and worry. In large part, she expected tragedy rather than maternity. This anticipation prevailed despite her constant communication with the foster mother whom she knew was caring lovingly for the child and who reported to her on the child's constant developmental achievements.

Margaret informed her patients of her upcoming departure but did not specify the reason. She did acknowledge to them that she was going abroad and did not know exactly when she would return. She recognized that she was being vague not only out of any careful thinking about the impact of that information on her patients out of a desire to protect herself from broadening the circle of persons with whom she would have to share any negative outcome of her trip. She wanted to perceive her work as a sanctuary.

At the same time, as she saw some of her patients exhibiting more regressive behaviors prior to her open-ended departure, she felt pangs of guilt. Yet, she was so distracted with planning for the trip that she was unable to give her feelings their due in sessions. The fertility treatments, which preceded her adoption efforts, made her lack of control was painfully evident, a sense that she transferred to the adoption situation. Her sense of uncertainty was intensified by certain elements of her present circumstance such as her dependency on a foreign government capable of reversing its decisions. It was also augmented by intrapsychic such as the guilt Margaret felt in relation to the adoption. She realized that the foster mother had become very attached to the child. As is the case in adoption, her new tie was predicated on another person's loss (Rosenberg, 1992). The sense of uncertainty was a self-inflicted punishment attached to her perception of herself of taking the child from the foster parent and from the biological parents as well.

Margaret was motivated to find means to reduce her apprehension and sense of powerlessness in a venue in which she did have control: her work with patients. Her means of achieving control was to refrain from sharing any hint of this project with her patients. In this way, she ensured that she would be spared facing a possible loss of a child in her work with patients. Other therapists might use information about the adoption in other ways to increase their perceived control over the adoption, for example, by sharing the information with certain patients and not with others based on their own needs, not the patients.

Margaret used the defense of compartmentalization to reduce her adoption-related anxiety. Another defense that some therapists might summon is denial, entailing a failure to recognize the indefiniteness of the process by developing plans for their departure that are unwarrantedly concrete. For example, an adoptive therapist might tell patients that he will be abroad for a period of 1–2 weeks. His doing so would be a defensive obliviousness of the many factors that could delay his return.

Whereas therapists have defensive reactions not to disclose the upcoming adoption, they might also be motivated, consciously or unconsciously, by the legitimate aim of sparing the patient gratuitous distress. As we have discussed in earlier chapters, it is relatively uncommon for pregnant therapists in the first trimester to reveal the fact of the pregnancy to the patient. Many therapists state that until they have completed successfully the first trimester or amniocentesis, they do not feel sufficiently secure with the pregnancy to introduce it into the patient's life. Until the adoption is finalized, the adoptive therapist might feel much like the pregnant therapist in her first trimester. Because (realistically or unrealistically) the potential challenges to the adoption might seem so great, the adopting therapist might legitimately worry that the announcement of the impending adoption might introduce an unnecessary complication into the treatment.

As the therapist brings the child into his or her home, another set of reactions might emerge that are tied to the societal value of adoption in contrast to biological birth.

Vignette 7.3

Rose's adoption of her son proceeded smoothly. Only 2 months after she and her husband contacted her adoption lawyer, a child became available. They were told that in 3 months, the child could become a part of their family. However, after her husband and Rose gained custody of the child, the birth mother had 6 months in which to assert parental rights and regain custody of the child.

Although the adoption appeared to be progressing well, Rose found herself to be fettered by a constant stream of worries. She thought continuously about the possibility of the birth mother's changing her mind. She ruminated over the caseworker's visits, and whether the caseworker would find her to be fit. At the same time, she noticed she was holding in feelings of irritation toward her colleagues, some of whom expressed skepticism about the adoption. They referred to studies showing the mental health difficulties of adoptive children. She also felt wounded by her impression that her colleagues made more of a fuss over pregnant colleagues. She combed her memory trying to recall what presents others in her work environment had received from coworkers. From this review, she concluded that she had been sorely shortchanged. She privately noted that the excitement that had existed in relation to her co-workers' pregnancies simply was not evoked by her transition to parenthood.

In her work with her patients, Rose noticed two respects in which she departed from her typical behaviors in sessions. At times she was distracted, being preoccupied with the many threats to her adoption. This heightened distractibility continued after her son's arrival for several months. In addition to contemplating obstacles to the adoption, Rose fantasized a great deal about what the baby and her new life would look like. Rose was also cognizant of engaging in an unusually high level of self-disclosure related to the adoption. She had informed patients of the adoption because she planned to suspend her professional activities for a 4-week period. After the announcement, some patients would periodically ask her about it. She found that she would elaborate to an unusually high degree providing details far beyond the patients' questions. In several instances, she thought she detected puzzlement on the faces of her long-term patients, who seemed to be registering that this was a departure from her usual stance.

In fact, Rose's behaviors show some similarity to those of pregnant women. Her diminished attention is highly characteristic of the pregnant therapist in the first and third trimesters. Both types of expectant parents are in the process of assimilating an event whose enormity in a person's life is incalculable. Distraction is an expected outcome. At the same time, each expectant state provides a somewhat different stimulus for distraction. Whereas the pregnant therapist has physical symptoms to divert attention from work, the adoptive therapist has the many impediments to the adoption to preoccupy her.

Rose's increased level of self-disclosure is also akin to changes in the demeanor of pregnant women. As we discussed earlier, during the pregnancy of the therapist, the real relationship is accentuated and becomes a therapeutic force in its own right. For adoptive therapists, this change can also occur. Yet, Rose felt that other elements drove her communications to her patients about the adoption. On analysis, Rose recognized that the self-disclosure was related to her questioning of the reality of her relationship with her child. Was she really a parent? Was the child truly hers?

Rose's self-doubt about her authenticity and legitimacy as the child's mother might have led her to desire others' affirmation of her in this role. Her insecurity was seen in her engagement in comparisons of the attentions she was accorded versus those given to pregnant women in the workplace. Indeed, her sense that her adoption was a lesser event than a biological birth might have been genuinely rooted in the perception of others. The pronatalist value that exists in many societies does not extend to adoption (Wegar, 1997), but to the contrary, leads it to be stigmatized (Brabender & Whitmore, 2013), a phenomenon known as *adoptism* (Steinberg & Hall, 2000). For a pre-adoptive couple, adoptism can exist not only in the community-at-large but also in one's own family. Perhaps Rose's insecurity was also intensified by family members' lukewarm responses. As Ramirez (2000) stated, "Grandparents, aunts, uncles, cousins will be asked to transform their notions of 'blood relatives.' Can the absence of key physical characteristics be overcome and the baby become 'one of us'?" These contextual factors might have led Rose to seek her patients' recognition of the adoption, a recognition that was cultivated by her extensive narration of unfolding events.

A particular occupational hazard for adoptive therapists such as Rose is the high likelihood of some colleagues' knowledge of studies investigating the mental health status of adoptive children. Some of these studies carry significant methodological problems, such as the over-sampling of clinical populations of adoptive children. Although adoptive children do show high frequencies of *minor* adjustment problems relative to their non-adjustment counterparts, they do not show a greater tendency toward severe psychopathology (e.g., Borders, Penny, & Portnoy, 2000; Irhammer & Bengstsson, 2004). However, what colleagues who proffer advice might not know are several findings from the literature. First, difficulties that are ascribed to adoption have their roots in other problems, such as early malnutrition, trauma and other negative circumstances (Brodzinsky, 2011). Second, characteristics of the adoption, such as the age at which the child is adopted, affect whether the child has difficulties and the extent of those difficulties, with adoption at younger ages associated with a lower risk of adjustment problems of various sorts (Shorey, Nath, & Carter,

2013). Third, the characteristics of the adoptive parents and the dynamics of the adoptive family make a great difference in adoption outcomes. For example, Simmel (2007) found that relative to pre-adoptive risk factors, the adoptive parents' readiness to adopt accounted for more of the variance in children's short- and long-term outcomes. Kriebel and Wentzel (2011) found that those adoptive parents who are highly responsive to their children could compensate for maltreatment of the child occurring prior to the adoption. Such empirical findings are potentially useful to the pre-adoptive therapist in responding, internally or externally, to colleagues.

Nonetheless, the cumulative toll of others' questioning of the therapist's adoption can be considerable. It can lead that therapist to feel neglected, abandoned and devalued by those around him or her. These impressions can be even stronger if the adoption accentuates other ways (being single or having a diverse sexual orientation or gender identity) in which the therapist might be different from the mainstream. They can also be intensified or lessened by patients' reactions to the adoption. Wagner (2000), on announcing that she was in the process of adopting a baby, observed in her adult patients very limited reactions. She noted that her patients' minimal responsiveness contrasted vividly with that of patients described in the therapist pregnancy literature. Wagner also attested to special sensitivity to the reactions of clients who had been adopted. Particularly deflating were sessions in which patients talked about their unhappiness over being adopted and their yearning to be reunited with their birth parents. These feelings, however, dissipated after Wagner became an adoptive mother.

Patient Reactions

Patients might react to their discovery of the therapist's adoption, to changes they detect in the therapist as a consequence of the adoption, or some combination of both. Similarly to patients' responding to a therapist pregnancy, responses to adoption are rooted in the patient's own dynamics. One patient might idealize the therapist for rescuing a child-in-need, perhaps a response to the patient's own longing to be rescued. Another patient might be focused on the therapist's assumed infertility, a reflection of the patient's own sense of defectiveness (Saakvitne, 2000). Still another might be focused on competitive strivings with the adoptive child. However, such reactions often are complex in that they frequently involve multiple dynamic elements and are also shaped sociocultural notions concerning adoption. We see this complexity next.

Vignette 7.4

In the weeks preceding her departure, Heidi was aware that her 30-year-old female patient, Patrice, had noticed Heidi's agitation during the session. Heidi, preoccupied with the adoption, at times found herself being eager to have the sessions come to an end. She manifested this eagerness by her frequent glances at the clock. Patrice would respond by looking at the clock herself. However, neither Patrice nor Heidi would acknowledge the instances of clock-monitoring.

Two weeks before her departure, Heidi told Patrice that she would be traveling abroad. Heidi indicated that although she anticipated it would be a period of 1 week, she could not be sure. Patrice accepted this uncertainty with no overt reaction. As it turned out, the adoptive trip went smoothly and Heidi returned to her first session with Patrice 1 week after she arrived in the country with her child. Heidi then informed Patrice about the adoption. Although Heidi rarely disclosed personal information, she reasoned to herself that because hers was a home office, Patrice might hear or even see the baby. Heidi reasoned that it would be better to demystify any changes that Patrice would encounter.

Heidi was startled by Patrice's response. Patrice began to sob. She said she must be going crazy, but she felt hurt because the therapist never revealed to her she was trying to adopt. She expressed happiness for Heidi, but the revelation just made her realize that she knew so much less about the therapist than she thought. She elaborated that although she felt a sense of closeness to the therapist, she now understood that this sense was illusory—in fact, the therapist was a stranger.

In the months that followed, Patrice explored the duality in her feelings toward the therapist—the contradictory impressions of being at once close and distant. She connected her experience with Heidi to that with her mother, a self-depriving woman whose almost extravagant attention to her children's needs made her an inaccessible figure. Her ability to identify her longing for the greater closeness was borne out of her disturbing reaction to her knowledge of Heidi's adoption of a baby.

The patient's discovery of the therapist's adoption of a baby differs from the discovery of a pregnancy in that the latter is based on a more gradual, progressive stimulus. Because of these features, the patient being treated by a pregnant therapist is likely to know about the impending event, the birth, at least several months before its occurrence. However, while the visual stimulus (the therapist's body) is changing, the constancy of its presence demands the patient's attention. The awareness of the therapist's adoption can be abrupt and might follow the child's entrance into the therapist's family. It is therefore more evocative of feelings of surprise and even shock (such as those experienced by Patrice) than a new awareness of a therapist's pregnancy. In a paradoxical way, the news can jolt the patient into recognizing the asymmetry of the relationship: by obtaining this one very significant piece of information, the patient might realize how much information he or she lacks. Although such a realization can be distressing, it can also provide an opportunity for learning. Patrice's illusion that the sharing of experiences between her therapist and her was reciprocal was probably a result of defensive activity. Through denial and other mechanisms, Patrice spared herself the perception of a facet of her relationship with the therapist that unconsciously reminded her of frustrations with her mother. The unexpected news penetrated Patrice's defenses and thereby paved the way for her engagement in an exploration that had not occurred earlier in treatment.

Patrice made good use of Heidi's revelation. Her ability to do so was due to the strong therapeutic alliance that was in place and her commitment to mentalizing her own affective reactions. Earlier in the book, we describe how the patient's level of ego functioning bears on the capacity of the patient to reflect rather than to act on reactions to the therapist's pregnancy. In the case of news of the therapist's adoption of a child, particularly when this information places in question the patient construction of the relationship, those individuals organized at the borderline and psychotic levels might not respond with Patrice's level of containment. The adopting therapist might witness the array of acting-out behaviors that have been documented by pregnant therapists on the patient's discovery of the pregnancy, as is seen in the following vignette.

Vignette 7.5

Sharon, a woman in her mid-twenties, was not a patient with whom Kaya chose to relate the fact of the adoption, because intuitively Kaya felt that Sharon "could not handle it." In fact, Kaya reasoned to herself that no purpose would be served by Sharon's ever knowing about the adoption. However, shortly after the adoption occurred, Sharon did hear about it—her medicating psychiatrist, thinking she already knew about the adoption, informed her of this event.

Sharon's initial response was to send an unusually large, stately bouquet of flowers to Kaya, who imagined it to look more like a funeral arrangement than anything celebratory. Sharon spoke with rapture in the session about the therapist's goodness: Kaya was, quite obviously, trying to do a good deed—save a child in just in the same way that the therapist was saving her. However, this period was short-lived. Sharon quickly moved into a different emotional posture in which she attacked Kaya relentlessly. The attack was precipitated by Kaya's last-minute cancellation of a session due to her child's sickness. Although Sharon was not told the reason for the cancellation, Sharon immediately guessed that it had something to do with Kaya's attending to her child's needs. She was livid that she would be relegated to second place.

In the weeks that followed, Sharon railed against Kaya in myriad ways. In her view, Kaya could do nothing right. One of her enraged states consummated in the comment, "You can't even have your own baby." Accompanying her expressions of anger were frequent absences, which she later made no effort to understand. After the third time Sharon suggested that Kaya was defective based on her presumed fertility status, Kaya wondered aloud if it would have been easier for Sharon were the therapist to have had a biological child. Sharon responded quickly, "Yes, it would have been better all around. Then, if I were to get pregnant, I wouldn't have to worry that you would resent me for it." Sharon reflected further, "And I wouldn't have to worry that my treatment is screwed up because you couldn't have a child of your own." Earlier in treatment, Sharon frequently expressed worry that problems of the therapist, unknown to her (the patient), might affect her treatment.

The direct discussions of Sharon's reactions to the adoptions effected a shift in Sharon's emotional state. Absences and tardiness diminished. A melancholy mood supplanted Sharon's fury. Sharon expressed feelings of being rejected by Kaya with increasing clarity. Why did Kaya need to adopt a child? Why did the therapist not adopt the patient (a remark she made with some ruefulness but the therapist felt the underlying yearning was genuine)? It became evident that the patient's discovery of the adoption led to an experience of loss on the part of the patient. The adoption and recognition of Kaya's subordination of some professional responsibilities to her child's welfare challenged Sharon's fantasy of a special relationship with Kaya. So, too, did the manner in which Sharon learned of the adoption. The dissolution of the fantasy ushered in a crushing sense of loss against which the patient defended by first trying to establish an identification with the cherished child and then, by seeing the therapist in wholly negative terms.

The theme of abandonment that emerged in Sharon's treatment is one that—as we have repeatedly seen—characterizes the material of patients of pregnant therapists. In both adoption and pregnancy, the therapist is entering a new and all-encompassing relationship, which has many qualities that the patient–therapist lacks. Furthermore, in both adoption and pregnancy, disruptions in treatment can and usually do occur because of this new relationship. Given these factors, feelings of sadness and a sense of exclusion are naturally evoked by the patient's knowledge of the therapist's life changes.

Yet, a feature distinguishing pregnancy and adoption is that whereas pregnancy establishes a woman's fertility, adoption calls it into question. The patient of the adopting therapist must grapple with the meaning of the therapist's possible infertility. Knowledge of the adoption activated in Sharon a view of the therapist as being imperfect or flawed. However, her focus on this aspect appeared to be a defense against her frustration and distress in having her fantasy of an exclusive tie to the therapist challenged. She might also have been using the presumed infertility as a means of ridding herself of her own feelings of self-dislike and even hatred. To expunge these feelings, she aimed to evoke them in Kaya by highlighting what she saw as Kaya's vulnerabilities. Other patients might see the infertility as a magical realization of their hostile wishes toward the therapist.

Clinical Decision Making and Adoption

This section explores the practical topics of (a) recognizing the factors bearing on the therapist's decision about the degree of disclosure about the adoption,

(b) reckoning with the uncertainties of the adoption process, and (c) managing the therapist's reaction in a way that will be helpful to both the therapist and his or her patients.

The Disclosure Decision

In facing the decision of whether or not to share information about the adoption with the patient, the pre-adoptive therapist should comprehensively consider the positive and negatives features attached to such a communication. On the positive side, the therapist's informing the patient of the adoption might help to demystify any irregularities in the treatment caused by the adoption. For example, suppose the therapist needs to introduce a hiatus in the treatment because of her imminent departure on an open-ended trip. Knowledge about the reason for the trip rather than total ambiguity is likely to be less distressing to the patient. It is certainly true that ambiguity might stimulate the patient's associations that in turn would enrich the treatment. Still, it might also be the case that the departing therapist is not available to explore the associations thoroughly as they emerge.

Once the child has arrived in the family, a benefit of the patient's knowledge of this change is that under this condition, the therapist might feel greater comfort in making the necessary allowances and accommodations for his or her child as the child is getting settled into the family. In the pregnancy literature, it has been noted (e.g., Bashe, 1990) that therapists retrospectively see themselves as not having made sufficient provisions for their pregnancies (e.g., not taking an adequate amount of time off before and after the delivery). It would seem that in an adoption situation in which the patient was not informed that an event of enormity was taking place, the therapist might not feel sufficient entitlement to suspend work activities to the necessary extent.

On the negative side, the disclosure of the adoption might entail a departure from the therapist's usual stance toward self-disclosure. This boundary alteration could induce anxiety in the patient who might feel a new uncertainty about where the boundaries lie. Particularly if the self-disclosure is seen as being gratuitous, the relaxation might activate a perception of the therapist as narcissistic or competitive. Alternatively, some patients might welcome the boundary relaxation and see this disclosure as an invitation to ask a wide range of personal questions. Other patients might be incited to test the therapist's tolerance of other boundary violations (such as tardiness, absence, or the untimely remittance of payments), a phenomenon that has been observed in relation to pregnant therapists.

Because the literature on the adopting therapist is in its infancy, we cannot yet tell how the characteristics of the patient are likely to affect the way that the disclosure of the adoption is experienced. In the authors' own experience of announcing an impending adoption, female patients responded more intensively than males in conformity with the pregnant therapist literature. Wagner

(2000) underscored the importance of the individual's own adoptive status. As mentioned previously, the responses of adults were muted. However, her child and adolescent patients who had been adopted responded very intensively. Most idealized her and some expressed a longing to be adopted by her. Hopefully, in the future, clinical data will be obtained on whether there are broad developmental differences among children, adolescents and adults in how they respond to the therapist's adoption of a child.

If the therapist decides that the patient will be informed of the adoption, a question that arises is when this communication should be made. Four points at which the therapist might consider making the revelation are the following: when the therapist decides to embark on adoption, when a child is assigned, when the adoption is immediately approaching, and when the child has entered the family. The advantage of notifying the patient early on is that the patient and therapist will have a longer period to explore any issues that are activated by the announcement. For patients who have attachment issues or who connect to adoption in some special way (e.g., are adopted themselves), a lengthy, non-interrupted period of exploration might be essential to the patient's growth. A longer period of notice also provides plentiful opportunity to formulate a plan for any hiatus in the treatment. The disadvantage is that early disclosure opens the therapy to the twists and turns of the adoption process. The introduction of the adoption of an early point in the process might also be an emotional hardship to the therapist who thereby loses the work venue as a respite from the issues associated with the adoption.

Grappling With Uncertainties

The uncertainty of the adoption process has implications for how to prepare the patient for any disruption in treatment the process instigates. In short, the patient must be apprised of those uncertainties that have direct effects on the treatment. A major uncertainty that is likely to affect the patient is the timing of the adoption. If it is true that the therapist might be called away virtually at any moment, the patient's knowledge of this possibility will be a protection of the therapeutic alliance. With some types of adoption, it might not be possible to forecast the length of the therapist's departure. For example, as discussed earlier, a trip abroad that might be planned to last a week could be extended over a considerably longer interval. Also, some children will have difficulties settling into the family (Tasker & Wood, 2016), and the therapist might take a longer period to help the child adjust than anticipated. Patients are likely to benefit from the knowing that temporal uncertainty exists with respect to any adoption plans.

Apart from the information that is disclosed to the patient, the therapist ought to take into account the degree of uncertainty in his or her development of specific plans for patients. Suppose a therapist intends to use the services of a substitute therapist during a maternity or paternity leave, a practice pregnant therapists use particularly with those persons who cannot tolerate a lapse in the sessions. The therapist protects both the patient's and his or her own well-being by making these plans well before the leave to prevent a stressful scramble for coverage at the last moment. Likewise, if a patient is involved with an alternate treatment provider who can step in during the therapist's absence, it might be useful to apprise this professional of the adoption plan early so that he or she could be poised to step in. The professional might even be able to make subtle shifts in his or her relationship with the patient that will aid the transition. For example, a medicating psychiatrist who purposefully refrained from delving into non-medication issues in order to maintain clarity of roles might broaden the range of topics discussed with the patient in the sessions.

Perhaps more difficult than coping with the logistical uncertainties is the task of addressing the affective uncertainties, the apprehensions over the completeness of the bonding processing both before and after the child enters the family. As Tasker and Wood (2016) found in their prospective study of six adoptive couples, the sense of uncertainty can remain at least as long as 6 months after the adoption has been completed. Probably no better antidote to the stress adopting therapists feel even after the child has entered the home is participation in a network of other adoptive families (Brabender & Fallon, 2013). Some therapists might feel a self-consciousness about this type of participation, but it is nonetheless likely to be useful. Especially helpful is communication with parents who are at a later point in the process. Many parents will attest to having had confusing, ambivalent feelings about adoption during the waiting period, only to have them resolved in a positive direction as the child becomes a member of the family and as the parent interacts with the child on a daily basis. Still, research (Foli, 2010) suggests that some adoptive parents expect themselves to be super-parents whose excellent skills preclude the emergence of difficulties. For therapists who treat children and adolescents, the emergence of adjustment problems can be a challenge to professional self-esteem. A therapist who discovers that uncertainty, ambivalence and an array of parenting challenges are exceedingly commonplace and do not auger poorly for eventual success in the child's adjustment are likely to have greater empathy for patients' parenting issues and enjoy greater well-being.

Managing Other Therapist Reactions

Beyond uncertainty, the therapist is likely to have a variety of other reactions that are stimulated by the adoption process. However, factors particular to the adoption situation (e.g., the societal value of adoption, the lack of visual change in the therapist, and others' eagerness to avoid introducing a topic that might engender anxiety in the therapist) might hinder the therapist from recognizing his or her own adoption-related reactions and how they might be influencing his or her work. The lack of external prompts requires that the therapist take considerable initiative in attempting to mentalize his or her own adoption-based reactions that might have significance for therapeutic work.

How can the therapist pursue a commitment to identifying and addressing adoption-related reactions in therapy sessions? In Chapter 3, we made recommendations to the pregnant therapist concerning how her reactions might be beneficially explored both during and after the pregnancy. Because a number of these recommendations pertain to expectant parenting rather than pregnancy per se, the pre-adoptive therapist is likely to find them useful. As noted, while many readings on adoption are available, the literature base focusing on the adoptive therapist is negligible. Likewise, in one's immediate environment, supervisors or psychotherapists having direct experience with adoption might not be available. However, adoption is sufficiently common among professional people to enable an adopting therapist willing to go outside of the confines of his or her own organization, to find a supervisor with relevant personal experience. Certainly lack of personal experience does not preclude a person in these roles from being helpful to an adopting therapist. At the same time, an adopting therapist might wish to investigate the attitudes that candidates in these roles have toward adoption that could be informing their work. For example, a supervisor who subscribes to the notion of the inherent supremacy of biological parenting might place undue emphasis on the adopting therapist's sense of loss in not being a biological parent, to the neglect of other issues that could be far more critical for any particular pre-adoptive therapist.

Single Parents

The single parent family is a common family structure in today's society. According to the 2009 American Family Survey, 35% of all of the women who gave birth in the past 12 months were never married, widowed, or divorced (U.S. Department of Commerce, 2009). The number of single mother households is considerably greater than the single father households by roughly a 5:1 ratio (U.S. Department of Commerce, 2010). Nearly 56% have a single child and 85% have two or fewer children (U.S. Department of Commerce, 2010). The trend seen in the United States exists more broadly in the Western world (Cairney, Boyle, Offord, & Racine, 2003).

Single parents are not a homogeneous group. One major source of difference is in the circumstance that led an individual to become a single parent. For many, single parenthood is a consequence of another major life change such as divorcing a spouse or the loss of a spouse due to death. In this case, the status of being a solo parent was not a choice. The subgroup upon which we focus in this chapter is composed of those individuals who actively decide to become single parents. This group, which is relatively new and increasing in numbers (Parke, 2013), is composed in part of individuals who might have been unable to find a suitable partner. For women in particular, the presence of the biological clock might galvanize a decision to move ahead toward parenthood lest this opportunity be missed. For others, a wish to be a parent without the complications of an intimate relationship might motivate this choice. Women in this latter group might pursue parenthood using a variety of means such as adoption, engagement with an acquaintance who has no aspirations to parent, or use of assisted reproductive technology (Harmon, 2005). Knowledge about single fathers by choice is just emerging (Golombok, 2015).

Challenges

The obvious challenge for the single parent is the responsibility of managing the full array of parenting tasks alone. Gailey (2010), who interviewed adoptive parents in various family configurations, described the immense weariness that solo adoptive mothers often report. For some, the weight of responsibility is so great that the effort is to manage tasks from moment to moment rather than seeing into the future. Solo parents by choice typically look to other important people in their lives such as parents, siblings and close friends to provide caregiving assistance. Nonetheless, knowing that ultimately the responsibility falls upon them alone is daunting. Moreover, the single parent is deprived of the collaborative problem solving that co-parents enjoy. When problems arise, the solo parent has only his or her perspective and the range of solutions occurring to him or her. Less opportunity exists to validate perceptions. Although other figures can certainly be helpful, both their investment in and opportunity to interact with the child is typically less. The single parent also has significant economic stress. Even if the parent enjoys a healthy income, the worry exists that were that income stream to be blocked, the family would be without resources. The single parent is also challenged in pursuing an adult social life and is thereby placed in a circumstance of longing for adult companionship. As Akhtar (2016b) notes, social deprivations could lead the mother to foster the child's excessive dependency on her.

Family Strengths

For all of these issues, the single parent family possesses certain strengths. As Parke (2013) notes, particularly in the case of women, these individuals are often older and well-educated. A second common strength is the capacity to develop a community network and use the resources of the community. The solo parent does not have the luxury of turning inward in the way that the traditional nuclear family does. By the child's witnessing the parent bringing others into the family and establishing relationships of mutuality with them, the child has the opportunity of internalizing this important skill. A third factor is that solo parents are spared the particular type of stress that is rooted in the differences that can arise with a co-parent in childrearing philosophy. Fourth, it stands to reason that children in a single-parent family do not have the luxury of absolving themselves from sharing household duties. R. D. Parke (2013) writes, "some children develop an ethic of care, whereby they become aware of their mother's stress and respond by attending to her emotional needs and actively participating in the household duties" (p. 74). Finally, in Gailey's (2010) interviews of adoptive mothers in different family structures, she found that single parents "were the most consistently appreciative of the strides their children had made and how close they felt to their children" (p. 136). Richards and Schmiege (1993) note that single parents also appreciate themselves as they recognize their own capacities to manage the stressors listed above of solo parenting.

Issues for the Therapist

Family literature—empirical, clinical and theoretical—is expanding in response to the increased prevalence of the single parent family structure. Nonetheless, it has not developed to a point to include specifically therapists who are single parents. Still, we believe that many of the themes articulated by prospective and current single parents apply to therapists who are making this transition, with special twists pertaining to the therapists' professional lives. These themes are reflected in the next vignette.

Vignette 7.6

Sylvia, a clinical psychologist, had dated several men during graduate school, but she was primarily focused on her studies. She had a series of long-term relationships through her late twenties and thirties. She and her psychotherapist had for several years been exploring the factors underlying the dissolution of these relationships. Although Sylvia continued to be hopeful that such a relationship would be part of her future, she felt very doubtful that she would be successful in establishing this type of relationship during her fertile years. "After all," she reasoned, "What assurance is there that any future relationship would not end up like the others?" She began to seriously explore the possibility of becoming a single parent. She broached this option with her therapist. After saying that the research clearly indicated single-parent families do not fare well, he immediately interpreted this plan as a means of avoiding the creation of a lasting intimate tie with a man. Sylvia was surprised that he mentioned the research findings because it was something he had never done before. Discouraged, Sylvia put the matter on hold for several months.

Sylvia discovered that the idea of having a child outside of marriage continued to resurface in her mind. She was having lunch with a very close friend, Joy, who had been abandoned by her husband when her son was 2 years old. Joy was the solo parent for her now 7-year-old son. Sylvia disclosed that she was contemplating moving forward with the plan of becoming a parent. Joy proceeded to provide Sylvia with a full account of the experience of being a single parent. She talked about the many frustrations and anxieties, such as her everyday realization that it was "all on her"—the notion that ultimately, she must rely on herself to make sure problems were solved. She also spoke of her financial worries, her gnawing apprehension of what would happen to her family if she lost her high-paying job in administrative social work. She also admitted that her anger toward her former spouse was ongoing, and she needed to be careful not to displace it onto situations at home or at work. However, she noted that despite all of the tribulations, she found her role as mother as the most fulfilling involvement in her life. She said the gratifications of parenting her son more than offset all of the difficulties. She also said that she would be available to Sylvia for assistance along the way.

Sylvia expressed curiosity about whether co-workers had any response to her parenting situation. Joy responded that those who had been present within the agency at the time her husband left her seemed to be quietly understanding of her situation. They often attempted to accommodate her needs as a solo parent. However, she found that newer co-workers, upon learning of her parenting status, sometimes responded with condescension, and at times asked invasive questions about the circumstances giving rise to her status.

Sylvia eventually decided that she was going to use assisted reproductive technology to have a child. She had investigated adoption with various agencies and found that very little latitude existed in the characteristics of the child she might adopt. Upon making this decision, she informed her family members. Her mother was excited and indicated that she would make herself available for childcare when Sylvia needed to be working. Her father provided a more muted response. Sylvia assumed he had some negative reactions to the plan but was being careful not to express them. Sylvia's aunt was clearly disapproving of Sylvia's pursuit of parenthood in this way. She made comments such as "A child needs a mother *and* a father" and "You have to think of the child, not just of yourself."

This vignette highlights various themes that are characteristics of the experiences of prospective single parents. One salient feature is that the single parent is likely to encounter negative reactions from the very beginning of the process and throughout the development of the child. According to a study conducted by the Pew Research Center (Wang, Parker, & Taylor, 2013), public reactions toward solo mothers specifically appears to be somewhat less negative. In 2007, 71% of respondents indicated that solo mothers represented a big problem whereas in 2013, this number shrunk to 64%. Nonetheless, public reaction continues to be quite negative. In this vignette, the therapist's hasty interpretation of the meaning of Sylvia's consideration of this parenting possibility might have been an example of a prejudicial reaction. If so, it is very unlikely that he would see it as being such. Like so many responses to stigmatized groups, the discriminatory reaction is rooted in a societal valuation of a particular group. Both the internalization of this valuation, as well as the responses that emanate from it, typically have a major unconscious component. Her aunt's reaction was more clearly a response based upon a perception of a single parenting family being an inferior type of family. In criticizing Sylvia as being selfish, it contained a direct expression of aggression toward her. Another manifestation of the societal view of single parenting was Sylvia's discovery that the routes to her parenting were more limited than those for other groups. For instance, prospective single mothers who seek to adopt are often directed to older children with special needs (Gailey, 2010; Harmon, 2005).

However, as in this example, the responses from others are unlikely to be homogeneously negative. We saw that both Sylvia's friend and Sylvia's mother presented themselves as allies in this process. Sylvia's friend's reaction is characteristic in that it is often individuals who share one's family structure or parent within some non-traditional structure who are most able to provide support. The quality of support is also important. Others who can provide a realistic appraisal of some of the challenges of single parenting abet the prospective single parent in anticipating the means of overcoming these challenges. Fortunately, single parenting is sufficiently common that any parent in this circumstance will likely find individuals in his or her social and professional environments who are so situated. However, single parenting has not grown rapidly for individuals in the higher echelons of education (Ellwood & Jencks, 2001). Therefore, someone like Sylvia might have difficulty finding another single parent who is also a professional person in his or her work environment.

Sylvia's therapist referred to the research on single parents. His broad statement has some congruence with research studies that have been done on single parent families. A review of the research by M. Parke (2003) suggests that children from single parent families do suffer some disadvantages relative to children in two-parent families. For example, children in single parent families tend to perform more poorly in academic contexts than children in two-parent families and are more likely to drop out of school (e.g., Amato, 2001). These problems seem to be greater in single father than single mother families (e.g., Downey, 1994). However, three caveats might be made concerning the conclusion that single parent families have poorer outcomes. The first is that single parent families are far from a homogeneous group. The category on which we are focusing, single parent by choice, is represented poorly in the literature. Second, children in single parent families do not seem to differ from those in dual parent families with respect to serious psychological outcomes (M. Parke, 2003). Moreover, the literature has identified particular positive outcomes in single parent families. For example, Richards and Schmiege (1993) conducted qualitative interviews with 60 mothers and 11 fathers who were functioning as single parents. They found that the vast majority could articulate strengths of their family structure. Key among these were parenting skills (e.g., helping children cope and fostering independence), family management (e.g., being well organized), and personal growth ("succeeding despite having many doubts," p. 281). Finally, some cross-cultural evidence exists that in countries in which economic resources are allocated more evenly between dual parent and single parent families, greater parity in children's outcomes is present (Pong, Dronkers, & Hampden-Thompson, 2003). To return to our vignette, we might note that the therapist's stating the research with such a remarkable lack of equivocation suggests that something beyond scientific interest was in operation. Indeed, as in the case of other non-traditional families (as we saw with adoptive families), research can easily be used (particularly by therapists and other human services professionals) as an opportunity to express in a seemingly objective way, a highly personal opinion about the value of a social structure.

Another fairly common feature is prospective single parents' sense of having their personal boundaries crossed in the work setting and elsewhere. The prospective parent is called upon to field a variety of questions that are not posed to expectant parents in a traditional family structure. Such questions include: Do you know who the father is? (in the case of a woman using assisted reproductive technology); Why don't you use a sperm bank? (in the case of a woman adopting); Does this mean you are not interested in a committed relationship? (in the case of all prospective single parents regardless of their means of building a family). Naturally, different individuals will have varying comfort levels with such questioning and different levels of openness to sharing personal information. All prospective parents benefit from knowing that this type of questioning is nearly inevitable.

For therapists, invasive questions can stimulate annoyance just as they do in the therapist's other interpersonal venues. However, the implications are different in that the therapist's negative reaction can create a disruption in the alliance. The therapist might respond to his or her sense of violation by withdrawing from the patient in an effort to protect the self from the patient's inquisitiveness. Moreover, when the patient, in response to the therapist's establishment of a boundary in what personal information is shared, experiences frustration, his or her sense of alliance with the therapist can be strained. The risk of the latter is greater if the therapist has been highly disclosing about personal details (we saw an example of such a shift in Chapter 3) before this transition. The patient can easily experience such a shift as a betrayal or rejection. Judicious self-disclosure entails setting a level of disclosure that the therapist can maintain across the treatment. Otherwise, the therapist might easily be setting the conditions for therapeutic ruptures. As Henretty and Levitt (2010) counsel, based on their extensive review of the therapist self-disclosure literature, therapists are well served by formulating self-disclosure principles to guide their communications rather than responding on an ad hoc basis. We discuss this point further later in this section.

Not only the *level* of self-disclosure but also the *content* of the information the patient gleans about the prospective parent-therapist is likely to affect the patient–therapist dyad. We see this phenomenon in the next vignette.

Vignette 7.7

Althea was in her fifth month of pregnancy and was beginning to show. She worked in a community mental health center in which she had a heterogeneous group of patients. Justine, a 40-year-old woman, had been seeing Althea for slightly over a year within the context of a supportive, psychodynamically oriented therapy. During one session that occurred over a year prior, Althea had acknowledged to Justine her single status as a way of communicating that certain of Justine's experiences resonated with her. Justine herself was single and lately was in the process of mourning her assumed loss of fertility.

In the current session, Justine said to Althea, "Congratulations!" Althea asked why she was being congratulated and Justine said, "I didn't know you were married, let alone pregnant! But I can see you are pregnant." Althea said, "Well, you're right about the second part—I am pregnant but I'm not married. I decided I wanted to be a parent, and I am single." Although she had communicated this information to several other patients who had taken it in stride, Justine did not. Justine said that she knew that "this kind of thing" was happening "more and more," but she didn't approve of it. The therapist attempted to explore Justine's disapproval further, but Justine said that although she disapproved of what the therapist was doing, she wanted to spend the session talking about her own concerns. Not sure what other tack to take, the therapist accommodated her.

The therapist was worried that the therapeutic alliance had been damaged. She was surprised that Althea did not show any alteration in her regular and prompt attendance or her payment of fees. Occasionally, they talked about the upcoming maternity leave and the resumption of their work following it. Then, in one session occurring about 6 weeks after the disclosure, Justine talked about receiving a reprimand from her elderly mother and she noticed that she was not intensely upset about it in the way she normally would be. The therapist responded as she often did—with curiosity. She wondered what made a difference this time. Justine said that in the moment, a thought of Althea's flashed through her mind. She said to herself, "Althea is all right with herself, even when other people criticize her." The therapist expressed some perplexity, reminding Justine that she seemed to be upset about the therapist's status of being pregnant as a single woman. Justine said, "I don't agree with it. I don't think it's a good idea. But, really, it's not up to me what you do. But in a way, I'm glad you're doing what you want to do. And I think that's what I should do, too."

Justine might not have articulated all of her reactions to Althea's pregnancy or even been aware of many of them. However, the one reaction she recognized was her wish to identify with the therapist's self-determination. Perhaps Justine employed projective identification in developing greater tolerance of others' disapproval. That is, she might have unconsciously endeavored to have Althea experience what she feels in response to her mother's disapproval. Justine was then able to take within herself the equanimity that Althea manifested. Although Justine could well have been using her identification as a defense against other inclinations toward the therapist (for example, envy of the therapist's pregnancy), its spontaneous emergence and goodness-of-fit with the situation at hand suggests that it had some genuineness in its own right. Within the context of a supportive therapy, it might have been more important to underscore the patient's mastery of her mother's disapproval than to unearth elements against which Justine was defending.

Therapists who are prospective or new single parents can expect responses from their patients that are reflective of (a) societal stances toward solo parenting, (b) the patient's own dynamics, and (c) what and how the therapist is communicating concerning her own changing status (the real relationship). We saw this in Justine's set of reactions toward Althea's pregnancy. Initially, Justine reflected the general societal value of traditional marriage as the appropriate context for childrearing. However, eventually, her own dynamic issues became more influential in her responsiveness to her discovery about the therapist. Her growth might have been in part due to the therapist's openness to Justine's negative reactions.

Practical Suggestions for the Therapist/Solo Parent

To enjoy fully the gratifications of expectant or new parenting, to achieve a stable sense of well-being, to maintain competence as a therapist, and to enhance that competence, the expectant solo parent/therapist should first of all recognize that questioning from others about the desirability of solo parenting will occur and is part of a societal value of the traditional family over virtually any form of non-traditional family. Knowing that such questioning is likely makes it less disconcerting when it occurs at work from co-workers and patients, and outside of work from friends and family.

Second, being a solo parent requires that an individual receive support outside of the home. Both single mothers and fathers tend to have greater involvement with their own parents than do mothers and fathers in traditional marriages, and single mothers also have a greater involvement with their siblings (Marks & McLanahan, 1993). Also support needed for the plethora of concrete tasks facing the single parent is crucial, the support of knowing what one is experiencing is also essential. Finding others who are in the shared circumstance of both therapists and single parents is likely to be a tremendously helpful resource. However, as noted previously, finding others in one's work or social environment who share this conjoint status might be challenging. It is here that professional associations and professional connections on the internet might expand one's social circle to include these similarly circumstanced individuals. Moreover, organizations exist that are devoted exclusively to the needs of single parents, such as www.choicemoms.org/. This organization offers reading lists, parent profiles, videos, podcasts and a bevy of other resources for single parents. Research suggests that mothers and fathers share many issues when it comes to single parenting, but also have distinctive issues. For example, Richards and Schmiege (1993) found that mothers worried about money much more, while fathers worried about the influence of their former spouses on the children. Such a finding suggests that it would be desirable for some same-gender connections to be established in the design of a support network.

Third, as in all expectancy conditions, self-disclosure should be handled with great care. In deciding whether or what to disclose to patients about one's parenting status, it is important to consider a variety of factors including the level of functioning of the patient, his or her dynamics, the length of time in therapy and the robustness of the relationship, to name a few. For every patient, it might be useful to develop a disclosure plan involving a consideration of all relevant factors. Roberts (2005) suggests that when making tricky disclosures, that is, sharing information that is likely to be provocative to the patient, employ "tentative transparency," which involves sharing with the client a small bit of information and then ascertaining the meaning the client makes of it before moving on. This way, the therapist can gauge the client's comfort level with each element and allow myriad client reactions to emerge. Additionally, Roberts counsels the therapist to deliver information in a sufficiently neutral tone that the client does not sense that a particular emotional response is expected from him or her. One can imagine a therapist saying with excitement, "Going to have a baby." This would call for nothing else but a celebratory response on the part of the patient.

Fourth, the disclosure of the single parent should include an acknowledgement of what this new role will mean for the therapy relationship. If it is a likelihood that the patient will have a greater number of cancelled sessions or less access to the therapist at off hours, these changes should be part of the discussion. Collaboratively, patient and therapist can identify ways to lessen any adverse effect the therapist's parental obligation will have on the therapist. For example, if Justine from our last vignette makes a very good connection while she was being seen by another therapist, Alfred, during Althea's maternity leave, it might be considered whether Justine would want to have a session with Alfred when Althea was unavailable. Within the context of a supportive therapy, such substitutions might not be highly disruptive.

LGBT Parents

According to data from Census 2010 (Gates, 2013), currently six million American children or adults have at least one LGBT parent.[2] Nineteen percent of same-sex couples under 50 years are raising at least one child under 18, with 27% of lesbian couples and 11% of gay couples parenting a child. If single parents are included in this mix, 48% of LGBT individuals are raising a child under 18.[3] Represented in this group are LGBT mental health professionals who raise children in various contexts—single parenting, cohabitation and marriage. Demographically, these families differ from families with heterosexual parents. LGBT parents are more likely to be racial and ethnic minorities. Their children are less likely to be their biological offspring or that of their partner, and more likely to be adopted or in foster care. Some LGBT parents serve as foster parents for children they ultimately adopt. One interesting phenomenon is a likely generational effect in terms of the routes LGBT individuals pursue in becoming parents (Parke, 2013). For example, Mirris, Balsam and Rothblum (2002) found that older lesbian and bisexual mothers (60 and beyond) were far more likely than their younger counterparts to begin their families in the context of a heterosexual relationship. This finding demonstrates the importance of looking at the ways in which a parent's multiple identities interact with one another—in this case, age and generation and sexual orientation.

To the best of the authors' knowledge, statistics on the percentages of LGBT mental health professionals who are raising a child have not been compiled. However, it is likely that they are at least as high as the percentage of parents in the larger LGBT population. In addition to having the same longing to parent that their counterparts in other occupations and disciplines do, mental health professionals often have the advantage of being knowledgeable about those social systems (e.g., the foster care system) commonly used by members of the LGBT community to build a family. Their comfort in working with these systems to realize their own personal goals can expedite the process of creating a new family.

Like all non-traditional families, those with LGBT parents have their own unique profile (Parke, 2013). Therapists who identify as LGBT and are either contemplating building a family or in the early phases of doing so would do well to know some of the special characteristics of LGBT families both to recognize and prepare for common challenges and to capitalize on the strengths in order to more easily meet those challenges. First we talk about the characteristics that apply to LGBT families in general, and then we consider the implications of these characteristics for the work of the therapist who has a diverse sexual orientation or gender identity.

Characteristics of LGBT Families

Strengths

In earlier chapters, we discussed how in heterosexual marriages the tasks of parenting, household maintenance and income generation remain somewhat specialized even though a shift has occurred in the direction of women's greater participation in the workplace and men's greater involvement in the family and the home. In contrast, gay and lesbian couples show less role specialization, as has been shown across various research studies (e.g., Farr & Patterson, 2013; Fulcher, Sutfin, & Patterson, 2008). This shared responsibility-taking in same-gender couples extends to the full range of childcare tasks and maintenance of the home (Farr, Forssell, & Patterson, 2010) and applies to both lesbian and gay male couples (Goldberg, Smith, & Perry-Jenkins, 2012). One exception has been found in lesbian couples who use donor insemination. In this case, the biological mother tends to be somewhat more involved in childcare, but not in housework (Goldberg & Perry-Jenkins, 2007). The generally equal sharing that occurs between gay and lesbian couples, which springs from an egalitarian philosophical base, has positive consequences for both children and parents. Children of gay, lesbian and bisexual parents are less likely to construct their life goals based upon gender stereotypes, as was shown in Fulcher et al.'s (2008) study with lesbian couples. It also protects each member of the couple from the extreme stress that results from balancing extremely high levels of responsibility at home and work.

Additional strengths include the supportive community that is available to LGBT individuals and couples who are raising a child and the willingness of LGBT individuals to take advantage of these and other supports (Morris, Balsam, & Rothblum, 2002). For transgender individuals, these supports have not been as available, although this circumstance appears to be rapidly changing. Also, individuals in the LGBT community are more likely to take advantage of psychotherapy when problems arise (Rothblum & Factor, 2001). Finally, but not exhaustively, sexual and gender minorities often learn to develop self-advocacy skills that they can employ on behalf of their children, and teach to their children (Padovano-Janik, Brabender, & Rutter, 2015). We discuss the importance of this facet further in the next section.

Challenges

Central among the challenges faced by LGBT families is the presence of stigma both in relation to the identity status of being a gender or sexuality minority as well as the status of being a member of an LGBT family. Long before the individual contemplates co-parenting within a same-sex relationship, that individual has experienced various types of stigma attached to his or her gender and sexual diversity. As Herek (2009) has pointed out, from *structural stigma*—those values and principles rooted in the ethos of a culture—other types of stigma follow. In his system, these include *enacted stigma*, actual acts of discrimination that occur in relation to a gender or sexual minority or their associates. *Felt stigma* concerns an individual's own perceptions and views of what evokes versus discourages the enactment of stigma. Finally, *internalized stigma* is the result of a process wherein an individual who is a target of negative social biases incorporates those biases into his or her own self-perception. All of these sources of stigma give rise to *minority stress* (Meyer, 2003), which is that stress above and beyond what members of the dominant members of society experience. This stress, and whatever coping responses the individual has marshaled to cope with them, are present before new sources of minority stress emerge related to building a family.

In June of 2015, the US Supreme Court required all states to recognize same-sex marriages. The ruling was necessary because factions of society were opposed to this core institution being available to individuals with diverse sexual orientations. Even after the ruling, many forces remained at work to undermine its implementation, as was seen in the famous 2015 case of Kentucky County Clerk Kim Davis, who refused to provide same-sex couples with marriage licenses. The fact that until recently, LGBT individuals were not able to marry in all states had enormous ramifications for LGBT families because it often denied legal parental status to one of the parenting partners, an example of enacted stigma. In the absence of a marriage, the individual's partner had no recognized claim on the child whatsoever, even after years of performing all of the functions a parent performs. How to be a parent without the legal recognition of being a parent created innumerable problems for the family. For example, if the parents were to separate, the parent who is unrecognized as such by the law does not have a protected tie to the child (Patterson, 2009).

A third challenge is the stigma that accrues to all members of an LGBT family simply for being this type of non-traditional family. Its early manifestation is when a married or cohabitating couple makes the fact known that they intend to create a family. Summarizing the objections to LGBT families, R. D. Parke (2013) writes:

> Early as well as contemporary critics of nonheterosexual parent families were and are concerned that the lack of a male figure or in the case of gay parents a female parental figure would disrupt gender role development, expose children to peer ostracism, and cause emotional and relational problems (Blankenhorn, 1995; Dobson, 2004; Wardle, 1997).
>
> (pp. 84–85)

Parke's summary of the research evidence to support these claims suggests that it is largely insubstantial. Rather, Parke's survey suggests that children raised in an LGBT home are comparable to their counterparts raised by heterosexual parents on such important variables as social and emotional adjustment, and academic success. Fedewa, Black and Ahn's (2015) meta-analysis produced similar findings.

Although prejudice against non-heterosexual and transgender individuals and families is declining, as suggested by their representation in the media, policy changes at all government levels and the lessened secrecy of those having a diverse sexual orientation (and to a lesser extent, gender identity), stigma remains. In contemplating forming a family and proceeding through the various stages of doing so, non-heterosexual and transgender individuals are likely to encounter enacted stigma of both covert and overt varieties. Not only are parents stigmatized but also their children. In a qualitative study of young adults who had been raised by lesbian mothers, most of the participants indicated that at some point during their formative years, their friends or classmates had teased them because of the identity status of their parents. When parents become aware of such untoward events, their own stress levels rise. Many LGBT families represent additional sources of diversity. Often, they are parenting within adoptive, single parent, or multi-racial families. For example, LGBT individuals are four times as likely to adopt as heterosexual couples (Gates, 2013). These factors will increase stigma and stress even further.

Although the compounding of stress factors can be daunting circumstances for parents, for many families, the stress is allayed with the parents' own knowledge and skill in coping with stigma. In the previously referenced study by Padovano et al. (2015), daughters of lesbian mothers said that even though they encountered teasing or bullying, their mothers had taken an active role through their childhood and adolescent years in teaching them how to contend with it. They described their appreciation that their parents did not dismiss reports of troubling events, but rather, used them as opportunities to cultivate their daughters' skills in coping with conflict situations. From the family interactions in relation to discriminatory experiences, the daughters consistently saw themselves possessing a robustness that otherwise might not have developed.

Issues in Psychotherapy

The vast majority of issues that we outlined in Chapters 3 and 4 pertain to therapists parenting within LGBT families as well as those doing so within heterosexual families. For example, we talked about the various thematic concerns patients introduce during the treatment such as dependency, envy and competition, and jealousy and sexuality. Each one of them can emerge in the treatment of individuals whether the therapist is from a traditional or non-traditional family. Yet, the LGBT therapist who is beginning a family will have an experience of working with patients during the expectant and early period of parenting that does have unique aspects.

First, the common themes are likely to develop or reveal themselves in distinctive ways. Second, the patient might learn about aspects of the therapist that were not previously known, and possibly different from what the patient assumed (Silverman, 2001). Consider the following vignette.

Vignette 7.8

Annette had been seeing Carlotta, a young woman of 19 who was herself a mother. Carlotta had engaged in unprotected sex when she was 17 and was very eager to assume a parental role. She said she would finally have someone for herself. The father was known but his involvement in his child's life was not sought. Her own mother, Stella, had had an almost identical parental trajectory as Carlotta's of being a single mother. However, Stella was a very committed grandmother and assisted Carlotta with childcare on a daily basis. Over her time working with Carlotta, Annette noticed that Carlotta did not derive gratification from Stella's relationship with her son. In fact, she seemed to have a resentful attitude, saying at times, "You never did that for me."

When Annette was in her fifth month, Carlotta asked her if she were pregnant. It caught Annette off guard because she thought she had masked her pregnancy with her clothes selection. She acknowledged that she was, and Carlotta appeared to take some pride in her ability to recognize Annette's state. Carlotta chatted brightly about the various enjoyments Annette would experience. In a somewhat more somber tone, she said that she hoped the child's father would give her more help than she received from her child's father. Annette said, "Well, the child will have another mother." Carlotta was silent for a moment, appearing confused. She broke it by exclaiming, "Wait a minute: Are you—you know—gay?" Annette responded affirmatively. Annette was relieved when Carlotta changed the topic. However, after Carlotta left, she regretted not exploring with Carlotta her reaction.

In the next session, Carlotta said that she felt "weird" about talking to the therapist. She had always imagined that the therapist had a husband. She wondered whether given that she's straight, should she have a straight therapist? How, she pondered aloud, could Annette help her with her problems with her boyfriend if she didn't like men and didn't suffer the troubles that men bring? She also asserted that she was "cool" with her therapist being gay, but thought she should treat people like herself. Interestingly, however, Carlotta presented no urgency to leave treatment and Annette blandly stated that they should keep talking about this issue.

In the subsequent sessions, Carlotta spoke about a series of sexual liaisons she had had, a marked change from previous behavior. She seemed invested in making her descriptions provocative, as if she were attempting to impress the therapist with her sexual daring. The therapist hypothesized aloud that Carlotta was trying to make it clear to both of them that it was boys she liked. Carlotta became extremely angry. She said that Annette was dense just like her mother, and walked out of the session, slamming the therapist's door. She returned 10 minutes later with a tear-stained faced. Annette said she realized Carlotta felt Annette did not understand her, but she was very glad she returned, and hoped Carlotta would help her to understand better. Carlotta talked about how each boyfriend dashed her hopes that she would finally feel secure and safe. It struck Annette that Carlotta was not looking for a mature relationship but rather, the soothing a caregiver provides a young child. Annette tentatively suggested that Carlotta was seeking from these men what she wished she could have received from her mother. Carlotta said with some shame that it was painful to see how loving Stella was toward her own child, and she simply did not believe she had ever received that type of caring from Stella. With some empathy, she described her mother as being "too hassled" to be the kind of caring presence she was with Carlotta's child. Carlotta then connected her mother's nurturing ways with her fantasy of how the therapist would be with her own child. Annette speculated that it might be painful for Carlotta to think about how Annette would be with her baby. Carlotta responded, "I would like to be that baby."

In the latter part of the last session described, we see the emergence of a common theme stimulated by the therapist's pregnancy—the theme of deprivation. However, the patient uses other elements within the relationship to defend against the pain attached to the client's sense of deprivation. Focusing on the therapist's sexuality and acting out sexually were both means of keeping frustrated longings for nurturance out of awareness. This is not to say that the therapist's revelation of her sexual orientation might not have aroused some questioning about her own sexuality. However, in this instance, the preoccupation with her own heterosexuality served as a shield against her awareness of her longings for the kind of nurturing from a caregiving figure that occurs very early in life.

Annette was astonished that Carlotta had noticed her pregnancy. In our research, we found that therapists are frequently surprised by a particular patient's capacity to discern their altered state. The consequence of being blind-sided is that the therapist is deprived of the space to formulate a response. Therapists in this circumstance can easily feel ambushed and retreat into a defensive posture. Whether Annette might have reacted more helpfully is uncertain, but at least she could have thought out various possibilities. One consideration is the desirability of the patient's finding out about the therapist's sexual orientation at the same time that he or she is learning that the therapist is having a baby. Both of these revelations have potential for stimulating a host of reactions from the client and at times, parsing out to what aspect of this juggernaut the patient is responding might be quite difficult. Even though Annette was able to work with Carlotta's complex response to the also complex stimulus Annette presented, in many cases, it might be far more difficult.

In an older analogue study, Atkinson, Brady and Casas (1981) found that gay men rated a hypothetical male therapist more highly if the therapist shared that he himself was gay, in contrast to either not disclosing sexual orientation or disclosing heterosexual status. For clients who themselves have a minority sexual orientation, finding out that the therapist, too, has a minority status on this dimension can be affirming (Henretty & Levitt, 2010). It stands to reason that were the patient to make this discovery after he or she was seen beyond a brief interval or somewhat incidentally as in this example, the patient might feel that the therapist had withheld a valuable source of support.

For some heterosexual patients, the therapist's disclosure of his or her sexual orientation can be reparative. Levy (1998) describes a case in which a woman had lived in a marriage with her secretly gay husband. The therapist's disclosure of his gay identity (although already conjectured by her) was very relieving. Whether the therapist separates these two disclosures, makes them together, or discloses only the expectant parental status and not the sexual orientation, we believe that these decisions need to be made judiciously and not on an ad hoc basis. However, such careful decision making rests upon the therapist's willingness to be open to the full range of his or her own feelings emerging in conjunction with those of the patient. It also demands a comfort on the part of the therapist with being known (Silverman, 2001), even amidst the vulnerability the therapist feels at this time. Without that willingness, the therapist can easily see a minimally disclosive stance as what best serves the patient's needs rather than embracing a continuum of disclosure from which to select a particular spot with a given patient.

Third, the patient's reactions to the therapist's revelation are likely to have layers of significance for the therapist that are rooted in the latter's own identity. The following vignette illustrates this point.

Vignette 7.9

George had been seeing Larry in the context of a humanistic therapy with feminist components. As an aspect of the latter, George was fairly self-disclosing with his clients on the notion that therapist non-disclosure promotes a hierarchical, authority-based relationship that could undermine the client's sense of agency. In consistency with this position, George had disclosed to Larry very early in the treatment his identity as a gay man, an identity that Larry shared. Larry, approximately 20 years older than George, had come into therapy to address the loss of his partner due to a fatal heart attack. Larry's relationship with his partner was different from George's relationship with his husband. Whereas Larry's relationship was not monogamous, George's was. Larry desired that any future relationship would also be characterized by non-exclusivity.

George and his partner were planning to adopt a baby boy in 8 weeks. Given his plan to take 6 weeks of paternity leave, he felt it was appropriate to reveal his plans to his clients. Larry congratulated George warmly when George shared his news. However, Larry came late to the two subsequent sessions, an uncharacteristic happening that George attempted to explore. Larry failed to return to treatment despite George's outreach efforts. George found himself worried and anxious about Larry's flight from treatment, so much so that it was interrupting his sleep. He shared his distress with his supervisor. Their explorations helped George to realize that he interpreted Larry's departure from treatment as a criticism not simply of his work but of him. He believed that Larry saw him as being co-opted by a heterosexual ethos. Part of George agreed with this perspective.

The supervisor facilitated George's evaluation of his interpretation against the backdrop of their shared knowledge of Larry's patterns in this and prior therapies. The supervisor hypothesized that the upcoming therapy hiatus was far more of a potent stimulus than George's family plan. They also considered the possibility of internalized homophobia—that George himself felt he might not be deserving of a family. Finally, George examined his own guilt over his perception of abandoning a sector of the gay community that had been very supportive of him during his coming out process. Although they didn't alight upon a single explanation, they agreed that the alacrity with which George interpreted Larry's behavior might point to some of his own conflict-ridden feelings stirred by the transition to fatherhood.

The supervisor in our vignette helped George through a process of exploring his reactions to the flight of his client, set off by his disclosure of his family plans. LGBT therapists and supervisors of those therapists are aided by the recognition that understanding some therapist reactions requires a grasp of the therapist's full identity context, including that relating to sexual orientation and gender identity.

When LGBT therapists are working with heterosexual clients, the negative reactions that clients exhibit in relation to the therapist's moving into parenthood might be seen as reflections of heterosexism and cisgenderism, and they might well be. Silverman (2001) writing from the perspective of a therapist who is also a lesbian observes, "The pregnancy and parenthood of a lesbian is not socially or culturally sanctioned. The public response to it may be discomfort, confusion or disapproval, causing increased feelings of vulnerability in the pregnant woman who is a lesbian" (p. 49). At the same time, it is important to keep in mind that many clients have a range of negative reactions to the therapist's status of awaiting a child regardless of that therapist's sexual orientation or gender identity. Any negative reaction that clients are currently exhibiting could be a response to their own dynamic issues, their prejudicial feelings about minority sexual orientations, their responsiveness to some aspect of the real relationship (e.g., not providing the client with sufficient notice of the therapist's absence), or some combination thereof. Therapists who encounter discriminatory reactions from their clients might be surprised at the strength of their own reactions in response. Although an LGBT therapist might have encountered such bias in treatment before, when it is extended to one's family, the emotions stirred are likely to be especially intense.

The literature on straight, cisgendered, heterosexual therapists treating LGBT patients is robust, but unfortunately that focusing on the reverse arrangement is extraordinarily slim. However, the accounts that are available provide suggestions for how client's manifestations of homophobia can be turned into therapeutic opportunities. For example, Iasenza (1997), a psychodynamic therapist who is also a lesbian, describes how the exploration of her male patient's extreme aggression toward gay individuals led to the uncovering of his sexual abuse over a 5-year period at the hands of an older cousin. In this case, Iasenza did not disclose her sexual orientation to the patient. However, she does demonstrate that treatment methods can be applied to it just as they can to any psychological problem and that the therapist can do so amidst have intense countertransference reactions to the attitudes the client is exhibiting. She observes, "Homophobia doesn't occur outside of a story lived. We don't all learn the same societal messages and become homophobes" (p. 22). Iasenza also highlights the importance of psycho-educational interventions. For example, the patient had incorrectly assumed that because the cousin preyed upon male children, the cousin must be gay. He also believed that because he had a sexual response to the cousin, he must be gay. In this case, the therapist's drawing critical distinctions was of great benefit to the client.

When an expectant LGBT therapist encounters homophobia and cisgenderism in patients, particularly during this developmentally sensitive period in the therapist's life, he or she would be well served by obtaining group or individual supervision from those who can understand the pain attached to the therapist's position. One contribution the supervisor might make is to help the therapist recognize that the client's demonstration of bias might represent for that client a therapeutic opportunity. For example, the supervisor might point out that helping the patient to mentalize the therapist's reactions allows that patient to construct a bridge between self (the patient) and others (the therapist), even as important identity differences between self and other are recognized.

Issues in the Workplace

The LGBT therapist's well-being at home and at work is highly affected by how peers and supervisors respond to that therapist's identity status. The therapist's sexual orientation and gender identity are likely to be showcased in the process of building a new family as others become interested in what that family structure will be and as they obtain new information incidentally. In the traditions of supporting an expectant parent (e.g., a shower), often the spouse or partner is included. How the site engages with the therapist's expectancy is likely to reveal to that therapist workplace attitudes toward his or her sexual orientation and gender identity.

The professional disciplines in which therapists are trained—psychiatry, clinical psychology, social work and so on—very explicitly articulate the values of tolerance for diversity. This has not always been the case. As Silverman (2001) points out, in the psychoanalytic community, diverse sexual orientations and gender identities were seen in pathological terms. Yet, in recent years, considerable change has taken place. For example, the American Psychological Association Ethics Code encourages psychologists to challenge their own biases as they emerge in the workplace (APA, 2002, Principle E). Such a value is likely instilled in the practitioner during his or her training. Yet, therapists remain members of society and as such, take in society's attitudes toward particular groups. Evidence exists that mental health practitioners do not escape this social transmission process, despite their training. For example, Crawford, McLeod, Zamboni and Jordan (1999) found that when psychologists were presented scenarios of a same-sex couple seeking to adopt a female child, they saw that couple as less qualified than a heterosexual couple. In a study of 187 social workers, Berkman and Zinberg (1997) found that the majority of participants exhibited heterosexist attitudes. Some suggestion that positive change is underway is suggested by the findings of a study by Camilleri and Ryan (2006), who used similar methodology to that of Crawford et al. They presented vignettes involving either gay, lesbian or heterosexual parents to undergraduate social work majors and asked them to rate various aspects. The participants rated the lesbian parents most favorably, followed by the gay parents and then the heterosexual parents.

The allegiance of one's colleagues to the ideals of their professions is likely to render any self-detected prejudicial attitudes at least somewhat unacceptable to them. Unless a colleague undertakes a thoroughgoing process of examining personal bias, it could well be submerged rather than eliminated, and expressed indirectly. For example, a colleague might say "your wife" after having been clearly told that the gay therapist has a husband. Upon correction, the colleague with some embarrassment might ascribe the mistake to a mere memory lapse. Then, the expectant therapist is in the position of wondering whether the lapse was benign or something more. If the causal factor was heterosexism, the question becomes whether it was consciously or unconsciously driven. The day-to-day ambiguities that such interactions create intensify the therapist's occupational stress, with stress levels already high due to the adaptation that expectant and new parenting requires. Moreover, in the midst of this ambiguity, it becomes difficult for the expectant therapist to know how to respond. Should this colleague be confronted, avoided, or still regarded as a possible source of support? Second-guessing also results, as the therapist wonders whether any internalized homophobia on his or her part is leading to suspicions about others' motives.

Typically, mental health professionals do not uniquely populate therapists' workplaces. In fact, some sites might have a majority of individuals from distinctly different disciplines. For example, a therapist might work in a small Employee Assistance Employment industry and be surrounded by many co-workers who are not mental health professionals. Even in those settings in which mental health professionals do predominate, staff members who perform secretarial and other support functions might have a major role in shaping organizational culture. In relation to this circumstance of interacting with a broader population of co-workers, the literature is somewhat more useful in helping the expectant LGBT therapist to identify factors that might influence his or her work experience.

For example, the Ragins and Cornwell findings (2001) point to the importance of organizational policies that explicitly prohibit discrimination based on sexual orientation, as well as sites that provide diversity training that includes sexual minority issues. Lesbian and gay employees perceive actual events of discrimination to be fewer at such work sites, have a more positive attitude toward the sites, enjoy greater job satisfaction, and show enhanced performance relative to workplaces lacking such policies and trainings. Relevant to the situation of the expectant parent is the finding that when partners are included in social events with co-workers, less discrimination is perceived. Although the direction of causality is unclear, one possibility is that as co-workers become familiar with the members of the lesbian or gay individual's family, biases relax. If this were the case, it might suggest that the employee's initiative in introducing others to his or her partner and child could have a salubrious effect on relationships. These investigators found that having a supervisor with a diverse sexual orientation was valuable, but not as much so as enjoying the protections of a workplace that outlaws discrimination.

Research (e.g., Lewis, Derlega, Griffin, & Krowinski, 2003; Szymanski & Chung, 2003) exploring LGBT well-being in the workplace suggests that workplaces vary greatly in their abilities to support or undermine the psychological status of LGBT individuals. Taking a particularly great toll on LGBT individuals are those settings in which LGBT individuals feel that it is necessary to mask their identity statuses in order to maintain employment (Pillinger, 2008, as cited in Davidson, 2011). It stands to reason that the enterprise of building a family and the workplace accommodations it requires would only augment this stress. Moreover, this same enterprise could make it more difficult for sexual minority employees to continue to camouflage their sexual identities. Therefore, in the process of seeking employment, individuals representing sexual minorities should attend carefully to issues of workplace climate before making a commitment to an organization. Indeed, all therapists in the process of seeking employment should ascertain the compatibility of a given site with their long-term family goals.

General Recommendations

1. Expectant and new parent-therapists who are in the process of creating a non-traditional family can expect in their treatment of clients many of the same issues that therapists in traditional families face, but also some special ones.

2. The mere fact of being a parent in a non-traditional family, irrespective of the type, is likely to evoke responses from the client. The therapist should expect that these responses might well be connected to the client's seeing the therapist as unconventional, a person who is going against the grain. The therapist can expect that based on the patient's dynamics, the tonality of the reactions might be positive or negative, but either can serve as a gateway to understanding better the patient's inner life.

3. For all forms of non-traditional family, the therapist might encounter overt or covert discriminatory responses, the anticipation of which might lessen their effects on the therapist. Likewise, other client reactions will be more specifically linked to the therapist's particular type of non-traditional family. For example, the prospective parent of the adopted child will be subject to the common attitude of the primacy of biological connections. The therapist should use supervisory resources to process painful reactions and to consider how these events in treatment can be used as therapeutic opportunities.

4. The therapist's expectant parenthood creates an opportunity to be more fully known by the client and whether this opportunity is beneficial or detrimental

to the client is at least in part shaped by the therapist's own comfort in being known.

5. Therapist self-disclosures should be handled with care and on an individual basis. Although not always possible, the therapist should anticipate early on in treatment what kinds of self-disclosure the vicissitudes of the therapist's life might require and organize the treatment accordingly.

6. Sites vary greatly in their accommodation of different family and individual identities. This variation should be one basis on which the individual seeking to establish a non-traditional family makes employment decisions. Attention to the climate of the setting, especially in relation to prevailing attitudes toward individual differences, is crucial.

Notes

1. A great deal of controversy surrounded the process by which some of these adoptions occurred. For example, some adoptions were so expedited that a thoroughgoing effort was not made to ascertain whether parents actually survived the earthquake (Thompson, 2010).

2. Because of issues with respect to disclosure of sexual orientation, these statistics likely underestimate the prevalence of same-sex families (Gates & Cooke, 2011).

3. The statistics Gates reports are taken from four data sources: the General Social Survey, 2008/2010; the Gallup Daily Tracking Survey, June–September 2012; Census 2010 (released in 2011); and the 2011 American Community Survey.

CHAPTER 8

Developmental Status of the Patient

The developmental status of the patient is an important focus of the expectant therapist for two reasons. First, the therapist's expectancy has a different symbolic significance depending on the developmental tasks that a certain period presents to a person. For example, in the latency-age child (beginning around 6 years) who is commonly focused on subliminatory activities (behaviors that enable a child to express repressed impulses in ways that will be acceptable to the self and others), the expectancy might be seen as a creative act or an achievement. The preadolescent experiencing an eruption of sexual drives might attend to the possibly shocking discovery that the therapist, too, is a sexual being. Second, the resources a patient has to address any given issue vary with changes in developmental status. The therapist's good judgment about what resources a patient possesses will figure prominently in deciding on a course of intervention. For example, the pregnant therapist must decide whether to continue to see patients until she goes into labor or to provide them with a pre-announced termination date. Very young children frequently have extreme difficulty grasping the notion of a lengthy treatment hiatus: a long separation is a permanent separation (Browning, 1974). For them, setting both a concrete departure and return date might help the child to grasp that the separation is only temporary. An adolescent or adult patient is more likely to grasp the finite aspect of a treatment hiatus. Therefore, the patient might be able to tolerate some ambiguity in the dates defining the therapist's sabbatical.

In most of the other chapters of this book, we focus heavily upon the experiences of those individuals in the middle of the developmental continuum, that is, adulthood. In this chapter, we look at the responses of children, adolescents and the elderly in relation to the therapist's expectancy. For these developmental periods, characteristic behaviors and themes, therapist reactions and intervention strategies are outlined. When we talk about developmental status, we often use the convenience of specifying age ranges. However, we recognize that the correspondence between age and developmental status is rough, with some individuals exhibiting precocity and others immaturity relative to their peers. Still, because development takes time, in general, the clinician can have different expectations for adolescents than children, and for adults than adolescents. These expectations, especially when borne out of the clinical realities the client is presenting, can help the therapist to plan treatment based on developmental status.

Treating Children

On the whole, the literature on the therapeutic ramifications for treating children and adolescents during pregnancy and other expectancy conditions is extremely lacking. The four studies that we reported in the first edition of this book continue to be the only ones available specifically on these populations (see Schmidt, Fiorini, & Ramires's 2015 review). In a few studies since that time (e.g., Shaw & Breckenridge, 2014; Wolfe, 2013), the pool of therapists who were interviewed during or following their pregnancies included individuals who treat children. A limitation of the existing research is that studies are confined to therapists within North America (Schmidt et al., 2015). Furthermore, much more has been documented about children's reactions to their therapists' pregnancies than any other expectancy condition such as expectant fatherhood.

When children acknowledge their first conscious recognition of the pregnancy varies from child to child. Some children will uncannily reveal their awareness of it at the end of the first trimester or the beginning of the second (Ashway, 1984). In some instances, their awareness precedes the therapist's willingness to acknowledge her state, a disparity that will be discussed at the end of this section. Other children fail to acknowledge any awareness of the therapist's pregnancy into the third trimester and must be explicitly informed of it. Callanan (1985) reported that 6 of the 14 child patients she was treating appeared "oblivious" to the pregnancy until she revealed it to them in the third trimester. Like adults, many children give evidence of unconscious recognition before conscious awareness occurs. Whereas with adults, this evidence often appears in their dreams and derivatives, in children, it might manifest itself in play and drawings.

The session in which the therapist and patient together acknowledge the pregnancy is an extremely important one from a diagnostic standpoint. Ashway (1984) wrote the following about her work with child patients during her pregnancy:

> It was my impression that from these initial first encounters with the perceived pregnant therapist could be drawn some conclusions about the patient's general psychodynamic issues and conflicts, intensity of drives, defense mechanisms, and ego strengths. In much the same way that a patient's first reported dream is often a summary of relevant psychodynamic issues, the initial session in which a patient discovers the therapist is pregnant is often a crystallization of ongoing psychological struggles in general.
>
> (p. 9)

Although Ashway's comments could also extend to adult patients, the fact that for children, the issues that are brought up by the pregnancy are ones that have greater immediacy (i.e., temporal proximity to the life experiences giving rise to the issues), both the defenses and the underlying impulses against which the defenses are exerted might have greater salience than for adults.

Very commonly, children respond to the explicit recognition of their therapist's pregnancy with some defense to diminish the impact of the pregnancy and the feelings and impulses it stimulates. The two defenses most commonly observed are denial and displacement. Denial is a defensive trend that Browning (1974) noted in the first article specifically devoted to children's and adolescents' responsiveness to the therapist's pregnancy. In the article, she described how each of three children she treated developed their own unique form of denial. For example, a 7-year-old boy said he was going to order the therapist diet pills to make the pregnancy go away. Other children will simply behave as if the therapist had never mentioned the pregnancy, such as the 7-year old girl described by Miller (1992), who failed to show any pregnancy themes in her play. At the same time, her play became more constricted and bland, suggesting the avoidance of an important issue. This patient also insisted to her mother that the therapist's delivery of the baby would not involve the therapist's absence from the clinic.

As a number of child therapists (e.g., Browning, 1974) have observed, a defense that often emerges after denial crumbles is displacement, which involves the child's shift in attention from the therapist's pregnant abdomen to another body part that is unrelated to the pregnancy. For example, after learning of the therapist's pregnancy, Browning's 6-year-old male patient began to take great interest in the therapist's hairdo. He also claimed that her eyes and teeth had become enlarged, a possible projection of his own hostility over the pregnancy. In another case example (Miller, 1992), a four-and a half year-old asked his pregnant therapist if she would remove her shoes so he could examine her feet.

Another commonly observed trend is the child's tendency to regress on learning of the news of the pregnancy. Frequently, the regression entails an intensification of the presenting symptoms. Paluszny and Posnanski (1971) described how an 11-year-old boy resumed the angry outbursts that brought him into treatment, outbursts that had previously abated on his establishment of a trusting relationship with the therapist. Beyond symptomatology, the child might become preoccupied with the themes and conflicts of an earlier developmental or psychosexual stage than that in which the child was working prior to the pregnancy. For example, Ashway (1984) described a 10-year-old girl, Ruth, who had been enraged by the discovery of her therapist's pregnancy and was driven to leave her therapist's office a mess after each session. Her behavior represented wishes to obtain control and to leave her messy feelings of anger with the therapist, issues suggesting a regression to the anal stage. The regression of any given child can be due to the pregnancy's stimulation of issues of a particular stage that were never resolved. Alternatively, the child may regress to an earlier period that he or she associates with conflict and mastery.

The progression of the pregnancy and the therapist's interpretive efforts work against the child's continued defensiveness. As the pregnancy comes to be more explicitly acknowledged by the child, concerns about abandonment and feelings associated with this concern are likely to surface (Browning, 1974; Byrnes, 2000; Miller, 1992; Nadelson et al., 1974). Anger, fear, sadness and guilt are all likely to be present but at varying levels from child to child. As delivery nears, increased access to specific fantasies (such as the fantasy, often motivated by both hostility and guilt, that the therapist is going to die in childbirth), become more accessible. In contrast to adults, children seem to be far less focused on Oedipal-level issues and less inclined to bring material of an explicitly sexual nature (Miller, 1992). However, connected to the maternal transference is a sibling rivalry issue (i.e., that the birth of the "sibling" will bring about the loss of emotional supplies from the mother). Although this reaction may be seen in children with or without siblings, a child's specific experience in this area will color his or her reactions to the therapist's unborn child. For example, an only child who can use only fantasy as a basis for imagining the losses to be endured on the arrival of a competitor may have a more catastrophic view of sibling arrival than a child who has had the actual experience.

Children are able to make use of the surge in previously unconscious material in several ways. The first is that children derive benefit from experiencing the therapist's tolerance for psychological contents that had been barred from consciousness previously. Often their own intolerance has been internalized from the reactions of early relationships with family members and the pregnant therapist provides a very different model to internalize. For example, Ashway's (1984) Ruth was unable to communicate her painful feelings to her narcissistically preoccupied mother in relation to the birth of her sister when she was 3 years old. The mother, on the report of the father, either physically or emotionally abused Ruth or ignored her altogether. In therapy, Ruth was able to express her rage and her wish that the baby might vanish. In contrast to her mother, her therapist facilitated and accepted this expression of feeling. Through this process, Ruth was able to accept a part of her psychological life previously repressed. This inability to accept these thoughts and feelings was critically connected to the severe anxiety and extreme insecurity that brought he into treatment.

The therapist not only accepts what the child produces but also helps the child to understand the emerging material through interpretation. More specifically, the therapist assists the child in seeing how expectations about present caretakers (specifically, the therapist) are influenced by past experiences. For example, with the therapist's assistance, Ruth realized that she feared that the mother would "stop caring or did care less for her when her mother was pregnant with Ruth's younger sister" (Ashway, 1984, p. 11). By Ruth's recognition of the connection between her mother's rejection of her and her expectation of the rejection from the therapist, she was helped to adjust her anticipations of others in the direction of reality. Moreover, the specific articulation of fantasies often mitigates fear and enables their more active testing by immediate experience. For example, by identifying a fear of abandonment, the child is assisted in its lessening when the therapist actually returns from her maternity leave.

Whereas some children's therapeutic work is catapulted by the therapist's pregnancy, others' work is relatively unaffected and still others' work is hindered, as evidenced by the child's deterioration either in terms of symptom pattern, ego functioning or both during the therapist's pregnancy (Nadelson et al., 1974). Some of these are individuals who cannot tolerate the therapist's pregnancy. According to McGarty (1988), individuals who have lost a caretaking figure might, in some cases, be adversely affected. A child who recently lost a parent could find a significant treatment interruption so traumatic as to fail to profit from the therapeutic processes outlined earlier.

Although many of the reactions described in this section are negatively toned, genuine positive feelings are also manifest. In fact, Byrnes (2000), who interviewed 24 therapists who worked with child clients, found that whereas all of the reactions documented in the literature were noted, the predominant reactions observed by the therapists were ones of excitement and anticipation.

In some cases, patients fail to show improvement over the course of the therapist's pregnancy because of the therapist's countertransference. Most therapist reactions discussed in Chapter 4 can be evoked in the psychotherapeutic treatment of children. However, certain reactions are likely to have particular strength, and these are discussed in the next section.

Common Therapist Reactions in the Treatment of Children

As stated in Chapter 3, a vital differentiation for the therapist to make is whether a given reaction is rooted in the real relationship, the therapist's dynamics, the child's dynamics or some combination thereof. An example of a reaction based on the real relationship is a therapist's taking on a new child patient without having adequate time to forge a therapeutic alliance or be useful to that child before the therapist's departure. Noting that a reaction is based upon the real relationship is useful in feeding into broad-based clinical decisions. For example, the therapist in this case might decide to refer the child to another therapist.

Like those reactions of the children they treat, therapists' reactions tend to center on abandonment. If the child feels that he or she is being abandoned, the therapist is likely to see herself as the abandoning agent. Because of both the centrality of this theme for the child and the therapist's perception of child's vulnerability (relative to adult patients), therapists are prone to feel keenly guilty about a child's treatment disruption. Moreover, due to the recency of critical loss events in the life of the child, the therapist has a more vivid sense of subjecting the child to a repetition of past traumas.

Therapists have a variety of strategies for resisting the complementary identification with the depriving object in the child's life. One common strategy is to be excessively gratifying by failing to provide appropriate limits and to maintain the usual boundaries within the sessions. For example, therapists might have difficulty ending sessions on time. Sometimes this difficulty in establishing a limit will extend to the maternity leave itself, with the therapist making unrealistic promises about a likely return date or phone contact during her absence. Another strategy is to interfere with, or fail to facilitate, the child's expression of feelings in relation to the departure by, for instance, offering hollow reassurances (e.g., "You'll see: The time will fly by until I'm back"). Still another strategy is to neglect to announce the pregnancy altogether. As discussed earlier, many children will refrain from bringing it up themselves (Callanan, 1985).

Another common therapist reaction concerns the therapist's sense of competence. Most therapists—except those who do not plan to return to professional work after delivery—have some anxiety about their capacities to juggle the responsibilities of home and office. Women naturally question whether they can be good mothers and therapists simultaneously. It is in relation to this anxiety that the child patient's criticisms of the therapist have particular potency to create disturbance in the therapist (Nadelson et al., 1974). Relative to adult patients, child patients are likely to be identified with the therapist's unborn child. The child's accusations of the therapist's insufficiencies, especially as they pertain to the therapist's pregnancy ("You are ruining my life by having this baby"; "You already pay more attention to the baby than to me"), are likely to sting. As Nadelson et al. (1974) pointed out, it is as if the therapist's child-in-the-womb is speaking through the child patient.

Up until this point, the countertransference reactions described in this chapter were examples of complementary identifications. Concordant identifications with the child patient also occur. The sense of emotional and physical vulnerability of the therapist is a well-established consequence of, and accompaniment to, any pregnancy. For example, Leifer (1980) interviewed 19 pregnant women and found them to be more concerned about death and more conservative in their actions than at other times. The therapist might find an identification with the vulnerability of the child disturbing not because it evokes guilt, but rather because it resonates with the therapist's own sense of fragility at this time. The therapist might project her own vulnerability onto the child and thereby see this quality in exaggerated terms in the child, while missing signs of the child's resilience. The therapist might even intensify the child's sense of vulnerability (in the form of a projective identification) by either failing to discuss the pregnancy or downplaying any negative reactions the child might have to it. The therapist could initially reveal the pregnancy to the parent rather than to the child, thereby avoiding direct communication. These behaviors convey to the child that he or she is too weak to address this very issue.

The therapist might also ward off a sense of vulnerability by failing to modify aspects of her interaction with child patients that could pose an undue physical hardship for her. Generally speaking, psychotherapy with children requires more physical exertion and agility than it does with older adolescents or adults.

The therapist might have to make significant modifications in how she interacts with her child patients, for example, substituting checkers for Twister (see the case example in Callanan, 1985). However, the ability to do so requires some tolerance for the inevitable physical limitations of pregnancy. While the failures to make the appropriate modifications might be the result of the wish to deny limitations, it might also be due to the previously discussed need to diminish the guilt associated with the perception of having abandoned the child patient. As we can see in the following vignette, the association between guilt and the acknowledgment of physical limitation was clearly drawn by one of the therapists we interviewed who was expecting twins.

Vignette 8.1

In my work with a 7-year-old girl, I could no longer play a favorite game of rolling a ball back and forth across the length of the therapy room and under a chair. The patient told me that her father couldn't play ball with her at home because he had cancer and was at times hospitalized for treatment . . . Initially, I felt sad and guilty that I could not give her the opportunity that she wasn't getting at home which, under ordinary circumstances and previously, I could easily provide. In retrospect, I was glad that I was able to tolerate the guilt. The patient without this activity began to talk more about what it was like for her to have a sick father, how she worried about him dying, and how she cried alone in her room.

The therapist's ability to tolerate guilt created a valuable therapeutic opportunity for her child patient. It also enabled the therapist to see that the play provided the child an opportunity to deny and compensate for the loss she suffered in relation to her ill father and the concomitant sadness involved.

The preceding discussion concerns the therapist's countertransferences during pregnancy. On return to clinical work, the therapist could find her reactions to working with the child patient even more powerful. Unless the therapist takes a relatively protracted maternity leave, the therapist will be conducting her professional life at the same time that she is mothering an infant who has not yet stabilized physically or emotionally. A therapist who is fatigued and overwhelmed could have difficulty in summoning the resources to respond to the enormous needs of child patients. All the maneuvers that were described earlier that therapists might use to deny a sense of vulnerability or to lessen anxieties about competence might be used at this time.

A more specific dynamic arises when certain child patient behaviors remind her of those behaviors in her infant that are most vexing. A child's demanding behaviors during the session can remind the therapist of the infant's hourly demands for feeding in the night. Because negative feelings toward the child patient might be experienced by some therapists as less threatening than negative feelings toward their infants, the child patient might serve as a displacement object for the therapist, thereby preserving the infant as the all-good object. Intense angry feelings for the child and any defensive maneuvers that are devised to quell these feelings, such as withdrawal, denial or reaction formation, are likely to hinder the therapist's effectiveness.

The therapist is also vulnerable to feeling guilt over time spent with the patient in his or her status as someone else's child. Such feelings are unlikely to be eliminated by the therapist's recognition of reality factors that necessitate that she work during this period. As the stimulus for such therapist guilt, the child patient might elicit anger from the therapist, which might be defended against in a variety of ways, such as the therapist's failure to establish appropriate limits within the treatment. The therapist might displace this anger onto other figures, such as the child's parents, teachers or other persons providing treatment to the child. Of course, hostility toward the child's parents might not be a displacement but a genuine reaction to the parents' behavior. Experiencing the innocence and defenselessness of one's own child within another could engender angry feelings in a therapist who is working with children who were abused or neglected by their parents in their infancy.

Therapist reactions are positive as well as negative. Shaw and Breckenridge (2014) interviewed a group of therapists, most of whom saw both children and adults. The therapists reported that the experience of parenting brings more empathy and a lessened tendency to judge negatively. The therapists also observed that their work in therapy helped them to become better parents by raising their awareness of particular skills such as affect regulation that would be helpfully cultivated in their children.

A summary of some common therapist reactions in treating child patients appears in Table 8.1.

Treatment Strategies With the Child Patient

The Announcement of the Pregnancy

The earliest decisions confronting the pregnant therapist typically concern the announcement of the pregnancy. The therapist must decide whether, when or how to announce the pregnancy.

Some circumstances might exist in which the pregnancy never becomes acknowledged within the treatment, the most typical of which would be a short-term patient treated in the therapist's early pregnancy. A therapist might decide to refrain from making the disclosure because doing so could derail the treatment focus, would stimulate the surfacing of issues that could not be addressed properly in the time frame provided, or both.

However, most practitioners agree that either in a longer-term treatment or when the treatment extends into the period of the pregnancy when bodily changes are manifest, the therapist should take some initiative in presenting the pregnancy to the patient if the patient shows no sign of detecting it on his or her own (Callanan, 1985; Simonis-Gayed & Levin, 1994). Moreover, given that

Table 8.1 Common Countertransference Responses With Children

During pregnancy

- Feelings of guilt over a sense of having abandoned child patients
- Worries about one's competence in mothering
- Excessive attunement to the child's vulnerability
- Resentment over the demands of treating child patients
- Fear that maternal absorption is depriving the child patient of sufficient care and attention
- Uncertainty as to how to answer the child patient's often rather direct questions

Upon return to work
- Guilt over spending time with someone else's child
- Missing the child while at work
- Frustration and felt fragmentation in relation to the responsibility of attending to children in two venues
- Continued worries that obstacles in treatment of a child portend difficulties in parenting.

even after the pregnancy is acknowledged, most child patients will put up a host of defenses, defenses that must be dismantled before the defended-against material can be addressed, considerable time is almost always a necessity. Time is also required to prepare the child for the upcoming separation, a preparation that was often lacking in most of the traumatic losses some child patients endured. What the therapist must balance is ensuring that the child has sufficient time to discuss the issues evoked by the pregnancy but also has the opportunity to discover the pregnancy on his or her own. Most writers on this topic have seen the end of the second trimester or beginning of the third trimester as the period when this disclosure would be made. Byrnes (2000) found that most child therapists reveal their pregnancies in the second trimester. Based on their work with their children, Simonis-Gayed and Levin (1994) argued in favor of waiting until the beginning of the third trimester, because doing so

> allows time for the client to project thoughts onto the therapist and gives the client time to project thoughts onto the therapist and gives the client time to process associations to the pregnancy without having to deal with the reality of the pregnancy itself.
>
> (p. 199)

However, a factor that might dispose the therapist to move up this disclosure is the possibility of premature delivery, particularly in the case of high-risk deliveries.

In some instances, a child's deterioration in functioning due to his or her tacit recognition of the pregnancy might necessitate that the therapist accelerate the disclosure of the pregnancy. Shrier and Mahmood (1988) described the case of a 2-year-old boy placed in a therapeutic nursery. The child had presenting symptoms of aggressive and disorganized behavior. Over the course of his treatment, he improved considerably. However, during the sixth month of the therapist's pregnancy, his aggression toward others surged dramatically. When he was observed making dolls pregnant by stuffing toys under their clothes and hitting them, it was decided that this was the stressor affecting his behavior. After the therapist discussed the pregnancy with the child and allayed some of his fears in relation to it (such as being rejected), he resumed his higher level of functioning.

Perhaps a more difficult situation is that wherein the child patient intuits the pregnancy at a very early point (e.g., within the first 3 months) prior to the time the therapist is ready to reveal the pregnancy either to the child or even to the other staff within the setting. A number of factors need to be balanced here. On the one hand, the therapist does not want to state any untruth that would undermine the child's trust in the relationship. Certainly, for example, the therapist should refrain from denying the pregnancy in any obvious or subtle ways. Neither should the therapist discourage the child's questioning by conveying that a question is somehow off limits. However, for a number of reasons, the therapist might not choose to affirm the child's observations or to answer directly a child's question. The therapist could legitimately consider the personal and professional consequences that would ensue by making this early disclosure (Haber, 1992). The therapist might also be concerned about the fact that acknowledging the pregnancy would necessitate acknowledging a miscarriage should one occur, and the therapeutic impact of the latter event must be weighed. The therapist might want to announce the pregnancy when more details are in place concerning the therapist's pregnancy leave. For example, a therapist deciding whether to quit work or merely take a maternity leave might want to have made the decision before informing the child of the pregnancy.

The therapist will be aided in formulating an effective intervention by developing an understanding of the child's motivation for either asking the pregnancy question or making the observation long before most others can. Is the child responding to an underlying fear of abandonment? Is the child expressing an oedipally based wish to be intimate with mother through the tool of intuition? Is he or she revealing a hypervigilance about a possible competitor? Whether or not the pregnancy is affirmed at this time, important interpretive groundwork can be laid concerning its significance to the child patient.

A final decision the therapist needs to make is how to announce the pregnancy if the child has not yet given indication of being aware of it. Here we make a somewhat different recommendation for children than what we offered for adults based on the clinical material both groups tend to offer. The reader might recall that with adults, we suggested that the announcement of the pregnancy be separated from that of the maternity leave because adults appear to respond to them differently. Because of the prominence of abandonment themes for children, the pregnancy and leave are part and parcel of the same event. Therefore, we recommend that with a child population, they be presented together. Failing to address the separation creates ambiguity that is likely to induce unnecessarily intense anxiety in the child, anxiety that could have a detrimental effect on the child's current level of functioning and even perhaps on the motivation to continue treatment. Although recognizing that the very young child will have extreme difficulty grasping this information, the therapist should be as specific as possible about the parameters of the separation. In some instances, the therapist might wish to announce the separation prior to announcing the pregnancy. One of the therapists we interviewed began to see a 9-year-old female patient early in her first trimester. This child had recently lost her therapist of 1 year. Her mother was currently being hospitalized for psychiatric reasons. The therapist felt it was important to anticipate the interruption in the treatment at the outset. However, she also felt that discussing the pregnancy at this time would be premature. Therefore, she merely told the child that after a certain number of months, she would be away for 2 months but would then return. It was not until the middle of the therapist's second trimester that the reason for the interruption of the treatment was discussed.

The parents are likely to have their own reactions to the therapist's pregnancy, and sometimes these reactions are actually more intense than those of the child patient. Some parents project their own reactions to the pregnancy onto their children. For example, one therapist announced the pregnancy to a 6-year-old girl who was in treatment with her. The child went running out to her mother in the waiting room in a jubilant fashion yelling, "Mommy, Dr. X is pregnant." The mother made a congratulatory comment. However, the next day, the therapist was surprised by the mother's phone call in which the mother in an angry tone said to the therapist, "How could you do this to my daughter?" How to deal with these reactions needs some careful thought. For instance, should the therapist continue to allow the parents (and in this instance, the mother) to use the child as a medium to express their own feelings of loss or abandonment? Or should the therapist attempt in a session with the parents (or this mother) to help them explore their own feelings about it? In this particular case, the mother had been sent to live with a grandmother when her younger sibling was born. This mother was ultimately able to articulate the connection she made. However, some parents will be unable to gain insight, and might act on their affections and projections by discontinuing their child's treatment, bringing the child sporadically, impinging upon the child's protected space with the therapist, and so on. The therapist must be in sufficient communication with the parents to garner information about these reactions (in addition to what the child can provide) to understand how these reactions might pose another stressor for the child.

As a practical point, parents might be more likely to notice the therapist's pregnancy than a child (Wolfe, 2013). If it is important to the therapist that she be the person who reveals the pregnancy to her child patient, it might be necessary to call the parents in at an early point, reveal the pregnancy, and stress the importance of allowing the therapist to make this communication.

Finally, the therapist should give careful consideration to how office staff communicate with parents and children. It is very common for office staff to be questioned about the therapist's situation (Simonis-Gayed & Levin, 1994). Office staff might be perceived as more disclosing than the therapist. Moreover, talking to the staff enables both the patients and parents to avoid any embarrassment that would result from an error in their inferences about the therapist. Given the likelihood of such inquiries, the staff should be given strategies for their responses that will provide the therapist with maximal control over any information that could have therapeutic impact and to enable direct exchanges between therapist and patient about the relevant issues (e.g., I don't think I should speak for Dr. Jones. Perhaps you could ask her.").

Following the Announcement

In an earlier section, it was described how the announcement of the pregnancy is typically succeeded by the resurrection of defenses and the ultimate surfacing of issues relevant to the pregnancy. However, quite often children are unable to establish the link between the emotions that are experienced in the session and the events—past, present and future—that are provoking them. For example, a small child might come in enraged at the therapist for failing to have a particular toy available, with little notion that the reaction has anything to do with the pregnancy. The invaluable contribution of the therapist is to draw this connection, always being careful to base it on clinical material the patient is presenting rather than on the therapist's pre-existing formulations. However, the therapist can stimulate the emergence of this material by having play materials evocative of the topic of pregnancy and its related themes. Among these might be dolls representing different family members including babies. Simonis-Gayed and Levin (1994) described how one child was assisted in enacting the delivery scene through use of a toy ambulance and hospital.

At this time, children commonly engage in three types of behavior that challenge the typical boundaries of the therapy: question asking, touching and gift giving. We address each area not to provide rules of practice but rather to offer points of consideration as the therapist develops an intervention plan that is consistent with her ongoing work with the child.

QUESTION ASKING

The therapist can expect children to ask a great number of direct questions about many aspects of the pregnancy (Miller, 1992), in fact, because for some children, this time might be the first when they clearly realize that the therapist has a life outside of the relationship with them. It also could even be their first up-close encounter with someone who is pregnant. The child in the face of this novelty could be inspired to ask many personal questions, which in turn could overwhelm the therapist. To diminish the likelihood of being taken off guard and answering a question in a way that poorly serves the treatment, the therapist should develop a strategy about how questions should be handled. Specifically, the therapist should decide what types of questions should be answered directly and the level of detail in the therapist's response. The plan should be tailored to the individual child. Among other factors, the therapist should consider carefully a given child's level of frustration tolerance in view of the fact than an unanswered question is often experienced as a deprivation. One of Wolfe's (2013) interviewees described using the child's questions as a springboard to helping the child explore his or her own early days. She reported,

> There was one client where we got out his baby album and we looked at all the pictures from when he was a baby, and mom reminisced about what that was like, and spoke to him about what kind of baby he was.
>
> (p. 60)

Of course, if treatment is occurring within a larger treatment setting, it might not be possible to have a disclosure policy that is adapted to each individual patient. For example, Callanan (1985) wrote about how a question posed to her by a 14-year-old boy was formulated by an entire class of a partial hospital program. In speaking to him, she was addressing the group. As Wolfe's child therapists noted, some children have little interest in the pregnancy except in how it affects them. These therapists observed that the parents were far more interested than their children in the details of the pregnancy.

The therapist can expect to obtain questions in two areas, both of which receive a lesser degree of interest from adult patients. The first is the therapist's childcare arrangement (Miller, 1992). In some cases, this focus reflects the child's identification with the unborn baby, an identification that leads the child to wonder, "How well will I be taken care of?" In other instances, the focus reflects a fear that the baby will usurp the child's time with the therapist. In fact, children often fantasize that the baby will be present in the therapy sessions. This idea might not be an altogether unpleasant one for the child. It might express a wish to achieve a union with the therapist through co-ministering to the baby and represent a solidification of identification with the therapist. For young girls, this longing might signal the crystallization of gender identity. The second area concerns the process of the delivery of the baby. Underlying the discussion of the mechanics of birth is oftentimes a worry about whether the therapist or the baby can survive the event (Paluszny & Posnanski, 1971). This fear could be based entirely on rational considerations. What adult has not at some time pondered how amazing it is that a baby could come forth from a woman? On the other hand, this concern could be a consequence of the child anger toward either the baby or the therapist. It also might be the child's way of punishing him or herself for having angry feelings toward the baby or therapist.

Touching

The child patient is more inclined than at other times to initiate touching the pregnant therapist, especially her abdomen (Miller, 1992). Although the primary driver of the pregnancy is curiosity about the baby, other motives could be present as well. For example, this behavior might be due to the child's desire to be reassured that the therapist is present, a desire stimulated by the therapist's pending departure. It might also be due to the intensification of maternal transference. As Miller (1992) wrote describing her own patients' reactions, "Perhaps because the therapist looked more like a 'mommy person,' children's intense neediness for contact with their own mothers at any level burst into physical expression in their interaction with me" (p. 634). Certainly, touching in psychotherapy is a behavior that must always be given careful consideration by the therapist. Therapists who work with children on a regular basis will no doubt have had to develop a policy in relation to this area. Although some might encourage the child to express actions in words, others might permit some touching but emphasize the importance of the child's obtaining permission before crossing this personal boundary (Miller, 1992).

Some children's touching is of an aggressive sort. The therapist is of course threatened by this behavior out of an understandable fear of harm coming to her baby. It is important that the therapist makes an initial determination of the realistic risk within the situation. At times, the therapist might eventually recognize that she exaggerated the risk of harm due to the projection of her own anger. In other instances, where the potential for danger might be great, it would behoove the therapist to take the necessary safeguards. For example, one of the authors in treating an anorexic preadolescent inpatient assessed the danger to be considerable based both on the patient's threats and a history of acting out against other staff. The therapist was careful to see her on the unit in a room that was accessible to other staff and used a seating arrangement giving the therapist an unobstructed path to the door. The therapist must be alert to any internal pressures leading her to deny vulnerability and thereby neglect to take critical precautions. If children have difficulty managing their aggressive impulses within the session, they should be encouraged to express them in relation to the therapist's toys rather than the therapist's person or possessions (Ashway, 1984). A child unable to do so should be transferred to another therapist at least temporarily. In this regard, therapists should exercise care not to succumb to workplace pressures that might discourage them from taking appropriate self-protective actions.

Gifts From the Child Patient

A very different behavior from physical attacks on the therapist is that of presenting gifts to the therapist for either herself or the baby. Frequently, the children have made the presents themselves, and in our view, the therapist should rarely refuse such a gift. Declining a child's offering has great potential to be narcissistically damaging and might be taken as a rejection of the child him or herself. However, although the gift might be accepted, it is important for the therapist to keep in mind that both the fact of the gift and its particular nature will be imbued with significance in relation with the child's current feelings toward the therapist and baby. The exception to this statement is if the gift is entirely the parent's idea, in which case it is likely to be reflective of the parent's dynamics (and perhaps the child's as well). Ashway (1984) described how the 12-year-old child she had treated in long-term therapy (previously mentioned in this chapter) presented her with a pair of booties for the baby before the therapist left for her maternity leave. The booties were an ambivalent offering reflecting both nurturant feelings associated with providing someone warmth as well as more aggressive feelings associated with kicking. Some children would benefit from exploring the dual aspects of the gift. However, whether or not the therapist chooses to unpack the symbolism of the gift, the awareness of the gift's meaning will help the therapist intervene sensitively.

Planning the Leave

If the pregnancy is going to result in the interruption of treatment, as it usually will, the therapist should present the leave at an early point and be as specific as possible about its beginning and ending (Simonis-Gayed & Levin, 1994). At the same time, the therapist should prepare the child for the possibility that these dates might be altered. The therapist does well to keep in mind Naparstek's finding (1976) that a large number of therapists in her survey felt that they had set a premature return date and many returned merely out of a sense of obligation. Clinical exigencies do need to figure into leave planning, but the therapist's parental responsibilities and emotional needs during this period must be given adequate weight. Ashway (1984) points out that too much eagerness on the mother's part to reassure the child about a particular return date might be due to a countertransferential wish to avoid the child's negative reactions.

For many young children, a protracted absence is felt to be a permanent loss (Miller, 1992). For this reason, many child therapists have some contact with the child during the separation either through phone calls (Browning, 1974) or writing. The latter might take the form of an exchange of letters, email or simply an announcement about the birth of the baby and health of both mother and baby. This latter notification might be particularly important for those children who fear that the therapist or baby might die during delivery. For some children who require continuous treatment in order to maintain an adequate level of functioning, use of an alternate therapist might be critical. If so, the alternate therapist might provide the child with any information about the original therapist from which the child could derive benefit. For children who are well along the road to achieving object constancy, a transitional object, provided by the therapist, might be sufficient for the child to maintain the image of the therapist in her absence. For example, if the child has produced a special painting during the sessions, the therapist might suggest that she hang it on her wall and use it to remind herself of the therapist's eventual return. In some cases, it might be preferential to have the child continue with the alternate therapist rather than to subject the child to another transition.

Treating Adolescents

The study of adolescents and their therapists during the latter's expectancy is relatively neglected in the literature, and what is available are only anecdotal accounts. This inattention is unfortunate given that adolescence is the period that sees the often-intense emergence of the young person's sexual impulses. The adolescent shares with the therapist the capacity to become a parent. Hence, this period is rife with potential identifications for the therapist to explore. Within the literature, some case examples and testimonies from therapists have enabled the construction of a picture of the issues and themes that are likely to emerge for this developmental group as the therapist awaits his or her child. However, again, what limited material exists in the literature is heavily slanted toward the pregnant therapist in relation to other expectancy conditions.

Behaviors and Themes

The literature suggests that for adolescents (years 13–21), distinguishing the patterns of males versus females is particularly crucial to adequately characterize their responses. However, although patterns characterize the populations, they are not necessarily descriptive of the individual client's responses. As on most psychological variables, the distributions of behaviors of males and females greatly overlap (Brabender & Mihura, 2016), and most writers agree that in this domain, we have much more to learn about gender differences (McGourty, 2013).

Female Patients

In general, adolescent girls do not show the high level of defensiveness that characterizes the responses of children. The features that seem to be especially prominent in this age and gender group are excitement about, and keen interest in, all aspects of the pregnancy, birth, and early life of the child. Fenster (1983) reported that the realization of pregnancy stimulates myriad questions, many of which have to do with the well-being of the mother and baby. In the older female adolescent, the interest extends to topics such as how the therapist plans to juggle work and family and the reactions of the newcomer's older sibling (Brouwers, 1989).

The curiosity reported by Fenster's therapists was also noted in the a sample of group psychotherapists who were treating adolescent patients, most of whom were female (Fallon, Brabender, Anderson & Maier, 1995). The leaders of these adolescent groups reported nurturant behaviors on the part of members toward their pregnant therapists. For example, one leader of an inpatient group described how the adolescent members recognized that she was having difficulty walking in her last trimester. If a task needed to be performed that involved walking (such as contacting another staff person on the unit), the members would spontaneously perform it. The goodness-of-fit between the therapist's need and members' responses suggested that the latter were borne out of genuine caring rather than defensiveness (e.g., a reaction formation against angry feelings).

Another related feature is patients' enhanced access to positive affects. An advantage of working with adolescents (as well as children) is that their positive expressions are not as fully tainted by social conventions, and are therefore more trustworthy. One of our interviewees described how she had been treating an 18-year-old college freshman woman for about 6 months when she announced the pregnancy to her. The patient had been attempting to separate from her parents and come to terms with her mother's mental illness. During latency, the mother developed severe emotional problems, requiring the patient to assume a parental role. She had a very vague recollection of events occurring prior to her mother's illness. When the therapist revealed her pregnancy to the young woman, it evoked a memory of her mother's description of the day the patient was born, a day the mother had portrayed in the most positive terms possible, "It was sunny and bright. The birds were singing and the flowers were blooming." In the sessions that followed, the patient seemed to have a heightened recollection of her childhood, which contained many happy memories. She proceeded to mourn the mother she once had, thereby enabling her to accept the mother she currently has. In summarizing the patient's gains, the therapist wrote, "These memories and the mourning process facilitated her separation from her parents and enabled her to explore her own growth and identity."

Vignette 8.2
A 17-year-old girl had been seen for 2 months in individual therapy, first as an inpatient on an adolescent unit and subsequently as an outpatient. She had a history of promiscuity and most recently had a string of episodes of running away from home to live with her drug-addicted boyfriend.

The patient had been shocked when she was informed of the therapist's pregnancy at the end of the seventh month. She responded with congratulations adding, "Wow, I never noticed a thing!" She then quickly moved on to lament the restrictions her parents placed on her as well as their unwarranted disapproval of her boyfriend. She continued with therapy for another month, during which time she admitted no particular reaction to the therapist's pregnancy. She terminated precipitously a month prior to the therapist's leave.

This patient used various mechanisms of flight to avoid the pre-oedipal longings for dependency that emerged in her relationship with the pregnant therapist.

The first mechanism was denial: the patient did not recognize the pregnancy when most others had. The second was flight into heterosexual romantic pursuits. The third was avoidance, with the patient leaving the treatment just as she had so frequently left her parents' home.

The juxtaposition of enthusiastic avoidance and avoidance suggests that for the adolescent girl, the therapist's pregnancy brings to the surface an existing conflict. As with all adolescents, the adolescent girl experiences of resurgence of dependency impulses at the very time she is called on to separate more fully from her parents and construct a separate identity, especially in relation to her mother. The different responses of adolescent girls to the therapist's pregnancy might be seen as different ways of resolving this conflict. The adolescent girl who immerses herself in the therapist's pregnancy is achieving a compromise between various need states. Her interest in this aspect of the therapist's womanhood enables further consolidation of her own female identity. In identifying with a figure of authority other than her mother, she is achieving some separateness from her and thereby, fashioning her unique identity. Through her identification with the baby, she is able to safely gain some indirect gratification of her dependent longings. By expressing a wish to participate in the baby's care by, for example, babysitting the therapist's baby, she is gratifying, in a projective identificatory way, the wish to be "babied" herself.

Despite the gratifications experienced in relation to the therapist's pregnancy, this occurrence also inflicts on all patients, including the female adolescent, many privations (e.g., the loss of perceived exclusivity of the therapy relationship, the lack of continuity in the treatment due to the maternity leave). All of these factors can and do elicit anger from female adolescents. In some sense, their presence is propitious: a fundamental task for the adolescent girl is to come to terms with her very early positive and negative representations of her mother in order to construct a complex and realistic image of the mother figure. Both the satisfactions and deprivations of this period enable the accomplishment of this task. Just as the baby can tolerate negative images of the mother through the experience of the more preponderant positive images, so, too, can the adolescent girl accept unpleasant aspects of the therapist's pregnancy because of their concurrence with the pregnancy's enthrallments. The intrapsychic and social payoffs of this accomplishment are considerable. As Blos (1985) wrote, "The future capacity for, and pleasure in, mothering are, to a large extent, facilitated by the mature female's unconflicted and open access to the integrated good and bad mother images" (p. 167).

However, as was suggested earlier, adolescent girls devise other solutions to deal with the challenge of the therapist's pregnancy. For some, pleasurable experiences in relation to the therapist's pregnancy might not be possible because the mother–infant image is too fraught with pain, associated as it might be with past traumatic experiences of deprivation. In such instances (e.g., the one reported in the prior case illustration) frequently, a rather total flight into heterosexual acting out occurs. It represents a compromise formation, at once providing fulfillment for tactile hunger and disguising the infantile character of the longing

(Blos, 1985). Others might flee into asceticism, often accompanied by eating disorders that emphasize the restriction of oral intake. Vandereycken and DeKerf (2010) found that 39.1% of the eating disordered patients they surveyed indicated that the therapist's pregnancy stimulated their own fear of becoming fat.

For many adolescent female patients, an alternation between relatively direct experiences of pleasure and pain, and acting out, can be witnessed. It is for this group that the therapist's interventions are critical to ensure that the acting out does not escalate into termination, pregnancy or both, and that the potential opportunities for growth are realized.

Male Patient

Within the literature, far less attention has been given to the male adolescent's reaction to the therapist's pregnancy. This is an unfortunate lacuna because, relative to the female patient, the male patient is likely to find the therapist's pregnancy a more challenging event. It presents the male patient with various threats to his well-being without offering the enchantments it provides the female patient. Like the female adolescent, the male experiences the intensification of passive sexual strivings as a natural part of early adolescence. Yet, relative to the girl, these strivings are far more unacceptable and generally elicit a more extreme defensive reaction (Blos, 1985). Hence, the infantile identificatory opportunity that the therapist's pregnancy provides to all patients is repugnant to many heterosexual male adolescents. Equally unacceptable are his own feminine procreative strivings because they are strivings never to be realized and are at odds with his burgeoning masculine identity. The therapist's pregnancy also invites the emergence of these strivings. At the same time as his anxiety increases about the emergence of forbidden parts of himself, so too does his anxiety intensify about the therapist. Corresponding to his perception of himself as passive is his view of the therapist in her pregnant state as aggressively overwhelming.

How the therapist's pregnancy is experienced by the adolescent trans men, trans women and individuals who do not place themselves within the gender identity binary is important and in need of study. However, insofar as the therapist's pregnancy readily brings up loss as well as gains in a person's life, it provides considerable opportunity for the exploration of the client's reactions. For example, the adolescent transgender man who is having gender affirmation surgery in the future might nonetheless grieve the loss of the capacity to bear a child. A transgender man who retains a physical capacity to bear a child might identify with the therapist's expectant state, an identification that could easily be missed if the therapist assumes, like many do, an equivalence between child bearing and femininity. It is crucial for the therapist to recognize the diversity of attitudes and longings that transgender persons have toward biological reproduction (Walks, 2013). Her pregnancy serves as a natural stimulus for a conversation about bearing children that the client might not have explored in therapy previously. What such a conversation could reveal are important aspects of a transgender man or woman's self-representation and their degree of fluidity (Riggs, 2013). For example, is the masculine identity of the transman compatible with breastfeeding?

Because the previously described self and object perceptions are so threatening, heterosexual male patients and some transgender male patients attempt to avoid reckoning with the pregnancy altogether by failing to notice it consciously. Concurrently, references to the pregnancy might occur in the form of derivatives, for example, the male adolescent might talk about his or her friends' sexual exploits. Once he is apprised of the pregnancy by the therapist, the male adolescent frequently experiences intense shame and embarrassment that he did not notice this change on his own. However, rather than these painful feelings leading to an exploration of the significance of the pregnancy, the patient is more likely to become defensive, often in an extreme way. He is prone to respond with a defensive style that emphasizes acting out, particularly in relation to aggressive behaviors. Within the sessions, he might be oppositional and querulous. If the therapist has the audacity to suggest that some of his reactions are due to the pregnancy or the upcoming separation, she is likely to be greeted with disdainful incredulity. As the adolescent advances in age, his defenses might take the form of an absorption in stereotypic male interests. Widseth (1989) described the behavior of a male college student whom she treated in a counseling center during her pregnancy

> a particularly complex and troubled senior with whom I was working twice a week to enhance a sense of continuity between the sessions, never allowed an opening for me to make any transference interpretation about his reaction to my pregnancy. He spent the last semester of our work together talking about mystery novels, computer hide-and-seek games, and the anthropology of early mankind.
>
> (p. 18)

Brouwers (1989) found a similar pattern of denial and avoidance in the male college students she treated.

Therapist Reactions in the Treatment of Adolescents

Many of the countertransference themes that were identified as emerging in the treatment of children in response to the therapist's pregnancy also arise with adolescents. Guilt in relation to a sense of having abandoned the adolescent patient and anxiety about the adequacy of one's future parenting as reflected by one's skill as a therapist are commonly present. Of course, the therapist is often more able to rely on the adolescent patient's capacity to verbalize. Therefore, the physical challenges of the pregnancy are less likely to require a modification of activities within the treatment, thereby enabling the therapist to avoid any countertransference reactions that might attend such modifications. On the other hand, when fears of the patient's aggression arise in the treatment, they are likely to be more intense for the pregnant therapist, given the adolescent's greater potential for physical destructiveness relative to that of the child (Vanier, 2001).

Some of the therapist reactions that arise tend to be connected to the different relational patterns exhibited by male and female clients. With girls, the often unremitting questioning about the pregnancy can evoke weariness, frustration and impatience. The questioning might also elicit pleasure if the therapist sees her patient as working to consolidate aspects of her own identity. If other patients are ignoring her pregnancy in obvious defensiveness, the adolescent girl's questioning might be refreshing. If prior to the pregnancy, the therapist had assumed a traditional psychoanalytic exploratory posture toward the patient's questions, then the therapist can easily feel guilt over the departure from a stance of neutrality. Her guilt is likely to be further intensified if she perceives it as a consequence of her own narcissistic preoccupation. The literature suggests that therapists have a great fear during pregnancy that they are excessively focused on themselves and would be prone to interpreting their behavior through this lens.

Therapist reactions to the patient also tend to center on the feelings the therapist has toward her body, especially in the third trimester. To the therapist bearing her own cumbersomeness, the more lithe adolescent bodies evoke envy and wistfulness about her more youth incarnations (Rosen, 1989). The multiparous therapist, for whom pregnancy might have lost some of its novelty and charm and whose body has been affected by past pregnancies, might experience this reaction with particular acuteness. Like both male and female adolescents, the pregnant therapist is undergoing physical changes that she cannot control. Vanier (2001) wrote about the horror a male adolescent experienced in the anticipation of the outcropping of pubic hair. The pregnant therapist, too, might have particular expectations about physical changes—especially those associated with labor such as the breaking of the amniotic sac—that could be especially disturbing. The therapist's communication of a concordant identification with the adolescent's lack of control might lead the sensitive adolescent to inhibit the discussion of such concerns.

To male adolescents, common countertransference reactions are responses to the avoidant behavior described earlier. For some therapists, a *quid pro quo* response occurs wherein the therapist mirrors the patient's disengagement from the relationship. The therapist might simply accept the patient's resistance, doing little to help the patient to recognize the issues evoked by the pregnancy. In some instances, the therapist's withdrawal might be a vehicle for expressing hostility. In other instances, it might be a genuinely protective response due to the therapist's perception of, and identification with, the patient's fragility. Therapists might collude with patients because of their wishes to avoid talking about some particular area related to the pregnancy, such as their own sexuality

(Pielack, 1989). In Chapter 7, we discuss how therapists with diverse sexual orientations might be hesitant to talk about the pregnancy because it could lead the client to learn about the therapist's minority status, a complication in treatment if the client or the client's parents is likely to have a strenuous response to the latter. In contrast to an avoidant stance, some therapists attempt to implode the patients' (at least seeming) indifference through vigorous confrontation and interpretation.

Once again, the correspondence between the patient's response and that of the larger treatment unit might lead the therapist to have stronger or weaker reactions to the patient. If the treatment context in which she works minimizes the pregnancy, as is often the case (Auchincloss, 1982; Schneider-Braus & Goodwin, 1985), the therapist is likely to have a more strenuous response to her male patient's similar response. If critical figures in her life also respond in the manner of the male patient (e.g., a husband who does not share her enthusiasm about the pregnancy), she is likely to find her patient's behavior more discomfiting.

In addition to these gender-specific responses, other therapist responses might occur in relation to either the adolescent's behavior or the material the adolescent presents, regardless of whether the patient is male or female. One type of response concerns the therapist's pattern of identifications. The primiparous therapist in particular might undergo a shift from a high level of identification with the adolescent's position vis-à-vis his or her parents to an overidentification with the parent's point of view. For example, the therapist might have a new understanding of restrictions the parent places on the adolescent and be less sensitive to the patient's feelings of being trapped, controlled or both. As Widseth (1989) argued, ultimately this greater understanding of the parental perspective helps the therapist to acquire "a more complex, objective stance" (p. 20). In the short run, however, it might lead to some confusion as the patient senses the alteration of the therapist's outlook. Consider this example given to us by a therapist:

Vignette 8.3
I saw this 13-year-old boy with multiple problems of aggressiveness with siblings and parents. He originally wanted to see a female therapist because he got along better with his mother than his father. Initially, he evoked a sad feeling in me when I reviewed his life and problems. Over the course of the pregnancy, I found myself wondering how I would deal with a child who was aggressive. I think he felt my empathy shift from him to his mother. At one point, the patient asked to discontinue treatment. In a family meeting, the mother verbalized it for all of us when she said, "He feels like you'll take my side."

In regard to both male and female adolescent patients, the therapist might experience some envy of the adolescents' relative freedom from responsibility, particularly the responsibilities that the therapist has assumed (Rosen, 1989). This feeling might lead to lapses in empathy. For example, the therapist might find the adolescent's complaints about the ups and downs of a romance to be vacuous or trivial. Intermixed with the envy is frequently a kind of nostalgia on the part of the therapist for her own youth, when she was able to think only of herself.

Treatment Strategies With the Adolescent Patient

The treatment recommendations described in the last section on child patients, concerning such topics as when to make the announcement and how to handle the separation, apply also to adolescent patients. In this section, the focus is on the two major subgroups of adolescents that were identified earlier: the *highly involved and under-involved adolescent*. Although young women and men are more likely to fall into the highly involved and under-involved groups, respectively, this gender assignment is by no means invariable.

Highly-Involved Adolescents

With the adolescent who is highly involved in the therapist's pregnancy, the therapist will struggle with a set of boundary issues. Probably, the biggest challenge is how to respond to the many questions that are asked. In making a decision, the therapist should take into account two pieces of information: (a) why the patient is asking the question and what meaning the answer would have to the patient; and (b) why the therapist is (or is not) giving an answer.

The common motives that adolescent patients have for asking a question fall into the following categories: information, identification, intimacy and inhibition of negative affect. Particularly young adolescents might see the therapist's pregnancy as an opportunity to gain enlightenment where confusion presently exists. If the therapist appears to be forthcoming in providing responses to some trial questions, the adolescent might eagerly seize the opportunity to have illuminated a hitherto mystery-shrouded area. In deciding whether to provide the sought-after information, the therapist must determine if this is the best venue for the adolescent's obtaining the information, how an educational focus will facilitate or hinder other therapeutic processes, and how this therapist activity could alter the adolescent's expectations about what provisions he or she is likely to receive from the therapist in the future. The therapist might then decide to provide the requested information or to help the adolescent to recognize specific domains of confusion about conception or the birth process and to identify possible resources for obtaining accurate information. It is important to have some understanding of how the parents of our child patients feel about the dissemination of this information. For example, one of the authors had a preadolescent girl who had many questions and misconceptions. However, the family was quite religious, and when the matter was discussed with the parents in a separate meeting, they expressed concern that any discussion about conception and childbirth would stimulate their daughter to act on her sexual impulses. They precipitously terminated the daughter's treatment.

In adolescent girls, especially, the wish to identify with the therapist accounts for many of the patient's questions about her pregnancy. The identification-seeking adolescent will ask questions with a less technical cast and be more focused on the therapist's subjective experience than the information-seeking adolescent. The therapist can assist the patient in consolidating a sense of identity by directly answering at least some of her questions (Fenster et al., 1986). By conveying a sense of pleasure in her pregnancy and happy expectancy, the therapist facilitates the adolescent girl in developing associations to her own feminine identity that are positive. In some cases, this experience might compensate for past negative associations the adolescent girl developed in relation to her mother's pregnancies. For example, a girl who observed her mother undergo a difficult, discomfort-fraught pregnancy, or one who had many aspects of her mother's pregnancy hidden from her, might think about motherhood in negative terms only. She might go on to either repudiate motherhood as an aspect of her identity or internalize it negatively. The therapist provides an antidote to these earlier experiences not necessarily by answering each question in a reflexive fashion but by having an attitude of inclusion (i.e., one in which the therapist's pregnancy is recognized as part of the adolescent girl's experience).

Sometimes, the adolescent's motive is to achieve a sense of closeness to or intimacy with the therapist. When this motive is exerting its influence, the content of the therapist's response is not so important as the fact that the therapist has elected to answer a personal question. The therapist's willingness to do so gives the patient a sense of union with the therapist. In other cases, the interest in the therapist's pregnancy that the questions imply could be a flight into activity to hide negative feelings that the pregnancy evokes. The patient's disregard for the specificity of the therapist's answers as well as the rapidity of the question-asking might betray this motive. In some cases, the therapist will feel under siege, suggesting that the questions provide an outlet for the patient's hostility.

As Fenster, Phillips and Rapoport (1986) have argued, it is in this instance that the therapist must be especially attentive to the dynamic underpinnings of the question-asking. It is critical that the therapist not convey that the patient's negative feelings about the therapist, the pregnancy, or the therapist's baby be sequestered from treatment. To facilitate the patient in recognizing negative feelings, the therapist should seek to identify the specific fears that lead the patient to avoid expressing hostility directly. Is the patient concerned that expressed hostility will damage the therapist or her baby? Will the hostility so offend the therapist that she will no longer be available to the patient, or will the therapist retaliate in some other way? Does the patient fear a precipitous loss in self-esteem? The identification of the fear (with or without reassurances that it is unwarranted) can go a long way to helping the patient operate less under its dominion.

Although question-asking will be the most common challenge faced by the therapist of the highly involved patient, other challenges will occur. For example, during the therapist's maternity leave, the patient might initiate frequent contacts with the therapist. After the therapist has returned, the adolescent might request that the baby be brought to a session or might offer to babysit for the therapist. The patient might merely request to see a picture of the baby. Certainly, any circumstance that invites the establishment of a dual role relationship (as in the circumstance of the patient qua babysitter) should be avoided. Other issues that are more equivocal should be dealt with through the same kind of process that was used in relation to the therapist's decision whether or not to answer questions. In general, however, the therapist should be clear with the adolescent patient about where the boundaries lie in terms of what will or will not take place within sessions.

The Under-Involved Adolescent

Again, the intervention problem the therapist faces could be conceptualized in terms of boundaries. Whereas the therapist of the highly involved patient must seek to ensure that appropriate boundaries exist, the therapist of the under-involved patient must consider whether boundaries are sufficiently permeable to permit an adequate flow of information between patient and therapist. That is, given that the patient has demonstrated a resoluteness not to grapple with pregnancy-related material, should the therapist interfere with the patient's defensive activity, and if so, how? When this defensive activity derives from a fear of merger between self and others, it is crucial that the patient be accorded the necessary psychological distance to feel safe (Alperin, 2001). The same carefulness should be accorded patients who might have endured trauma in relation to an earlier pregnancy (e.g., their mother's postpartum depression after the birth of a sibling). To the extent that the defensive activity represents a reasonably healthy adaptation to core developmental problems, the patient's defenses should be permitted to operate. For example, it is extremely common for boys in their early adolescence to distance themselves from their mothers, and especially from whatever elements she manifests that are perceived as part of her femininity (Blos, 1985). Any attempts to interpret the wish to achieve union with the pre-oedipal mother or the wish to be pregnant himself are likely to have a regression-promoting effect in cisgender males.

Yet, although the therapist might wish to support some repression, assisting the patient in coming to terms with certain reactions in relation to the pregnancy might serve the psychological growth of the highly defended adolescent patient. Within each adolescent patient's psychology, certain elements related to the pregnancy will be tolerated better than others. For example, a patient who responds to the pregnancy with exhibitions and bravado might tolerate considering how he feels some hostility toward the therapist's husband but not how the overt competitive might be a cover for developmentally early longings to merge with mother. For another patient, it might be possible to discuss his irritation at the disruption in the treatment (necessitated by the maternity leave) but not his primal sense of abandonment. By focusing on issues that are experience-near, the therapist can use the pregnancy to foster the under-involved patient's acceptance of his or her psychological life without stimulating the patient in a way that would be harmful. It would also spare the therapist from delivering an accurate but premature interpretation that would be helpful at a later point in treatment (Rosen, 1989).

With the under-involved patient, the therapist should exercise some care to remind the patient of any relevant realities concerning the pregnancy as it affects the treatment. For example, if the patient fails to mention the upcoming maternity leave, the therapist should warn the patient of its imminence. In this way, the therapist provides an invitation to the patient to offer any reactions to the pregnancy that the patient can identify and also avoids colluding with any denial on the part of the patient.

Treating the Elderly Patient

Behaviors and Themes

The topic of the pregnant therapist treating the elderly is virtually a neglected one, even though the elderly constitute a relatively large segment of the population. According to the U.S. Census Bureau (2015), almost 15% of the population is 65 or older. Although several brief vignettes with elderly patients appear in the literature (e.g., Cullen-Drill, 1994), rarely are the elderly person's reactions discussed through a developmental lens. We make a foray into this topic with the hope of stimulating further discussion of it.

The elderly person, as has been discussed in the literature, has the developmental task of finding meaning in life to achieve integrity (Erikson, 1950). Although many process are involved in the construction of meaning, among these is life review, that is, a revisiting of earlier periods in life. In fact, reminiscence has been used as a major therapeutic method in the treatment of elderly patients (e.g., Meléndez Moral, Fortuna Terrero, Sales Galán, & Mayordomo Rodríguez, 2015). Pregnant therapists provide a powerful stimulus for both reminiscence in the short run and the achievement of ego integrity in the long run because they invite identifications with child and parenting phases of development.

Among the therapists interviewed for this project, many spontaneously commented that elderly patients distinguished themselves by the intense joy they expressed upon learning of the therapist's pregnancy and throughout the process. It appeared that the joy was particularly heightened for those persons who were able to access their own past rapturous feelings of being an expectant parent. The demonstration of caring and concern, often in the form of advice, was also common. For these patients, being in a position to be nurturant was itself of benefit.

Yet, elderly patients are likely to show the range of conflicts found in the general adult population. Cullen-Drill (1994) presented three cases of elderly individuals. Two of these cases are women, both in their eighties, who were able to confront issues pertaining to their experiences of abandonment in connection with a sense of having been displaced by younger siblings. Their exploration of these issues enable the lessening of painful feelings and in one case, the institution of very concrete change in the woman's life. By addressing the connection between her self-esteem and her perception that she had been abandoned by her mother, she was able to pursue a goal that had been in abeyance for a long time: doing volunteer work at a local hospital.

In Cullen-Drill's (1994) third case, a 64-year-old male patient who had developed an erotic transference toward the therapist reported having sexual fantasies about her. The patient had had significant early abandonment experiences by an alcoholic father. The mother had a series of sexual partners in the home. The therapist began wearing maternity clothes before she announced her pregnancy. During this period, the patient referred to her as "Sister Mary"—a likely denial of his sexual feelings toward her as well as his Oedipal vanquishing by another man. Soon after, the patient expressed a desire to leave therapy. The patient, however, felt some guilt about leaving the therapist, thereby projecting his feelings of abandonment. In this case, we see the emergence of significant Oedipal conflict as well as the use of Oedipal issues to cover up early abandonment issues. Unlike the female patients, however, this male patient did not stay in treatment to work through the activated conflicts, but left precipitously.

In the preceding case, the patient's concern about the therapist was more defensive than genuine. With an elderly population, because concern is a particularly prominent aspect of patients' reactions, the therapist's sometimes difficult determination is to what extent the patient's concern, even if genuine, is used as a mask for another set of feelings. The patient's capacity to come forth and express a complex array of feelings, as well as the absence of acting-out behavior, will be useful in this regard. By placing the range of feelings within the domain of what can be discussed by patient and therapist about the pregnancy, the elderly patient might go a long way toward achieving the integration that is critical for this developmental phase.

Therapist Reactions

Work with elderly patients during pregnancy is evocative of a distinctive pattern of therapist reactions. The nurturing efforts on the part of some elderly patients might constitute a role reversal that challenges the therapist's authority and her sense of efficacy as a caretaker herself. Particularly for primiparous women, feelings of resentment might emerge if the therapist has been the recipient of much unwelcome advice from persons in other realms of her life. The therapist might look forward to her professional hours as a time when she can feel in control and masterful.

The therapist might have an alternate response of enjoying the caretaking her patients provide. The therapist is at especially great risk for this response if needs in this domain are not being met by crucial figures in the therapist's life, such as parents and spouses. Furthermore, earlier in this text, we described how therapists see themselves as having a heightened focus on self. Having the patient focus on the therapist might be narcissistically gratifying and could prevent the therapist from recognizing any possibility that the caretaking has a defensive element. Certain ageist attitudes on the part of the therapist could also play a role. If the therapist fails to recognize the capacities of many elderly patients to do meaningful exploratory work, she might neglect to engage the patients interested in understanding aspects of the patient's caretaking that could be driven by motives such as the wish to avoid feeling abandoned by the therapist.

The topic of the therapist's vulnerability has come up repeatedly in the chapters of this book. Therapists who wish to deny their own physical limitations during this period might use their elderly patient's infirmities as projective identificatory vehicles. The therapist might unconsciously encourage the patient's focus on physical symptoms by unwittingly becoming especially attentive to the patient when he or she describes somatic complaints. The therapist might also refrain from making interpretations about possible psychodynamic components of these complaints, for example, failing to consider the patient's possible underlying motive for cancelling a session due to arthritic problems. Finally, the therapist might miss opportunities to help the elderly patient recognize his or her resilience.

One of the developmental tasks that elderly persons need to perform is an acceptance of the reality of death. This is an inherently difficult task for therapists to facilitate, in that it is a fate from which the therapist can escape no less than the elderly patient. Introducing the topic of the beginning of life can invite the emergence into the treatment of an existential framework that in turn precipitates a discussion of life's ending. To the extent that the therapist has anxiety in relation to death and its discussion within treatment, she might forestall the announcement to the patient of the pregnancy and might subsequently endeavor to focus on it minimally.

Treatment Strategies With the Elderly Patient

Although the therapist is cautioned to maintain a spirit of inquiry about all behaviors the patient exhibits during the pregnancy period, the therapist is also well advised to recognize that the patient's provision of emotional supplies to the therapist might be of great benefit to the patient at this time. For elderly patients in particular, the need to feel able to make a contribution to others is felt intensely. How satisfying it might be to the patient to provide an emotional gift to a person who has provided the same for the patient! Also worthwhile are the reminiscence activities that are provoked by the patient's learning of the pregnancy. For patients within a different age group, such activities might be defensive in many instances; for the elderly patient, they more typically represent a consolidation of life experiences that is inherent to this age. The therapeutic prescription, therefore, is for the therapist to feel the freedom to enter into the patient's story by showing interest, making reflective comments about the patient's feelings, and encouraging the patient to elaborate on areas that might demand further scrutiny. For example, it could be useful for the patient to delve into a discussion of decisions and past behaviors that might be associated with regret. In the case of some elderly patients, this exploration might uncover sadness over never having had the opportunity to have a child and regret about any decisions that led to that circumstance. In the case of others, it might entail an acknowledgment of insufficiencies in the kinds of parents they were. To the extent that the patient can at long last make peace with what occurred in the past, he or she can make strides in achieving the sense of wholeness and integrity that Erikson and Erikson (1998) described as a crucial accomplishment of this developmental stage.

The pregnancy of the therapist is a developmental stimulus for an all-important issue for the elderly individual: legacy and generativity. The pregnancy of the therapist raises the question in the individual approaching the end of life: "What am I leaving behind?" For the individual who has been childless, the pain is not simply the deprivation that has been sustained over life. It is also the idea that there is no one to carry on the legacy (Rubinstein, 1996). Upon interviewing elderly women who had either been childless or had lost only children, Rubinstein (1996) found that women tend to deal with their circumstances in complex ways. For some, childlessness at the end of life leads to a feeling of "lineal emptiness" (Rubinstein, 1996, p. 59). For others, a focus on social legacy, that is, the contributions one has made through professional or charitable activities, prevails. Still other women saw their legacy as existing through their ties to persons in their families who were like their children, for example, their siblings' children. The therapeutic opportunity for the pregnant therapist is to help the elderly patient regardless of that patient's circumstances to recognize those elements from his or her past that might serve as the material for legacy creation. The patient might also be assisted in seeing how positive ways of relating to others with the present, ways others could internalize, could be part of that individual's legacy.

In six of seven countries studied, elderly individuals who were childless were more likely to be living by themselves (Koropeckyj-Cox & Call, 2007). Moreover, some evidence exists that elderly childless individuals have weaker social networks than parents (Albertini & Kohli, 2009). The therapist's departure for maternity leave could be felt very deeply. Prior to her departure, the therapist might usefully help the patient to bolster in social supports in her absence.

Recommendations

Our overarching recommendation is that therapists think always about the developmental tasks that the client faces and the ways in which the pregnancy of the therapist facilitates or impedes the completion of those tasks.

1. The therapist treating children and adolescents should recognize that because these populations are in a period of being actively parented, these clients can easily evoke a variety of reactions on the part of all expectant parents as they imagine what kinds of parents they will be.
2. Therapy might benefit from the therapist's having a more flexible-than-usual attitude toward the boundaries established in treatment with individuals at both ends of the developmental continuum.
3. With children, in particular, decisions about disclosure of the expectancy should be coordinated with the parents.
4. With adolescents, the therapist should anticipate the potential for acting out, be alert to its manifestation, and show sensitivity to the different meanings it could have in different individuals.

CHAPTER 9

Diagnostic Status of the Patient

In this chapter, the personality structure, personality style and psychopathology of the patient are considered as these factors bear on the patient's reactions to the therapist's pregnancy. Based on their interviews of 22 primiparous therapists, Fenster et al. (1986) noted, "Sixty-one percent of the pregnant therapists interviewed maintained that diagnosis was the single most important factor in determining a patient's response to therapy" (p. 29). We would add that personality features, which often provide the foundation from which particular psychological problems develop, also crucially shape the patient's perceptions, cognitions, emotions and behaviors.

For our purposes, it is useful to think about diagnosis in a bi-dimensional way. Based on a nosological scheme developed by McWilliams (2011) and reflected in the *Psychodynamic Diagnostic Manual, 2nd ed.* (Linguardi & McWilliams, 2017; also see Lingiardi, McWilliams, Bornstein, Gazzillo, & Gordon, 2015), we consider developmental level of personality organization and types of character organization as separate and interacting dimensions enabling a comprehensive diagnosis of an individual. The *developmental level* characterizes the person's degree of pathology, level of individuation, and the maturity level of the person's customary defenses. The three levels of development are: normal to neurotic, borderline and psychotic, and each is discussed in turn. The *type of character organization* refers to the individual's personality style, including such features as prominent drive and affect states, ways of experiencing the world, customary self states, and typical modes of interpersonal relating. For illustrative purposes, we focus on two contrasting organizations that the clinician is likely to encounter: histrionic (or hysterical) versus obsessive-compulsive. However, many other styles (for example, dependent personality, psychopathy, narcissistic personality) produce their own patterns of patient/therapist reactions and interactions. We selected these two mainly to draw the reader's attention to the importance of personality style.

Developmental Level of Personality Organization

Psychotic-Level Person

Individuals organized at the psychotic level come to treatment with great confusion about many types of boundaries (Davis & Mill, 1999). For example, they are frequently perplexed about what exists within versus outside of themselves. They show a tendency toward *psychic equivalence*, wherein a thought is viewed as having external reality (i.e., if I think of a monster, there must be a monster) (Bateman & Fonagy, 2004). They are easily inclined to ascribe their own feelings and urges to other people. To lessen confusion and to create an environment for psychological growth, the therapist typically is fastidious in creating a consistent therapeutic environment for the patient. By establishing boundaries within the treatment in relation to time, place and role, the therapist offers the experiential base for the patient's constructing the internal boundaries that contribute to the formation of a more stable sense of the self and the other person (McWilliams, 2011).

Themes and Behaviors

The pregnancy of the therapist tends to erode some major sources of stability and predictability in the relationship. The constancy of the therapist's attention to the psychotic patient could be undermined by her inward focus or her absorption with physical complaints. Relative to patients at more mature levels of ego organization, psychotically organized individuals tend to have a greater sensitivity to changes in others partially because they operate less under the sway of abiding concepts of the other person. They can be more in the moment than others. They therefore do not make allowances for the other person when they discern moment-to-moment fluctuations in the other's behavior and appearance. That is, they take these fluctuations more seriously than a person organized at a more mature level. The psychotically paranoid persons who are capable of developing very fixed notions about the other person can represent an exception to this trend. In the typical case, however, the therapist might need to make alterations in the time or place of the meeting to accommodate the pregnancy. For example, one therapist in her advanced state of pregnancy could no longer walk around the hospital grounds—a practice that diminished the patient's anxiety about meeting with her—but was forced to see the patient in the more confined setting of an office. The specter of the maternity leave is also disorganizing to these patients. For them, the therapist's reassurance that she will return after an interval of separation has little meaning or soothing effect. More catastrophic still is the circumstance where the therapist is planning to terminate treatment altogether because of the birth of the child.

All of these instabilities introduced into the treatment might evoke no less than terror in these persons. If the therapist's constancy provided the glue to help the psychotic individual achieve some sense of tenuous identity, then the loss of that constancy could precipitate a fragmentation of the different elements of the self, a fragmentation that is experienced as the annihilation of the self. Manifestations of fragmentation include the greater presence of first-rank symptoms such as hallucinations and delusions, greater withdrawal and increased self-stimulation behaviors such as rocking back and forth.

The incapacity of the psychotic person to establish boundaries between feelings and actions makes the exploration of the former at best a challenging activity for the patient and therapist. The psychotic patient potentially experiences all of the painful feelings described in Chapter 2 in relation to the therapist's pregnancy. However, in contrast to patients at other levels of ego organization, the psychotic person has a more unshakeable conviction that the mere expression of these feelings can destroy the therapist or her baby (Rubin, 1980). Whether or not the patient manages to express negative feelings directly, the self-referential aspect of the patient's thinking could lead the patient to assume responsibility for any untoward event that might occur during treatment, such as the therapist confinement to bed rest during the pregnancy or the miscarriage of the fetus.

The psychotic patient's difficulty in distinguishing fantasy from reality leads the patient to embrace, often tenaciously, various untenable beliefs concerning his or her personal connection to the pregnancy. The patient might believe that he (or she) impregnated the therapist or that she (or he) is pregnant along with the therapist. For some, a sense of loss occurs when the patient discovers that neither is the case. For others, the notion of being pregnant might elicit horror. For example, Martindale and Summers (2013) write about the case of one psychotic woman who experienced her pregnancy as invasion by an alien. Some patients might think the therapist plans to give the patient the baby after the delivery (Comeau, 1987) or, less dramatically, that the baby will be a regular visitor in the session. Because of the blurred boundary between masculine and feminine identities, as well as the weakness or absence of the repressive defense, the therapist might find little gender specificity in the feelings or fantasies expressed. For example, whereas it has been found that in general, males do not express directly the longing to bear a child, psychotic men will find both direct and indirect means to exhibit such a wish. In one of the most extensive and richly detailed case studies available on the pregnant therapist's treatment of psychotic persons, Lazar (1990) chronicled the vicissitudes of the transference of a schizophrenic inpatient male whom she had treated for 1 year. She described his reaction several weeks after he learned of her pregnancy, "Mr. A took to walking around with a pillow under his shirt and he asked the staff for a bowling ball and a shopping cart to wheel around the unit" (p. 207).

Although the therapist is likely to witness the eruption of much primitive material due to boundary failures, the therapist is also likely to observe the patient mount some defensive effort against psychotic anxiety and the sense of annihilation accompanying it (P. Kernberg, 1994; McWilliams, 2011). For example, Lazar's Mr. A (referred to in the previous quote) had an intense skirmish with a large male aide on the unit early in the therapist's pregnancy and prior to the time the pregnancy had been acknowledged by therapist and patient. In discussing the event in the next therapy session, Mr. A described how he felt comfortable unleashing his hostilities on the aide because of his massive size. In the associations that followed, it became clear that he had much anxiety about directing his aggressive feelings toward the small-sized (and hence, vulnerable) therapist. The patient might have been displacing hostility stimulated by his tacit perception of the therapist's pregnancy on an object perceived to be hardier. This patient also went into a posture of extreme withdrawal from the therapist at various points to prevent the emergence of dangerous feelings and impulses within the treatment.

From an existential perspective, the psychotic-level person might be defending against the acknowledgment of certain realities that the therapist's pregnancy illuminates. Comeau (1987) wrote about how a 30-year-old schizoaffective male patient requested to leave a psychotherapy group in which he was participating during the therapist's pregnancy. He reported that he was experiencing auditory hallucinations telling him he was impotent. As he described his reactions to the pregnancy further, it became clear that one of the issues with which he was struggling was his realization that he would never have a family due to the severity of his illness and he was grieving this likelihood. Events in the lives of therapists that place them within the social mainstream might acquaint or remind chronic patients of what might never be for them. In addition to sadness, envy might also be evoked by the contrast between the therapist's relative normality and the chronic patient's symptom-fraught life.

Characteristic Therapist Reactions

The evident need and fragility of the psychotic-level individual evokes a parental response from the therapist (McWilliams, 2011). For the pregnant therapist, an admixture of positive and negative feelings accompanies this role. Often, the psychotic patient is able to give an expression of gratitude toward the therapist for enabling the patient to experience some sense of connection to the interpersonal world. The pregnant therapist is thereby likely to enjoy the positive feelings associated with the confirmation of her nurturing abilities, a confirmation that might be an antidote to anxieties that the therapist has about her eventual maternal role.

At the same time, the therapist can easily experience guilt in relation to the significance of the pregnancy for the patient's life and well-being (McGourty, 2013). The therapist might fear that any disattunement or absorption with herself during the pregnancy might be shattering to the psychotic-level patient. Will the patient, she might worry, sustain the trust developed earlier in the relationship sufficiently to endure the maternity leave? Is she, she wonders, subjecting the patient to the kinds of abandonment experiences that might have traumatized the patient early in life? These feelings are not unlike those that the child psychotherapist is likely to experience in relation to her patients' reactions to the pregnancy. Also, like the child psychotherapist, the therapist of the psychotic-level person is at risk for feeling overwhelmed by the enormity of her responsibilities to the patient, especially given that she is now assuming new responsibilities. She might even wonder whether it is possible to manage competently the demands of an infant and one or more severely regressed patients. Accompanying this questioning could well be a sense of aloneness, given that the therapist is typically alone in her position in any given setting.

Strategies for Intervention

From any theoretical standpoint, a goal of the therapist for the psychotic-level patient is to sustain the positive connection between patient and therapist during the pregnancy and postpregnancy periods and, possibly, strengthen it. In object relations terminology, the intrapsychic goal would be the maintenance of whatever network of positive representations had been constructed by virtue of the therapeutic work. The object relationist perspective would further hold that the therapist's pregnancy constitutes a threat in that it impinges upon the representational network with negative affects stimulated by the pregnancy. Stated more concretely, the therapist should be aware of the risk that the patient would have such anger, despondency, envy and so on in relation to the therapist so as to be unable to experience the therapist as a helpful figure and no longer able to see the therapy as a useful enterprise.

The therapist can augment the patient's positive representations while limiting the negative ones in many ways. Most importantly, the therapist should convey to the patient that negative feelings of all varieties in relation to the pregnancy are natural, and such feelings can be expressed safely in the treatment. To this end, the therapist might usefully employing a *clarifying interpretation* (Kibel, 1981), which involves acknowledging the validity of negative reactions. For example, the therapist might say,

> You became furious on the unit Saturday night because it has been so upsetting for you to learn that I am going to be having a baby. It is very understandable that you should have anger and confusion in relation to this development. It is important for us to discuss these feelings as we go on.

By taking initiative in pointing out the connection between the patient's experience and behavior, and the pregnancy, the therapist is normalizing the patient's experience and thereby reducing the toxicity of the feelings the patient is experiencing. The technique suggested here is akin to Horner's (1990) notion of *interpreting upward*, which involves a matter-of-fact labeling of primitive content and a statement of its connections to the patient's life experiences. Through such means, the therapist is reducing the overwhelming quality of these negative feelings by giving them a specific focus.

Whereas the preceding example shows one way in which the psychodynamically oriented therapist could intervene, most theoretical approaches have some technique for helping clients to cope with negative feelings. For example, within Acceptance and Commitment Therapy (Hayes, 2004), the effort would be to discourage the psychotic client's experiential avoidance but also to support the defusing of these emotional and cognitive reactions so that they are not experienced as part of the self (Bach & Hayes, 2002). Were, say, the client to have certain thoughts about the therapist's pregnancy that would strike most people as odd, the goal would not be to interpret them but to help the client to recognize that they are a few ideas among many ideas the client has about the therapist. Such a line of intervention would limit the potential of the ideas to be destabilizing and help the client maintain continuity of the self amidst the flux in treatment relationship.

McGourty (2013) points out that with a psychotic patient, risk management must be a focus, with the potential risks being to the patient, the therapist or others outside of the therapeutic dyad. As part of the risk management process, the therapist, she holds, should revisit the original therapeutic objectives and make any needed modifications that take the heightened risk of acting out into account. McGourty notes, for example, that the period in which the patient is reacting to the therapist's pregnancy might not be a time to do trauma work. Not only might the processing of traumatic experiences overwhelm the patient, but also the time before the therapist's leave might be insufficient to process them adequately.

As with all patients, the therapist must engage in decision making in relation to the announcement of the pregnancy, the degree of self-disclosure about the pregnancy, and the plan for the maternity leave.

Announcing the Pregnancy

The observation has been made in the literature that psychotic patients tend to sense changes in the therapist earlier than do other patients, especially relative to those organized at the neurotic level. Often because of the reality-testing deficits in this group of patients, they might have more difficulty than other groups making sense of their impressions that something is different about the therapist. What is ambiguous in the outside world, especially in relation to critical figures, is extremely anxiety-arousing. Therefore, it would behoove the therapist to be alert to early indications that the patient has some awareness of her altered behavior, appearance or status.

Once the therapist has sensed an at least preconscious awareness, several options present themselves. The therapist could neglect to acknowledge the pregnancy-related material. However, because thoughts about the pregnancy are likely to be evocative of great anxiety on the part of the psychotic patient, such unresponsiveness from the therapist serves only to prolong this state. The therapist might also disclose her pregnant state, which might provide a means for the patient to bind and channel any anxiety. It would also offer the patient a lengthy period in which to prepare for the eventual separation, temporary or permanent. However, two problems are attached to the direct acknowledgment of the pregnancy. First, if the therapist sees the pregnancy as a tenuous state, a fairly usual perspective prior to favorable findings from an amniocentesis or at least the passage of the first trimester, this sense could unwittingly be conveyed to the psychotic patient. Such a communication could readily destabilize the patient's tenuous sense of self. Still another alternative is to address pregnancy-related content without directly acknowledging the pregnancy. Balsam (1974) related the case of an 18-year-old schizophrenic male who excitedly talked about collecting milk bottles outside his front door. He then abruptly decried pregnant women for being "disgusting." The therapist, only 2 months pregnant, briefly considered revealing her pregnancy to the patient. Instead, however, she focused on helping the patient explore the connection between his seemingly disconnected thoughts about pregnancy and milk bottles. Ultimately, the patient was able to recollect that he had seen a woman in maternity attire retrieving her milk bottles as he was fetching his and had constructed a fantasy that he had impregnated her. Merely understanding the link in his thoughts allowed the patient to feel less agitated. Later, the impregnation fantasy did come up in regard to the therapist in her more advanced pregnancy when she had the physical manifestations of the pregnancy. She felt that the time of the discussion was more favorable than in her first trimester in that the patient's reactions were connected to a very apparent (to all) reality.

In a recent paper, McGourty (2013) describes the cases of five psychotic patients who were informed of their therapist's pregnancy. She notes that in all of the cases, a heightened level of risk was involved to the client or to others. In order to manage the risk level, she advises that adaptations need to be made in the treatment. For example, while the patient is grappling with the therapist's pregnancy and is anticipating the therapist's departure, she should consider exploring elements of the patient's traumatic past. She also makes the point that if the therapist is working within a cognitive-behavioral framework, it might be necessary for the therapist to integrate that model with elements of a psychodynamic approach in order to create the means for the client to work with the issues the pregnancy poses, such as rejection and abandonment.

THERAPIST SELF-DISCLOSURE

Many times in this text, we have pointed out that therapist pregnancy easily leads to a relaxation of the boundaries between patient and therapist. Frequently, patients feel a freedom to ask the therapist questions about herself that they would not have asked otherwise. Part of this confidence is due to the fact that the pregnancy leads the patient to realize that the therapist has a private life about which the patient knows little. Like other patients, the psychotic-level patient might be intrigued by this glimpse into the therapist's life and have his or her appetite stimulated for more information. Unlike many other patients, the psychotic-level person is unlikely to recognize the extent to which the material sought from the therapist is personal. Hence, the therapist should not be surprised, as one of the authors (VB) was, when a group therapy psychotic-level patient asked her, during her pregnancy, to discuss her plans about having a natural childbirth and breastfeeding. That pregnancy has a disinhibiting effect on some patients is seen in the fact that this patient had never expressed any curiosity about anyone in the group previously.

In responding to a psychotic patient's questions, the therapist should think developmentally. Largely, the patient is working to accurately assess and connect with the therapist as a real individual, a striving that creates a motive to learn about the therapist in a very concrete way. In the therapist's response, the legitimacy of the patient's need should be affirmed. Psychotic patients at times will make observations about the therapist's appearance and infer some aspect of the therapist's psychological state. The patient might say, for instance, "You looked really dragged out lately." Although the therapist might be hesitant to admit to negative feelings, it might be useful to consider that when such reactions are disavowed, the psychotic patient, still intuiting their presence, will see them as too terrible for the therapist to acknowledge. On the other hand, were the therapist to say, "You're right: I've been feeling quite tired this week," she would be showing that her discomfort is not so intolerable as to necessitate its banishment from their discussion (or perhaps her awareness). Moreover, her confirmation of the accuracy of the patient's perceptions makes more tolerable to the patient those occasions in which lapses in reality-testing are identified.

Answering Questions

The therapist might decide not to answer the patient's questions because she wishes certain information to remain private. The therapist's preferences about what information she wants to share has a legitimate place in the therapist's decision making. In the prior example, the author felt that her decision of whether or not to breastfeed was a very personal one, which she did not wish to share with the group. Nonetheless, she would be able to explore the multilayered meanings of the question itself. The decision not to disclose could also be made because the therapist feels certain information would be too stimulating or threatening to the patient. In such a case, a very direct acknowledgment of what types of information the therapist is or is not willing to share is likely to be less disturbing to the patient than subtle evasiveness. Specifying the boundary between the public and the private serves as an antidote to the fused notions about relationships held by psychotic persons (McWilliams, 2011).

Planning the Maternity Leave

The third problem is particularly knotty, given that the patient's achievement of the ability to experience individuals as existing despite their physical absence still lies in the future. Yet, several strategies might assist the patient in having a sufficient connection to the therapist through the maternity leave to maintain a relative sense of well-being and to be willing to resume work with the therapist on her return. The therapist might broaden the patient's network of positive images of self and others by fostering a positive institutional transference, a term coined by Reider (1953), encouraging the patient's use of other supportive relationships in his or her life, having an alternate therapist assigning homework during the maternity leave or any combination of these. Each of these is discussed in turn.

An *institutional transference* (Bolognini, 2006; Wellendorf, 1986) is the patient's formation of a bond with an organization, presumably that which provides the context of treatment. It often occurs quite spontaneously with chronic patients who are treated in the same facility year after year and might have regularly changing therapists with very different theoretical orientations. Sometimes it occurs defensively: the person attaches to the institution because attachments to actual people make him or her feel too vulnerable. By tapping into this institutional bond, the therapist can enable the stabilization of the patient during the maternity leave. The author (VB), who worked in an inpatient facility, had a chronic, isolated patient who regularly came to walk on the extensive grounds of the hospital when the therapist was on vacation. As her pregnancy leave approached, the therapist reminded the patient of the soothing effects of these walks. The therapist also supported the patient in committing to do volunteer work at the hospital, an involvement he continued after the maternity leave was over.

Frequently, chronic patients have other practitioners involved in their care (Bridges & Smith, 1988). Advising the other members of the treatment team of the imminence of the maternity leave, the patient's likely reactions to it and the patient's ability to profit from additional support is likely to help the patient through this period.

The use of an alternate therapist might be especially important when the maternity leave is long or the patient has a proneness to regression accompanied by acting out. McCarty, Schneider-Braus and Goodwin (1986) described a format they developed wherein pregnant therapists participated in group supervision and provided therapy for one another's patients during each therapist's maternity leave. The therapist's regular participation in the group supervision enabled the alternate therapist to be highly familiar with the dynamics of the case. Within McCarty et al.'s approach, conjoint sessions with the primary and alternate therapists were used at times, but were not a constant feature. However, in neither of the cases they document was the patient psychotic. With psychotic patients in particular, it is very important that such conjoint sessions occur. The psychotic patient is unlikely to associate on his or her own the alternate therapist with the primary therapist. Through conjoint sessions, the patient acquires the experiential base to forge such connections. His or her image of the nurturing therapist is thereby expanded to include the features of the alternate therapist.

Besides using figures other than the therapist during the maternity leave, the therapist can use herself as a resource by having some form of contact with the patient. Such availability is most likely to benefit those psychotic patients who have made some progress on the road to object constancy. Communications in the form of phone calls, email, or written notes help the patient to cull up the image of the therapist during the therapist's absence. However, a disadvantage of this strategy is that in the case of phone calls, the therapist, deprived of visual cues, might be more prone to make a misjudgment about the patient's condition or reaction. With any written communication, the therapist has no opportunity to witness the patient's response. The risks of the reduction in information are lessened when another professional is following the patient closely. In addition, crises might still arise and the new mother might not wish or be in position to manage them.

A final strategy is particularly useful with patients who are in the structured therapies so commonly implemented with psychotic-level patients such as social-skills training, a popular, evidence-based approach with this population (Granholm, McQuaid, & Holden, 2016). A regular component of these therapies is the assignment of homework between sessions. Whereas the usual function of homework is to increase the probability of the transfer of learning, the therapist can use it to help the psychotic patient to bridge the gap by providing a transitional object (Winnicott, 1965) during the therapist's maternity leave. The therapist can create assignments for the patient during the entire period of the leave. The homework book enables the patient to maintain a connection to the therapist even though that patient lacks the ability to cull up the image of the therapist during her absence. The homework book can come to represent the hope that the therapist will return in the same way that the infant uses a blanket to maintain a link to her mother and to soothe her during the mother's absence (see LaMothe, 2001, for an excellent discussion of Winnicott's conception of transitional objects). The patient can maintain a journal reporting on his or her progress on the homework. The patient who reads, executes and reports on assignments is reminded of the therapist's existence. Combining it with the previously discussed strategies can augment this strategy. For example, an alternate therapist could review and check on the patient's homework. The patient could also send a record of the homework to the therapist.

Borderline-Level Patients

The borderline-level of ego organization represents an advance over the psychotic level in that individuals in the former category have a greater capacity to recognize boundaries between systems (McWilliams, 2013). They can, for example, demonstrate some minimal cognizance of a boundary between self and others, words and actions, fantasy and reality and so on. Relative to persons organized at the neurotic level, they have a greater reliance on primitive defenses such as splitting, projection and projective identification. Yet, in contrast with psychotic persons, they are more effective in using these defenses to separate reliably good and bad self-object representations and to associate positive representations with one another. For example, in experiencing another person, they can realize that all of those positive qualities they perceive about that person are associated with one another rather than existing as discrete elements. The more stable representational structure that they enjoy relative to psychotic individuals provides for greater stability in their sense of self relative to their more regressed counterparts: whereas the psychotic person doubts whether he or she (or the therapist) exists, the borderline-level patient does not, for the most part. Nonetheless, associated with their use of primitive defenses is an inherent fragility. Any significant stressor, especially in the interpersonal realm, leads to the dissolution of the structure on which the borderline person's sense of well-being depends. Hence, the pregnancy of the therapist is generally a tumultuous period for the borderline patient in ways that are discussed in this section.

Themes and Behaviors

Some research suggests that borderline-level patients recognize the therapist's pregnancy earlier than do either psychotic or neurotic patients (Fenster, 1983). Fenster et al. (1986) explain this phenomenon as due to the extreme sensitivity of the borderline-level person to changes in the therapist, changes that occur during the first trimester of the therapist's pregnancy. The ability exhibited by higher-functioning individuals to screen out momentary fluctuations, to make allowances for little inconsistencies in the other person, is unavailable to borderline patients due to the absence of object constancy. However, this explanation applies even more so to psychotic persons. Although some tendency exists for psychotic patients to notice the pregnancy early, this trend does not appear to be as consistent as it is for borderline patients. Perhaps the psychotic person's access to primitive forms of denial permits him or her to ignore a reality with such potentially disturbing implications.

Once the therapist acknowledges the pregnancy, or in some cases even before, acting out frequently ensues. Bridges and Smith (1988) point out that even relative to other loss events, the therapist's pregnancy appears a particularly potent stimulus to acting out. Two studies suggest that relative to patients at other levels of ego organization, borderline patients are more likely to engage in destructive behaviors of various sorts. In Berman's (1975) study of acting out reported in Chapter 3, she found that whereas only one-third of her sample was at the borderline level, among these patients were two-thirds of the individuals who acted out during their therapists' pregnancies. They engaged in such behaviors as suicide attempts, unplanned pregnancies and violent acts. Fenster (1983) found that borderline individuals were more likely to terminate treatment abruptly during the therapist's pregnancy.

Why are borderline patients so much more likely to act out than patients organized at other levels? That they do so more than neurotics is not surprising given that neurotics access mature defenses for regulating their psychological lives. The psychotic patient, on the other hand, also lacks mature defenses while being beset by many of the intense affects and primitive impulses as the borderline patient. Yet, the borderline-level patient does not struggle with the psychotic patient's terror of having his or her existence placed in question. It is a terror that is always present for the psychotic patient but that is either awakened or intensified by the therapist's pregnancy. This terror frequently dominates the psychotic person's experience, making other reactions such as anger or envy less prominent. It induces a paralysis that is often at odds with acting-out behavior. Borderline-level patients' acting out is at least in part a consequence of their extensive and organized use of projective identification. Because this defense involves coercion of the other to experience the unwanted element, some response on the part of the therapist is necessary. Through projective identification, the borderline-level patient compels the therapist to hold that part of himself that feels abandoned (due to the pregnancy) by cancelling sessions. Moreover, the acting out is also likely to evoke worry in the therapist so that even in between sessions, the therapist is forced to experience agitated concern about the patient.

For most patients, the multiple losses that accompany the therapist's pregnancy stimulate the patient's separation anxiety. For the borderline-level patient, this issue is core. The borderline person is unable to have an experience of an object that is at once separate and available. Moreover, the sexual aspect that underpins the pregnancy might, via the patient's identification with the therapist, activate early trauma associated with sexual abuse, common in this population (Bateman & Fonagy, 2004). Intrapsychically, negative self and other representations overwhelm the individual, thereby causing him or her in one fell swoop to lose access to the good representations. The high level of activation associated with these conjoint losses overwhelms the individual's capacities to mentalize internal events (Bateman & Fonagy, 2004). It is thereby unsurprising that many borderline-level patients launch a major defensive effort. A regression back to a state of fantasized merger with idealized caregivers is common and leads to a variety of acting-out behaviors. The unplanned sex and pregnancies, and the flight into romantic relationships, frequently have as an underpinning the effort to realize the longing for symbiotic union with the therapist through another relationship.

The defensive effort to create the experience of merger with the therapist is at odds with reality and therefore founders. The patient's failure to achieve a sense of symbiosis amidst the many elements of separation associated with the therapist's pregnancy leads to intense negative feelings, most especially sadness. Yet, insofar as the sadness frequently evokes from others the nurturance that the patient is seeking, it partially provides the sought-after gratification. Envy will often accompany the sadness as the patient sees the therapist as filled up with something good. It often reveals itself in attacks on the therapist especially in the form of raising questions about the therapist's goodness. When envy does arise, as it often will, rarely will the patient have direct awareness of it, and therapist comments referencing envy will tend to be spurned (Spillius, 1993). Oedipal issues might also be present. For example, the patient might exhibit a heightened interest in the therapist's partner not only in the session but also outside, attempting to get information about this individual on the internet. In general, these manifestations will mask developmentally earlier issues that are likely to surface when Oedipal pursuits fail to produce the developmentally earlier gratifications the patient seeks.

Characteristic Therapist Reactions

Borderline-level patients are well known for their capacities to evoke intense therapist reactions, and these capacities are on full display during the therapist's pregnancy. Therapists and patients are likely to engage in enactments in which the patient acts in some manner to induce the therapist to assume a particular role, and at times, the therapist does the same (Frosch, 2002). When enactments occur, both parties are likely to have a sense of having reached an impasse, primarily because that which is blocking mutual understanding is the target of dissociation (Ginot, 2009). The unpacking of enactments holds tremendous potential for catapulting the treatment via a dramatic increase in empathy of therapist for patient, and patient for therapist (Ginot, 2009). The therapist is aided in the unpacking process by recognizing the kinds of enactments that pregnancy invites in the therapist–borderline patient dyad. The therapist benefits from recognizing that a primary dimension of the borderline individual's transference is extreme anger in relation to the therapist's failure to be the perfect caregiver that the patient was seeking. The primitive nature of the borderline-level patient's anger is highly evocative of fear in the therapist, whose sense of vulnerability is probably increased by the pregnancy. The therapist therefore might be particularly prone to walk on eggshells with such a patient—assuming the role of the anxious caregiver—and provide excessive gratifications in order to discourage the patient from unleashing his or her full fury upon the therapist. An example of excessive caution would be a failure to confront the patient on his or her contributions to enactments within the therapeutic relationship as well as on the acting out that is so likely to appear during the pregnancy. Excessive gratifications can take myriad forms, such as failing to end sessions on time, disclosing information about the pregnancy with no therapeutic intent, or allowing the patient to make excessive and necessary intrusions into the therapist's life outside of the sessions (phone calls, etc.). Some therapists, rather than containing their patients' disturbances, might regard the patient as lacking the resources to receive exploratory interventions and recommend psychotropic medication instead (Rothstein, 1999), thereby assuming the role of the detached caregiver.

Empathy for the borderline patient can be difficult to achieve because of that individual's rapidly fluctuating affect states and the extremeness of the negative feelings expressed (McWilliams, 2011). Unwittingly, the therapist might feel relieved when the patient is in a non-attacking, depressed, regressed state, and might respond with the most consistent empathy at these times. An especially disquieting dimension of countertransference is guilt when borderline-level patients do act out, given that the changed status of the therapist so clearly precipitates it. One therapist we interviewed reported that it was a great relief to her to be able to talk about the fact that during her pregnancy, two of her borderline-level adolescents also became pregnant. She said she had a painful sense of responsibility for these untoward occurrences but felt too guilty to discuss her reactions with colleagues. Guilt is also evoked by the attacks the patient makes on the therapist's commitment and integrity, attacks often prompted by the patient's envy, and intensified by a workplace that also sees the therapist's pregnancy as guilt-worthy (see Chapter 11). It can be useful for therapists struggling with guilt to know that both acting out and attacks within the sessions are common with this patient population.

Therapeutic Strategies

A therapeutic objective during this period is to increase the borderline patient's tolerance for separation by supporting his or her endurance of the many elements of separation that the pregnancy brings. Intrapsychically, this means that the individual is able to have an early experience of ambivalence involving the concurrent activation of positive and negative images of the therapist. It is achieved through the patient's recognition of the therapist's unbroken empathy with the patient through all of his or her pregnancy-intensified rageful states. Empathy enables the patient to maintain a positive tie in the midst of the negative feelings and creates a holding environment (Winnicott, 1945) in which such feelings can be safely expressed. The therapist is helped in achieving empathy by a clear developmental perspective from which negative feelings are recognized as necessarily emerging if the patient is to progress.

Despite any countertransference pressures to do otherwise, it is critical that appropriate limits be set at this time. Therapists who fail to maintain the structure of the treatment risk confirming patients' negative beliefs that the treatment cannot "hold" the patient. The patient gets validation for his or her belief that elements of that patient's inner life are toxic and therefore unable to be verbalized within the contained environment of the treatment. Such an unwitting confirmation promotes regression rather than progression to integration. Moreover, through the setting of limits (for example, limiting when the patient can call the therapist), the therapist provides her own need states their due, which ultimately safeguards her positive tie to the patient and offers a model of self-respect and containment for the patient to internalize. Furthermore, it challenges the denial of the therapist as a separate individual, a denial so common in patients with borderline pathology (Domash, 1984).

The problem, however, is how the therapist can safeguard the treatment environment and curb acting out. Baum and Herring (1975) found that the more therapists were aware of their countertransference, and the more active they were in encouraging patients to explore their reactions to the pregnancy, the less acting out occurred. Additionally, as Bridges and Smith (1988) suggested,

> On occasion, when a therapist knows a patient well, it is useful to comment in advance—by offering the patient a prediction of what forms the acted-out transference might assume and encouraging the patient to self-observe behavior changes.
>
> (p. 107)

These authors describe a case in which a pregnant therapist, on announcing her pregnancy, forecasted to a young borderline woman that she might feel a temptation to have unprotected sex in relation to the announcement. In this way, the therapist formed an alliance with the patient to protect the treatment and the patient during the pregnancy.

For some patients, it might be productive to collaborate with them in identifying links that the patient has made—perhaps initially unconsciously—between the therapist's pregnancy and past traumatic experiences. For example, a patient might recognize that her depression in reaction to the therapist's pregnancy might be rooted in her association to her mother's extended illness and hospitalization during her toddlerhood. Bridges and Smith (1988) noted that it is also useful to help the patient to differentiate between past trauma and the realities of the pregnancy. For example, the patient might assume that the birth of the child will make the therapist uninterested in the patient. Helping the patient to test this belief using the backlog of experiences with the therapist might be quite reassuring.

Finally, many borderline-level patients are likely to require a substitute therapist during the therapist's leave. Some of these patients will want to continue on with their new therapist, even after their original therapist returns. Those connections that are most alive for these patients exist within the here-and-now, even if other relationships might have greater longevity.

Neurotic-Level Patients

Neurotic patients distinguish themselves from psychotic and borderline patients on the basis, first, of their lesser degree of reliance on primitive defenses such as splitting and projection and their greater reliance on more mature repressive defenses that entail less submergence of the elements of their internal lives (McWilliams, 2011). Second, they have a capacity to regulate their affects, and third, they manifest an ability to reflect upon their experiences productively (Sugarman, 2007). As McWilliams (2011) wrote, "the neurotic-level client maintains some more rational, objective capacities in the middle of whatever emotional storms and associated distortions occur" (p. 57). Fourth, they enjoy a more continuous sense of identity, based in part on the prior abilities and the capacity to rest their self-esteem on their allegiance to values and moral codes rather than oscillating feedback from the external world. Fifth, generally, they can see the world the way others do.

Themes and Behaviors

All of these features described previously bear upon the neurotic patient's responses to the therapist's pregnancy. Relative to the other groups of patients, the neurotic patient shows a more mature stance in relation to this discovery, a stance that has features of complexity, moderation and realism. The maturity of the responses will be seen in the patient's expression of positive emotional states such as joyfulness and admiration alongside negatives states such as anger or envy. Frequently, patients will report an active sense of ambivalence about the pregnancy ("I feel happy for you but also envy you terrifically"). This ability to countenance internal conflict is a hallmark of neurosis. Reactions will also be more moderate. Neurotic patients are less likely to feel the kinds of intense feelings that press for immediate discharge, feelings that for lower functioning patients are driven by catastrophic fears such as "Now that you are pregnant, you are lost to me forever; only your child matters!" The responses to the pregnancy are more realistic: they do not exhibit the irrational and unshakeable convictions that are often seen in the psychotic patient and more occasionally, the borderline-level patient. Finally, they are likely to have many responses that have little to do with conflict. The joy, envy, admiration and other emotions might simply be authentic reactions from the individual's conflict-free spheres.

Yet, as has amply been illustrated in the literature, individuals organized at the neurotic level do have central conflicts activated by the therapists' pregnancies that are related to the difficulties they encounter in everyday life. The themes that emerge for neurotically organized patients are quite variable and encompass all of the transference themes outlined in Chapter 3. The reason for this variability is that the presence of a neurotic organization in no way precludes the importance of pre-oedipal issues for an individual. For some neurotic persons, the pregnancy might stimulate primarily pre-oedipal issues. However, the neurotic person will be able to address them with reflective resources lacked by persons at psychotic or borderline levels of ego organization. For other patients, the conflicts stimulated will be entirely Oedipal. For example, a given patient might feel the pregnancy as a defeat at the hands of an Oedipal rival. Still others will show a progression of themes from the pre-oedipal to the Oedipal over the course of the pregnancy and postpregnancy periods or even across multiple pregnancies that the therapist might have.

Characteristic Therapist Reactions

Relatively to individuals residing at a lower point of the developmental continuum, the therapist's responses to neurotic patients are on the whole more moderate. The therapist's unique reactions to this type of patient are likely to derive from the realistic aspect of the patient's emotional responses and observations of the therapist. The therapist might recognize that the patient is on target in noting that the therapist is tired, preoccupied, physically uncomfortable and so on. The greater realism of the neurotic's responses might dispose the therapist to feel more fully exposed than with other patients at other levels.

One defense that is available to the therapist is to exaggerate the contribution of unconscious factors to the generation of the patient's response while minimizing the stimulating the patient is receiving from the therapist. Bolstering this potential defense might be the therapist's recognition of components of the patient's response that are genuinely conflict-based. For example, a woman brought a blanket to the therapist as a baby present. The therapist immediately had an awareness of certain symbolic elements of the gift that tied to the patient's area of dynamic concern. The therapist vigorously drew the patient's attention to these elements, failing to acknowledge the positive affect associated with the fact of the gift. This therapist response is fairly atypical, however. Our research suggests that generally therapists will focus on the positive feelings and neglect other elements. That is, commonly the therapist assumes that all reactions to the pregnancy are within the realm of the real relationship. This bias occurs for at least two reasons. First, any distortion tends to be subtler and less exaggerated than in the case of patients at a lower level of organization. Therefore, it could be more difficult to see and present to the patient as worthy of exploration. Second, the therapist might have greater trepidation about inflicting a narcissistic hurt on the patient by calling attention to a defended-against response that is at odds with the pronatalist bias of the culture, a bias to which the neurotic patient might have greater sensitivity than individuals at level rungs of the ego-functioning spectrum.

Another pitfall is excessive self-disclosure about the pregnancy to the neurotic patient due to enjoyment over sharing this special experience with someone who is able to understand and even identify with the experience. That therapists derive satisfaction in talking about their pregnancies was seen in the pleasure many of the authors' interviewees expressed in participating in the interviews. Particularly when therapists have seen certain patients over a long period of time, the opportunity to enter this personal domain with high-functioning patients is tempting. Regardless of the motive, in so doing excessively, the therapist undermines the patient's capacity to elaborate his or her fantasies about the pregnancy.

Although a high level of self-disclosure might be due to countertransference, some emotional reactions to the normality of the neurotic patient's response to the pregnancy might not be. For example, one of our interviewees provided the following contrast between her two psychotherapy groups:

> In inpatient eating disorder groups, I began to be self-conscious about size and watchful for people's reactions to me physically. In my high functioning group, I was different because people were more attentive to me and how I felt and I appreciated this fact.

Particularly when therapists work with more disordered patients, an understandable relief, if not gratitude, is felt upon encountering more mainstream responses.

Strategies for Intervention

With neurotic patients, the therapist's pregnancy is an opportunity because it creates the possibility for new levels of conflict resolution in relation to Oedipal and even pre-oedipal struggles. A primary tool that the psychodynamic therapist can use is interpretation, helping the patient to recognize one or more elements of a conflict. The use of interpretation is highlighted in the following vignette.

Vignette 9.1
Maxine, a single woman in her mid-twenties and a grade-school teacher, initially expressed a sense of joy and excitement over her therapist's pregnancy. However, curiously, the patient quickly dropped the subject and made no further reference to it for several weeks. Maxine then began canceling sessions and coming late. Both behaviors were unusual for this patient. Maxine began to worry rather excessively about minor jocular comments having "hurt the feelings" of several of her students, even in the absence of any evidence that they were more than mildly affected. Occasionally, her concerns about her own verbal ineptitude led her to call in sick. She feared saying something that would be so provocative that it would jeopardize her career. Maxine was relatively able to resonate to, and elaborate on, the therapist's observation that the jokes about the children contained considerable hostility, albeit in muted form, and it was the fear of being punished for her hostility that worried her greatly.

In the next several sessions, the patient went on to talk about her ambivalent feelings toward children, and this exploration led to associations about her family and younger brothers specifically. She described her mother's evident adoration of and lenient attitude toward her male siblings. The mother was particularly idolizing of the brother closest in age to Maxine. Although she had been celebrated in her family for her keen wit, her sarcastic comments to her brother were so searing that she earned the reprobation of family members, particularly her mother. During the period of her exploration of this theme, she missed another session. In the session that followed, the therapist wondered aloud whether it had any connection with the feelings she had been exploring toward the children at school and her younger siblings. The patient responded that she felt a strong urge to cancel, but why she did so mystified her. The therapist said simply, "Perhaps it's because now there's a child in the room." The patient then recounted how in the several months in which she had known about the pregnancy, she was beleaguered by the incessant passage through her mind of insults toward the therapist and her pregnant state. Much like in her dealings with her students, she sought to flee when her hostility seemed too close to the surface.

In the months that followed, including well after the period of the maternity leave, the patient explored her jealousy toward the therapist's baby and her brothers (especially her near-aged brother) and her feeling of resentment toward her mother and therapist for giving birth to a competitor. She was able to develop greater tolerance for these affect states so that her maladaptive means of indirectly expressing them (the teasing and the flight behaviors) lessened greatly. She succeeded in gaining a more realistic perception of her brother's favored status. She came to appreciate that while in childhood her brother might have received an intensity of affection she was denied, as an adult her mother had a special relationship with and regard for her.

What distinguishes the neurotic patient's response to the pregnancy from the other groups considered is the capacity to engage in an alliance with the therapist in understanding his or her reactions to the pregnancy. Relative to borderline and psychotic groups, the neurotic patient makes a more active effort to provide material that will yield understanding and to respond to the therapist's interpretive efforts with a lesser degree of defensiveness. The neurotic patient's more stable sense of self helps the patient tolerate the recognition of the conflictual elements identified in interpretation. In the preceding vignette, once the affect of jealousy was isolated and labeled, not only was it relieving to the patient, but also the patient was energetic in uncovering all of the venues of her life where its hidden presence led to behaviors that were not in the service of the patient's long-term interests.

However, as this vignette also suggests, acting out does not preclude a diagnosis of some type of neurosis, a point that has been made previously (Bassen, 1988). This particular patient exhibited acting out both by her tardiness and absences from sessions, but also by her behavior outside of the group (i.e., the teasing of her students). However, the kind of acting out in which the patient engaged, characteristic of neurotics, is of a milder, less self-destructive variety than what is likely to be observed in borderline patients. One of our group therapists who ran a group composed of members with various types of neurosis provided an example. The therapist had transferred the group to her home during and following her pregnancy. When this transfer occurred, one member began to accept a ride to the group from another member, a behavior that violated a rule of the group. Because it represented no serious harm to the member or anyone else, the behavior lacked the interpretive urgency that the acting-out behaviors of borderline and psychotic patients can possess. The therapist had greater freedom to maintain a position of neutrality and to garner sufficient data to render an accurate and specific interpretation before calling attention to the acting out. Occasionally, however, the acting out will be of a more serious nature (e.g., unprotected sexual activity), necessitating a more immediate response from the therapist.

With respect to announcing the pregnancy, the factors of providing adequate time for exploring the meaning of the pregnancy and planning for maternity leave must be weighted for neurotic individuals as they are for borderline and psychotic patients. Various specific considerations apply in the case of the neurotic patient. By delaying an announcement, the therapist is giving the patient an opportunity to develop associations to early physical (and possibly psychological) manifestations of the pregnancy. These associations might be useful to the full elucidation of the patient's reactions to the pregnancy. Another consideration is the possible advantage of having the patient recognize the pregnancy on his or her own. Because neurotic patients do not habitually employ primitive denial, it is less likely that their non-recognition of the pregnancy will be protracted and extend into the later period of the pregnancy. What is particularly common for patients with many forms of neurotic disorder is to notice the pregnancy but inhibit comment on it. The therapist is then in a position to acknowledge what has already been registered by the patient.

With the neurotic patient, planning of the maternity leave is somewhat easier. The patient's very solid acquisition of object constancy allows the patient to hold on to the image of the therapist during her absence. Hence, substitute therapists or contact during maternity leave is often less necessary than for the more primitively organized patient. However, if, say, the neurotic patient is experiencing exceptional stress, it might well be useful to introduce supports during the leave.

The themes with neurotic, borderline and psychotic individuals are summarized in Table 9.1.

Personality Style

Knowledge of the patient's ego organizational level is invaluable in helping the therapist to recognize themes, identify therapist reactions, and plan interventions that are likely to be useful prior to and following the therapist's departure. Yet, such information is insufficient to tailoring the patient's treatment during these special periods. The expectant therapist also must grasp the patient's personality, that is, his or her typical characteristic conflicts, affects and impulses, temperament, modes of relating to others, and sense of self (Linguardi & McWilliams, 2017). Many different personality styles have been described in the literature, and it would be impossible within the limits of this text to do justice to all of them. However, in order to show the importance of personality style independently and as it interacts with level of ego organization, we focus on two contrasting styles: the obsessive personality and the hysterical or histrionic personality.

Themes and Interactional Style

The Obsessive Patient

The obsessional person is caught in a web of self-ambivalence, a continuous battle within the person between self-love and hatred for the self (Bhar & Kyrios,

Table 9.1 Common Therapist Responses Based on Developmental Level of Ego
Organization

Level of Organization	
Neurotic	• Sense of exposure in relation to patient's accurate perception of therapist's condition
	• Assumption that all patient reactions to the pregnancy are in either the real or therapeutic relationship
	• Excessive self-disclosure about the pregnancy
Borderline	• Anxiety in relation to patient's aggression leading to excessive gratifications or failure to confront acting out
	• Anger over the burden of managing patient's acting out during pregnancy
	• Fear that acting out will accelerate
	• Guilt over patient's acting-out episodes
	• Efforts to distance from the patient
	• Relief when patient assumes a more depressive posture
Psychotic	• Increased nurturing
	• Guilt over disruption of relationship
	• Fear concerning the safeguarding of trust
	• Anxiety about re-traumatizing the patient
	• A sense of being overwhelmed by the responsibilities of being a parent and caring for psychotic patients

2007; Kempke & Luyten, 2007). Both psychodynamic and cognitive-behavioral thinkers conceptualize this self-ambivalence as rooted in interactions with parents who are alternately loving and morally judgmental. The child internalizes both perspectives on himself or herself. To reduce the tension associated with this split, the obsessive individual shifts attention toward rational, linear cognitive processes—a world of rules where compliance brings freedom from harsh judgment—and away from emotions (Kempke & Luyten, 2007). Given that to the obsessive patient, reactions to the therapist do not appear sensible—after all, the therapist is not the patient's problem—minimizing such reactions is almost inevitable, particularly early in treatment. Of course, the therapist's pregnancy will not escape the patient's denial. In the patient's view, the pregnancy is irrelevant to him or her (except for a few limited features such as the disruption of treatment created by the maternity leave). Hence, emotional reactions are likely to gain neither awareness nor expression without the very active intervention of the therapist.

Yet, the obsessive patient is likely to be affected deeply by the therapist's pregnancy because of a very characteristic preoccupation with being able to regulate his or her internal and external world. The obsessive individual has an exceptionally strong need to control others (McCann, 1999), given that others are able to activate disturbing elements of the patient's internal world. The therapist's pregnancy is a radical demonstration of the patient's lack of control over this important figure in his or her life. The patient cannot control the fact of the pregnancy, the fetus' weekly presence in the session or the therapist's need to take a leave. The obsessive patient typically will have little power over finding out about the pregnancy because that person's narrow focus will prevent the person from registering and interpreting the physical cues of the pregnancy.

Some of the features of the obsessive patient's response will be similar to those of the narcissistic patient's reaction to the pregnancy. One important difference is that the narcissistic patient will often experience and express negative feelings about the fact that the therapist now has another focus in life. For the obsessive patient, it is not the loss of attention but the loss of control that is disturbing.

The felt absence of control predictably evokes rage in the obsessive patient. However, this affective response is anathema to him or her on several levels. It strikes the patient as irrational, reduces the patient's experienced level of control even further, and violates the individual's perfectionistic strictures. Probably more than any other type of patient, adherence to convention will lead the patient to strive valiantly to reflect the pronatalist norm of the culture. Any departure from this conventional behavior in the form of an expression of anger evokes extreme discomfort in the patient because to the patient, such departures have negative moral implications.

To avoid the terror and guilt that an acknowledgement of rage might bring, the obsessive patient is likely to launch a major defensive effort. The therapist will observe an intensification of those intellectual defenses that the patient used prior to the pregnancy. The specific manifestations will depend on the level at which the obsessive patient is organized. Psychotic and borderline-level patients will employ a defensive ancestor to isolation, a primitive form of denial, and appear schizoid-like in their reactions. The therapist might also observe an unbridled form of intellectualization. For example, the patient might launch into lengthy monologues about the population explosion, while adamantly denying any emotional reaction to the therapist's contribution to this problem. Concerns about such phenomena as world hunger might be the patient's derivative expression of his or her own sense of being deprived by the therapist. For the more neurotically organized obsessive patient, the defensiveness will take a subtler form. While attempting to manifest the conventionally expected—albeit woodenly expressed—good will toward the therapist, the obsessively neurotic patient will avoid the emotional ramifications of the therapist's pregnancy for him or her.

As noted, the anger that the therapist's pregnancy stimulates creates a crisis for the obsessive patient. He or she cannot have a conscious experience of anger without having to endure intolerable levels of guilt, particularly if the anger is perceived to be irrational or unjustified. One defensive strategy used by the obsessive person is making irrational anger rational through a process of displacement. Often, the obsessive patient will become preoccupied by rules given their strong connection between rule violation and guilt (Akhtar, 2016b).

For example, an obsessive patient might get irate over the therapist's tardiness to create an outlet for the less justifiable anger about the pregnancy. Anger arises as a particular problem for the obsessive patient if anything goes awry in the therapist's pregnancy. Events such as a miscarriage or a hospitalization lead the obsessive patient to worry about his or her contributions to this untoward happening. Often, exploration will yield the discovery that the patient sees his or her anger, or its manifestations toward the therapist, as a cause of the therapist's difficulties. For example, the aforementioned patient might ruminate that he was wrong to have bothered the therapist with his annoyance over her tardiness "in her fragile condition." Whether or not the patient is able to articulate such a connection, he might also attempt to assuage his guilt by solicitude toward the therapist. Extreme demonstrations of concern are helpful to the therapist because they reveal important areas to probe.

The Histrionic Patient

Whereas the overt response of the obsessive patient to the therapist's pregnancy is likely to be muted, in the histrionic or hysterical patient it hews toward the lavish (Davis & Millon, 1999; *PDM-2 Task Force*, 2017). Because the histrionic patient in general is inclined toward intense affectivity, any of a diverse set of feeling states—be they shared joy with the therapist or fear in relation to the maternity leave or disappointment that the therapist did not apprise the patient earlier—will be richly and fully expressed.

Yet, as with the obsessive patient, the histrionic person leaves much unexpressed. For the histrionic patient, what is likely to be very troubling is the set of sexual issues stimulated by the therapist's pregnancy. The pregnancy underscores that the therapist is a sexual being. From the standpoint of many psychodynamic writers beginning with Freud (Freud & Breuer, 1895), sexualization is a defensive and adaptive mechanism that arises out of the hysterical individual's dual fixation at the oral and Oedipal levels. Within the oral phase, the child experiences some deprivation from the mother whom she comes to devalue. With relatively intense longings for nurturance, she arrives in the Oedipal period, which provides another opportunity to obtain gratification for early needs. Her capacity to resolve the conflict between yearning for the father, and fear of and love for the mother is impaired because her earlier devaluation of the mother hinders her identification with her. On the other hand, she cannot renounce her mother because her early frustrated longings keep alive her need for her mother. She is therefore locked within a position of seeing males as being strong and powerful and women as being helpless and weak. At the same time, she senses that her own sexuality is a means of securing the attention of men. Hence, sexuality is an instrument for achieving an end, an enticement, rather than an end in itself. Her hostility toward, and fear of, men due to her perception of their far greater powerfulness, makes actual sexual interaction a most threatening prospect.

For the histrionic female patient, the therapist's pregnancy might be seen as the therapist's defeat of her on the Oedipal plain, a defeat that evokes her hostility and jealousy. At the same time, because the patient retains some identification with the therapist, she might experience vicarious fear that the therapist has engaged in sexual intercourse, the dreaded-of-all activities. The therapist's femaleness underscored by the pregnancy establishes her as an object worthy of denigration.

In short, the therapist's pregnancy invites the emergence of the histrionic patient's core conflicts related to dependency and sexuality. The elements contained in these conflicts are dangerous ones for the patient: the surfacing of disappointment in maternal figures as well as Oedipal longings stimulate concomitant fears of maternal and paternal rejection or loss that, in turn, invoke the mounting of a defensive effort. Whereas the obsessive patient commonly uses ideas to fend off affect, the histrionic patient uses repression and affect displays to defend against the linkages between ideas and their corresponding affects (Allen, 1977) or against more disturbing affects. For example, one histrionic patient became more visibly distressed in the weeks following her discovery of the therapist's pregnancy. She would have bouts of crying and would talk about the impossibility of her life improving even with therapy. Initial attempts on the part of the therapist to explore the possibility that the patient was having a reaction to the pregnancy were responded to with such comments as, "I have no idea . . . I just know I'm miserable."

The hysterical patient, particularly the female patient, is also likely to have complicated feelings in relation to the therapist's bodily changes. As McWilliams (2011) notes, hysterical patients, seeing their own physicality as a tool in winning others' admiration, associate sexual attractiveness with power, and often, masculine power. To the extent that the therapist's changing body shape is seen as reducing her attractiveness, the hysterical patient might perceive the therapist as having diminished power. Such a perception of the therapist as a weaker being is likely to arouse the patient's anxiety and possible flight to a therapist who is perceived as stronger and thereby, more able to help the patient. On the other hand, competition with female figures is common for cisgender women with this style. For histrionic trans women, the prominence of such competitive strivings is less clear. On the one hand, the therapist's physical changes might make her less of an object of fantasized sexual competition. On the other hand, the pregnancy might signify a victory over the patient to the extent that she feels the therapist received something she was denied. For heterosexual males, the pregnancy of the therapist might communicate that she is unavailable for seduction. Given that histrionic men tend to find power in their ability to seduce (Lubbe, 2003), such a development is likely to spawn bewilderment as to how to manage himself within the relationship: it raises the frightening prospect that it is not he but the therapist who is in control. For both male and female patients across gender identities and sexual orientations, a high level of responsiveness to social norms is likely to lead them to respond to the therapist's pregnancy with an overt display of warmth. As McWilliams (2011) noted, although the warmth might be exaggerated, it is nonetheless genuine. The greater problem is that it is likely to mask the more painful reactions the client is having.

Contrasting Therapist Responses

Particularly vivid are the contrasts between the therapist's reaction to the obsessive and histrionic patients during the therapist's pregnancy, contrasts deriving from the under-emotionality of the former and the over-emotionality of the latter. The lack of apparent emotionality of the obsessive patient frequently requires the therapist to be a container for the many affects warded off by the patient. The patient's bland dismissal of the importance of the pregnancy might evoke irritation from the therapist. The therapist can easily feel frustrated and ineffective in response to the patient's unflappable posture—even in the face of the therapist's best intervention efforts. The therapist might also feel shame and embarrassment when the patient conveys bafflement at what appears to be the therapist's narcissistic preoccupation, or horror at the messiness the therapist has brought into the treatment.

Some therapists, however, might find a relief in the obsessive patient's unresponsiveness to the pregnancy, particularly in its latter period when other figures in the therapist's professional environment might be preoccupied with it or having severe emotional reactions in relation to it. Time with the obsessive patient might be regarded as a kind of oasis, a space where a certain level of maternal preoccupation seems allowable. To preserve this space, the therapist might permit the patient's intellectualized discussion of other matters, a discussion that is likely to induce the therapist's eventual disengagement, if not boredom. Boredom might be both a realistic response to the patient's hollow discourse and absorption in details as well as a defensive reaction to her quid pro quo hostility. Alternatively, the therapist might make an aggressive resistance interpretation, bluntly labeling the patient's defenses as a way of ridding herself of anger and frustration (Ogden, 2001; Winnicott, 1945).

With the hysterical patient, disengagement is less of a risk than with the obsessive patient. The patient's intense emotions also evoke strong feelings from the therapist. Moreover, the patients' feelings are likely to cover a spectrum, ranging from effusive displays of concern for mother and child to extreme anger. For some therapists, the intense neediness of hysterical patients easily pulls for frustration, hostility, impatience and exasperation. At times, the patient's manifestations of emotion will appear inauthentic, more for purposes of display than anything deeply felt (McWilliams, 2011). Such an impression is conducive to the therapist dismissing the patient's reaction while not realizing that the patient's theatricality contains seeds of a genuine reaction. As McWilliams (2011) explains, the hysterical patient enlarges expressions of feeling as a means of counteracting fears about their manifestation. The therapist's dismissal of such expressions intensifies the patient's fears.

For patients organized at the borderline level, negative reactions on the part of the therapist are especially likely because the behaviors of the patient are more likely to be disruptive to the therapist's life outside of treatment. Anger and frustration are especially likely to be intense if the therapist's interventions do not diminish the patient's efforts to obtain more supplies from the therapist. On the other hand, the histrionic patient might provide an opportunity for the therapist to rid herself of any feelings of vulnerability and neediness that the pregnancy has activated. In identifying with the patient's expression of need, and attending to that need, the therapist can experience some measure of freedom from the need's grip. Under the sway of such a dynamic, the therapist is likely to see the adult patient as a child and treat him or her accordingly. The therapist takes the hysterical patient's show of helplessness at face value rather than seeing it as a flight from the anxieties that are stimulated by the patient's confrontation of adult issues. The therapist might reactively gratify the patient's dependent wishes because not to do so potentially intensifies the therapist's own sense of vulnerability and might evoke in the therapist feelings of being a bad, depriving parent, much as in the case of child patients (see Chapter 8).

Therapeutic Strategies

Just as the personality styles of the histrionic and obsessive patients contrast greatly, so too must the therapist's style vary with each type of patient in order for that style to be effective.

Obsessive Patient

Like most patients, the obsessive patient is likely to use his or her customary defenses in a more elaborate, exaggerated way in response to the therapist's pregnancy. Accordingly, the emotional range of the patient narrows upon discovery of the pregnancy. The therapeutic potential of this narrowing is that it invites the patient to see more clearly his or her defensive way of reckoning with emotional experience.

An early opportunity of this nature is likely to arise when the obsessive patient first learns of the therapist's pregnancy. In the authors' experience, it is not unusual for obsessive patients to fail to notice the pregnancy, necessitating that the therapist initiate the conversation. Following this communication, obsessive patients quite commonly are thrown into a state of shame over having failed to ascertain the pregnancy on their own. The experience of shame leads to withdrawal (Akhtar, 2016a), even if the patient comes forth with some conventional congratulatory comments. One customary means by which the patient withdraws is via a tedious review of all of the evidence available that directed the patient away from figuring out on his or her own the fact of the therapist's pregnancy (e.g., "Given these facts, it would have been impossible for me to realize"; "I knew you were looking heavier, but I reasoned that you were wearing heavier winter clothing; it is winter, after all"). Even those patients who do discover it on their own are likely to focus on whether or not the pregnancy could have been detected at an earlier point.

How the therapist works with these preoccupations should depend on the patient's time and progress in treatment, as well as his or her level of ego functioning. For either the relatively new patient or the patient operating at a psychotic or borderline level, it might suffice simply to agree with the patient that in light of the evidence at the patient's disposal, recognizing the therapist's pregnancy would have been difficult. In this way, the therapist avoids conveying that the patient violated some parental stricture. At the same time, the therapist might point out, gently and respectfully, how this second-guessing reveals the patient's needs to be omniscient and perfect, and what pain these needs create whenever life surprises the patient. For the neurotically organized patient, particularly one who has already made some progress in examining his or her obsessive defenses, a more ambitious line of intervention might be useful. The therapist might engage the patient in considering how both missing the cues about the pregnancy and lamenting over having done so suggest an effort to maintain a level of control over the inner and outer world to avoid his or her own self-ambivalence.

As the pregnancy and therapy progress, the therapist will note the patient's relatively low level of responsiveness to the pregnancy. For some patients, labeling the defensive maneuvers (such as philosophizing or ruminating) that protect that patient from being effectively present in the sessions is useful. For many others, creating a safe environment for the expression of affect is the most productive route. Although these objectives can be accomplished in many ways, we will mention a few. For the many obsessive patients who are sensitive to pronatalist cultural norms and the strictures of conscience, the admission of negative feelings toward the therapist might well be anathema. Yet, as discussed earlier, the obsessive patient might find greater ease in expressing negative feelings about perceived therapist imperfections that are ostensibly unrelated to the pregnancy and yet, are a displacement from the latter. For example, if the patient becomes vexed at a billing mistake, it might be perfectly evident to the therapist that the overreaction is caused by the mistake being embedded in the content of the therapist's pregnancy. Perhaps, the error is a symbol to the patient that other matters preoccupy the therapist. Yet, the therapist might do well to simply allow the patient to work within the metaphor he or she has created because movement to the pregnancy-related interpretation might only serve to strengthen the patient's resistance.

The therapist's engagement in a mild to moderate level of self-disclosure can also be useful for the obsessional patient. For example, if the patient observes that the therapist appears tired and the therapist agrees, then the therapist is showing the patient that fallibilities are tolerable and reactions to the pregnancy are fair game for patient–therapist discussion.

Finally, the therapist is aided by having reasonable expectations about what the obsessive patient can accomplish in achieving greater depth of expressed feeling during the pregnancy. For example, one of the authors had an obsessive patient who eventually said, "It irritates me slightly that my therapy will be interrupted because of this baby of yours." For this patient who had previously refrained from making even the mildest negative comment, this admission was immense. Had the author attempted to get the patient to attest to a stronger feeling (e.g., "Do you really mean 'irritates,' don't you really mean 'makes you angry'?"), the client would likely have felt guilt for having violated a societal rule of showing consideration of women during their pregnancies.

The Histrionic Patient

The two major challenges faced by the therapist in working with the histrionic patient are the patient's acting out outside of sessions and intense affect and enactments within the sessions. The former is of particular concern because such behavioral patterns might have long-term negative consequences for the patient. For the histrionic patient, acting-out manifestations might be diverse, but sexual acting out is especially likely. As was discussed for borderline-level patients, a useful therapeutic strategy is anticipating for the patient the likely temptation to engage in particular behaviors. Simultaneously, the patient should be encouraged to deploy an armamentarium of alternative responses, some of which the patient used in the past and others which may be new. As this repertoire is being developed, the patient is simultaneously being encouraged to appreciate and tap his or her own resilience (Robbins, 1998).

As the therapist is helping the patient to look ahead, he or she must take care not to be omniscient: the histrionic patient uses others' knowledge of her, particularly knowledge that she lacks, as evidence of her inferiority. The therapist can avoid the negative effects of such anticipatory statements by explicitly using the patient's past behavior as the basis for articulated concerns about the patient's near future. For example, the therapist might say, "We've seen in the past that when you've received unwanted news, you felt tempted to miss sessions. If you begin to feel this way again, it would be important for us to discuss it."

Not all histrionic patients act out outside of the sessions. Some will engage in affective storms within the session accompanied by the assumption of a helpless, dependent posture. Such individuals profit from interventions designed to move them beyond their global dysphoria to the identification of specific affect states, such as anger or envy. Often during this time, the patient will experience such a sense of threat that the patient's customary defense of dramatization of affect will appear in exaggerated form. This almost-caricatured version places the therapist in an excellent position to label the patient's histrionic maneuvers so as to enable the patient to feel more fully, a key goal in working with histrionic individuals. In doing so, the therapist must exercise care not to patronize the patient, a response that can readily result from the patient's exaggerated displays. As McWilliams (2011) points out, it is precisely the fear of having his or her emotional manifestations rejected that leads the patient to exhibit them with bravado. It is as if the patient is saying, "See: I am going to force myself to show you that I have this feeling despite my fearfulness." Any lack of respect on the part of the therapist will intensify the patient's fearfulness of showing genuine affect.

For some therapists, understandably, the patient's weak, depressed posture is more comfortable than his or her angry presentation. Not only is the patient likely to be more tractable in a depressed state, but also the therapist is able to enjoy the gratifications of being in a nurturing role, thereby providing the therapist with a foretaste of what is to come. The therapist's self-awareness of this bias is essential so that she can exercise care not to reinforce the former over the latter.

In therapies that are primarily designed to augment the patient's ego strength and coping capabilities, the patient's learning of the therapist's pregnancy might be followed by a lessened motivation to benefit from the structure of the treatment and the therapist's interventions. For example, patients in cognitive-behavioral therapy might fail to complete homework assignments in their efforts to identify automatic thoughts. Members of a mentalization group might balk at having to provide events within the group on which members can practice their mentalization skills. In Acceptance and Commitment Therapy, individuals might show an increased engagement in experiential avoidance. Patients in problem-solving therapy might manifest a constriction in brainstorming solutions to problems. On the appearance of such resistance, it could be useful to raise the hypothesis that the change in clients' behaviors is due to the announcement of the pregnancy. Each model of treatment explicitly or implicitly has the means to address such changes. For example, within cognitive behavior terms, the realization of the pregnancy evoked certain automatic thoughts associated with negative affects. Members are helped to see the potential of identifying these thoughts.

Recommendations

1. Our broad recommendation is that therapists think about the client's level of ego functioning in ascertaining productive ways to assist the client in responding to the therapist's pregnancy in ways that will maintain gains and even create the potential for additional progress.
2. With patients at the two lower rungs of ego functioning, risk management should be a major focus. In the case of psychotic individuals, therapists should consider carefully the prudence of taking on new patients within their caseload. For patients occupying the borderline level of ego functioning, the therapist should employ means to discourage acting out inside and outside of the sessions.

3. The patient's level of ego functioning will affect such factors as how and when the pregnancy is disclosed, how questions are answered in an ongoing way, and what plans are made for the maternity leave.

4. Because personality style also figures in important ways to what issues will emerge in relation to the therapist's pregnancy, the therapist's reaction to the patient, and the optimal interventions to advance the patient toward the therapeutic goals, therapists are encouraged to attend to this aspect, especially as it interacts with level of ego functioning.

CHAPTER 10

Multi-person Therapeutic Modalities: Group, Couple and Family Therapies

In earlier chapters, our emphasis, particularly in our examples and descriptions of patient and therapist reactions, has largely been on the individual therapy relationship; this emphasis reflects that of the theoretical and empirical literature at large. Certain, this bias does not do justice to the rich array of circumstances in which therapists expecting a baby practice. Not only are the modalities in the field various, but therapists in the process of building a family are especially likely to use modalities besides individual therapy. As is discussed in Chapter 11 on peer and supervisory relationships, pregnancies in particular are very common in women in the training phase of their professional lives. Many male trainees experience expectant fatherhood during their training years. Many common training sites place emphasis on macrosystem intervention such as group, milieu, community and family therapies, as well as various types of consultation.

Examining each modality in its own right is important for three reasons. First, the structure of the therapy can determine the issues that surface for both the patient and the therapist. For example, having peers in the group session accentuates certain issues to a greater degree than the individual therapy session lacking a peer component. Second, the management problems posed by pregnancy and other forms of expectant parenting vary from modality to modality as do the resources available to solve problems. For example, in individual therapy, by definition, the therapist's maternity leave requires that either the therapy will be interrupted or continued with another therapist. In group, family or couple psychotherapies, the presence of a co-therapist may do much to provide continuity during maternity leave. In fact, the co-therapist can use the hiatus as a therapeutic opportunity to assist the client in processing reactions to the other therapist's absence and life change. Third, different patient reactions and clinical decision making are likely to beget differences in the therapists' own cognitive and emotional responses. For example, the therapist whose group is being covered during her absence might be less likely to endure intense feelings of guilt than the therapist whose individual client has an actual treatment disruption.

We will discuss the phenomena attached to the pregnant therapist, the expectant father-therapist and the adoptive parent-therapist within multi-person therapies. As is the case with the literature at large, we know far more about the pregnant therapist than the latter two categories, and our chapter is weighted accordingly.

The Pregnant Therapist

Since the end of the 1990s, the literature on the pregnant therapist has broadened to include modalities beyond individual psychotherapy. A handful of anecdotal accounts of therapists' experiences leading a psychotherapy group while being pregnant has amassed (Anderson, 1994; Breen, 1977; Fenster et al., 1986; Gavin, 1994; Rogers, 1994). To see if trends emerge across therapists, we and our colleagues surveyed group, couple and family therapists on the clinical phenomena emerging during their pregnancies (Anderson, Fallon, Brabender, & Maier, 2000; Fallon et al., 1998). We conducted semi-structured interviews with 29 group psychotherapists and five couple and family therapists about their observations of their patients and themselves during each of the trimesters of pregnancy and their re-entry into the workplace. We also collected vignettes from therapists practicing multi-person modalities concerning events occurring during their pregnancies or their returns to work. Because all of our participants also conducted individual therapy, we invited them to make comparative statements of the two modalities vis-à-vis their pregnancies. We integrate here our own findings with other writings on multi-personal psychotherapies.

Group Psychotherapy

This section first outlines patient reactions and then therapist reactions to the therapist's pregnancy. Although this sequence occurs for expositional ease, recognizing the interconnection between these two sets of reactions, and their co-construction and embeddedness in reality elements, is critical for fully appreciating the dynamics of the relationship during this period. At the end of this section, we do include some observations about fathers who are group psychotherapists.

Patient Reactions

The reader will recall that in Chapter 3, the authors identified three reactions patients often have toward the therapist's pregnancy. They are issues related to: (a) abandonment, loss or deprivation; (b) rivalry with the therapist, baby, husband or some combination thereof; and (c) sexuality. Additionally, as discussed in Chapter 3, patients have reactions existing within the real relationship (i.e., reactions that have little or nothing to do with conflict or psychopathology). The question is, which of these various reactions, mostly identified in the individual therapy relationship, also emerge prominently in the group situation? Also, do particular reactions appear more conspicuously in the group than individual situation?

THE GROUP PSYCHOTHERAPY LITERATURE

Breen (1977) was the first to examine patient reactions to the group psychotherapist's pregnancy. She focused on the group members of her long-term, psychodynamically oriented, co-led group. The major area in which the group worked, Breen observed, was the third of the thematic areas mentioned: sexuality. The group considered varied aspects of sexuality including members' own sexuality, that of their parents, and the question of whether parents and children could acknowledge to one another their sexual selves. The male members responded to the topic of sexuality with content related to homosexuality. The pregnancy, she believed, activated a core conflict between their wish to show their sexual sides and their fear of being castrated by sexual women, particularly the therapist, for having done so. Breen also found that issues of abandonment, loss and deprivation were not particularly common in the experiences of members and less common than in those in individual therapy. She hypothesized the group situation is less evocative of dependency on the therapist than the individual situation because participants in the former can depend on one another and the group as a whole. She also saw the presence of the co-therapist—someone who could safeguard the group's continuity during her absence—as lessening the sense of members' loss. Sibling rivalry issues, she observed, were much less common among group members than individual therapy clients, presumably because group members face the demand of sharing the therapist on an ongoing basis. For individual members, having someone else (that is, the baby) attend the session was for the most part, an unprecedented circumstance.

Breen's observations have received partial support in the literature from therapists conducting groups from a group analytic perspective. Foulkes (1975/1986, p. 3), the founder of this approach, defined it as "a form of psychotherapy by the group of the group, including the conductor" who is the group analyst. Rogers (1994), another group analyst, provided confirmation for the importance of the topic of sexuality and the distinctiveness of men's reactions to this topic. However, in the group, the focus was on the therapist's sexuality and the evident fact of the therapist having a sexual partner. The men explored their potency and, in contrast to Breen's male members, showed a heightened attunement to the sexuality of the women in the group. Although Rogers saw the therapist's pregnancy as activating abandonment issues in some individuals, the activation of sexual issues in the group predominated.

Gavin (1994), also using group analysis, saw abandonment as a much stronger concern for the group during the therapist's pregnancy than any other. In her group, prior to her pregnancy, the group had been dealing with early dependency issues, but the pregnancy led to their intensification. As she described it,

By session five [following the acknowledgment of the pregnancy], group themes centered on the wish to be special to me, to be contained, coupled with intense fears of being swallowed, fears of engulfment, not having an identity, fear of being swallowed, fear of exposure, the need for boundaries, the lack of a father, self-hatred and lack of entitlement.

(Gavin, 1994, p. 66)

Unlike the aforementioned therapists, Gavin observed no appreciable thematic differences between the material produced by her group members and her individual therapy patients. Whether the differences in Gavin's observations and those of other therapists is rooted in differences in patient populations is a matter for future study.

The existing literature suggests that the themes that are of major importance in individual therapy also achieve ascendancy in the group setting. However, group writers seem to place emphasis on the prominence of sexual issues, particularly those associated with Oedipal conflict. Group therapists' reports of men subgrouping in the exploration of sexual identity and potency issues represent a departure from the individual therapy literature. Although the same issues concerning sexuality arise in both modalities, men in individual therapy show substantial inhibition in addressing them; in group therapy, men's expressiveness seems to be stimulated by the presence of others with related issues. Groups described in the literature have diverged from one another in the extent to which conflicts related to dependency and loss have dominated the group's life during the therapist's pregnancy. Whereas in Breen's (1977) group, these conflicts did not seem particularly salient, in Anderson's (1994) and Gavin's (1994) groups, the pregnancy led to an intensity of conflicts related to dependency and loss. In Rogers's (1994) group, the therapist's pregnancy seems to effect a shift from dependency to sexual conflicts.

OUR RESEARCH ON PATIENT REACTIONS

In the midst of all of the variability in prior findings, a clinician might wonder whether any trends exist in the dominant themes during the therapist's pregnancy or if the thematic emphases of any one group are more idiosyncratic than otherwise. To make this determination, one must go beyond the individual case study to the examination of a cohort of psychotherapy groups. This is precisely what we did through a study in which we interviewed 29 women who had experienced pregnancies while functioning as group psychotherapists (Fallon, Brabender, Anderson & Maier, 1998). These participants were obtained through notices in national professional meetings, letters of request to each affiliate group of the American Group Psychotherapy Association, and referrals from other volunteers. As Fenster et al. (1986) found, we observed that female therapists were delighted to have an opportunity to discuss this exciting period in their lives.

The therapists were varied in their orientations, although a psychodynamic orientation was predominant. Sixty-seven percent of the sample reported on their group experience during a first pregnancy. Participants ranged in age from 28 to 44 years with a mean age of 34.4, almost exactly the age of those interviewed by Fenster (1983). Therapist reports were based exclusively on outpatient groups (54%), a combination of inpatient and outpatient groups (23%), exclusively on inpatient groups (15%), and solely on partial hospital groups (8%). Most (78%) had a co-therapy leadership format. The majority of group members (64%) averaged a length of stay 6 months or longer. Most groups (74%) were mixed gender but over a quarter of the groups were all female. Tables 10.1 and 10.2 provide additional information about the therapists and the groups, respectively.

A semi-structured phone interview was conducted to glean from participants their own reactions during their pregnancies and return to work, and those of their patients. The therapists' comments were then analyzed for recurrent themes. Across trimesters and during the return period, the following thematic categories emerged most prominently: (a) abandonment, deprivation and loss; (b) sibling rivalry; (c) envy of the therapist, her husband, her baby or some combination thereof; (d) parenting; (e) sexuality; (f) information-seeking about pregnancy; and (g) positive feelings for the therapist. In the next sections, we focus on the themes as they emerged across five units of time.

The Three Trimesters

In the first trimester, group therapists perceived their members to be unaware of their pregnancies. Very few therapists announced the pregnancy at this time, and very few patients discerned it on their own. However, when an occasional member did recognize some alteration in the therapist, that member generally approached the therapist outside the group. For example, one therapist wrote,

> A very sharp woman in her seventies began to look at me strangely even in my very early pregnancy. Then, on one occasion, I had to give her something after the group session. She stood very close to me and asked me if I was pregnant. I told her I would address that later. I hoped I could keep her at bay until after the amniocentesis.

The wish of most group therapists (as well as individual therapists) was to avoid taking up the pregnancy with the group until the pregnancy seemed secure. This intent might have unconsciously hindered the therapists from recognizing any allusions to the pregnancy that do occur in the first trimester.

In the second and third trimesters, the majority of therapists saw members as producing material that was related to, and precipitated by, their pregnancies. In both trimesters, the most common theme was abandonment and related issues (loss, separation, etc.). The emergence of abandonment concerns was not limited to particular types of groups or patient populations but appeared across a wide spectrum of group therapies. For example, a therapist of a long-term incest survivor group described her members' reactions as follows: "Panic . . . fear of abandonment, and lots of anger were there. Members said to me, in effect, 'How could you do this? We need you!" The therapist of a long-term private outpatient group said, "It raised questions of group cohesiveness. They wondered, 'Can we take care of one another? Would I pick a substitute therapist good enough to take care of them?' " The therapist of a partial hospital group saw members expressing "a feeling that no one was available to them. There was no one to take care of them." It is remarkable how similar the language is among these different types of groups.

Although abandonment issues were prominent in both trimesters, differences were present between the two trimesters in how the thematic material unfolded. In the second trimester (which generally had greater thematic richness than either trimester one or three), abandonment reactions were frequently intermingled with the expression of envy and in some cases, explicit death wishes toward the therapist, the therapist's sexual partner and the baby. Members seemed to perceive this period as the safest one in which to express their negative reactions in their most intense, direct form.

In contrast, in the last trimester, members' anger seemed to recede somewhat. Perhaps the baby's more evident presence in the group and the imminence of the therapist's departure inhibited members' expression of their full ranges of reactions. In the third trimester, members directly attest to their fearfulness about the well-being of the therapist's baby (particularly in light of their past verbalizations of hostility toward the baby), and the therapist. However, even more striking is members' expression of concern and fearfulness about how they will tolerate the therapist's absence (despite, in most cases, the continuation of the group with the co-therapist).

With their lessened expressions of hostility toward the therapist and the other figures in the birth drama, group members found less direct ways of dealing with the negative feelings stimulated by this anticipated event. Unlike individual therapy, displacement is one defensive opportunity that group psychotherapy makes readily available, and the therapists in our sample indicated that their members took great advantage of it. The co-therapist and the substitute therapist (whom members may or may not have met) were the most common displacement objects. Members homed in on specific qualities of these figures that in their view suggest that their caretaking of the group would be deficient. Representative of this response was one group that became preoccupied with the co-therapist's condescending attitude at a time when they barely knew her. Sometimes, these sentiments were revealed in members' behaviors. One group, for example, responded to the pregnant therapist's interpretations with deference and thoughtfulness while dismissing the co-therapist's contributions out of hand.

Besides the co-therapist, other members of the group functioned as displacement objects for members' negative feelings. For example, one therapist observed that in her third trimester, a member expressed her rage toward, and mistrust of, the therapist for being pregnant. The members were horrified by this woman's attack on their therapist. They proceeded to scapegoat this member who left the group prior to the therapist's departure.

Reaction formation was another mechanism that members used to defend against their negative feelings toward the therapist in the second trimester, but even more so, in the third. Members would express heightened positive feelings that appeared to mask anger, envy or other negatively toned reactions. Many societies having a pronatal ethos, a collective value of women's maternity over other roles (Morell, 2000), provide a host of memes by which to give this defensive effort concrete form. Relative to other modalities, the psychotherapy group provides more robust opportunities to transform members' reactions into actions. Not uncommonly, group members organized a session-based baby shower for the therapist. This was an effective defensive maneuver in that therapists oftentimes were so disarmed and fearful of seeming ungrateful that they abandoned any effort to use this opportunity to interpret the meaning of the group-as-a-whole behavior. Other groups took measures to prevent the therapist from exerting herself (e.g., moving chairs into a circle for her prior to the group). Here, the therapists' relief at being freed of any activity that was difficult or onerous protected the patients' resistance. Other groups made regular inquiries into the health of the therapist and the baby. As discussed in Chapter 3, all of these manifestations could exist within the real relationship. However, the therapists we interviewed also felt that these behaviors occurred as a means to diminish members' anxiety over the intensity of their negative feelings toward a person on whom they depended. Just as in the case of the baby shower, therapists expressed regret that they did not plumb the multiple meanings of the group enactments.

Completing the trio of defensive maneuvers is acting out.[1] For the group members of our participants, acting-out behaviors were extremely common in the latter two trimesters. In the second semester, the incidents of acting out largely fell into two categories: behaviors related to attendance and sexual acting out. Attendance-related acting out took several forms: missing sessions, expressing intent to discontinue the group, or actually dropping out. For example, one therapist, the solo leader of an outpatient group, indicated that in the session following the pregnancy announcement, "People were shutting down and not talking. One member said, 'I need to be in individual treatment and not in group.' Strong feelings were expressed by three members (out of 5) about not wanting to come to group." Sexual acting out, occurring in 2 of the 29 groups, took the form of intensified promiscuity during this period. No incidents of actual pregnancies were reported because of this sexual activity. Other examples of acting out were unique to each group. For example, the therapist of an inpatient group reported, "[members] would express their anger by breaking the rules of the group. They would chew gum and leave the room to go to the bathroom."

In the third trimester, the types of acting out broadened. Once again, the primary area of acting out was in members' attendance. Other forms were sexual activity, suicidal gestures, and socialization outside of group sessions. The acting-out behaviors of the third trimester were generally of a more serious nature than those of the second trimester, an unsurprising finding given members progressively lessened expression of anger within the sessions themselves. The former were significant in that they posed a serious threat to the integrity of the individual, the group or both.

Our therapists noted a variety of member responses that appeared to belong to the real relationship. The pregnancy frequently catalyzed discussions about parenting in adult patients and questions about childbirth in younger group members. For example, in an outpatient private practice group in which all of the members were considerably older than the therapist, the discussion of her pregnancy led to pleasurable reminiscences about their own experiences with childbirth and childrearing. For a group of male patients, the therapist's pregnancy stimulated a conversation about the difficulties of balancing home and work responsibilities.

In many types of groups, the therapist's pregnancy evoked genuine positive feelings toward the therapist. Members also felt enhanced pride in their recognition of their capacities to give something back to the therapist. For female adolescent and young adult patients, the positive feelings toward the therapist were often accompanied by the wish to identify with the therapist. For example, as one therapist leading a group of eating-disordered patients noted, "C. is the most curious about me and my body getting bigger. She wants a real relationship with me. The pregnancy stirred up so much that she wants to know more about me." Patients want to know more about the therapist in part so that they can pattern themselves after the therapist.

From our interviews of female group psychotherapists who were pregnant while running a group, three conclusions can be drawn. First, group psychotherapists identify many of the same issues that individual psychotherapists, interviewed in prior studies, have described. Second, these issues are in the domain of both the therapy relationship and the real relationship. Third, group members' dominant concern, a concern about loss and abandonment, is the same as that of individual therapy patients.

To determine whether any differences exist between the modalities, our therapists who practiced both modalities were asked to make direct comparative judgments about the responses of their group therapy versus individual therapy patients (Fallon, Brabender, Anderson & Maier, 1998). To this end, the investigators designed a questionnaire that asked therapists to compare the intensity levels of 10 possible reactions. These included envy toward the therapist, feelings of being excluded, a sense of rivalry toward the therapist's husband, resentment that the outside world was intruding on the therapeutic relationship, hostility at having to share the therapist, fear of the therapist's sexuality, a desire to take care of the therapist, excitement and enthusiasm, and increased expression of same-sex attraction.[2]

Our therapist-participants were asked to indicate whether these reactions during the therapist's pregnancy were of greater, equal or lesser strength in individual therapy patients versus group psychotherapy members. Specifically, individual therapy patients expressed feelings of intrusion, envy toward the therapist, and hostility over having to share the therapist more intensely than did group psychotherapy patients. In the group setting, members expressed with greater intensity feelings of excitement and enthusiasm, as well as a wish to be caretaking of the therapist. Stated simply, the major modality differences that we found were that affect states that are commonly seen to be negative (e.g., anger, envy) appear to therapists to be expressed more intensely in individual psychotherapy. More positively toned affects appeared to be expressed more vividly in group psychotherapy. This trend held across theoretical orientations, experiences of the therapist, the primiparous and multiparous status of the therapist as well as the therapist's level of experience.

Several additional trends were revealed in the data. In individual psychotherapy the here-and-now focus increased, whereas in group psychotherapy no change occurred. In both individual and group psychotherapy, female patients were seen as responding more intensively than male patients. The dropout rate was not greater for group versus individual psychotherapy during pregnancy, the maternity leave and the early period of the therapist's return to work. However, the total drop rate across the periods was significantly greater for individual than group psychotherapy patients. On the whole, psychotherapists perceived individual psychotherapy patients as having more intense reactions to the pregnancy than group psychotherapy patients.

When all of our findings of group psychotherapists are taken together, a complex pattern emerges that can be summarized by the following statements. First, for both individual and group psychotherapy patients, the theme of loss and abandonment emerges more prominently than any other theme. This finding is highly consistent with the literature and suggests that most pregnant therapists should anticipate its presence in their group and individual therapies. Second, individual therapy patients react to the pregnancy more intensively particularly when negative affects are evoked by the pregnancy. As Breen (1977) suggested, this difference may be structural: due to the constant requirement placed on members to share time and attention in the group, group members might see the therapist's pregnancy as less of an incursion than do individual therapy patients. Third, perhaps because of the lower intensity of group members' reactions to the pregnancy, group members have greater room for the emergence of positive reactions to the pregnancy. Fourth, this disparity suggests that individual and group modalities each provide, not unique, but specialized opportunities for patients to do psychological work. Specifically, in individual therapy with the intense here-and-now emergence of conflicts related to separation and abandonment, patients have an opportunity to resolve these conflicts. In group psychotherapy, other conflicts related to sibling rivalry and sexuality also emerge with some prominence, as do reality-based issues concerning childbirth and childrearing. Members also seem to participate more fully in the joy of the therapist's pregnancy. Their opportunities to provide caretaking to the caretaker seem to be esteem-bolstering. An alternate interpretation of the therapist's perception that group members are more nurturing is that the group atmosphere itself provides support to the group psychotherapist—the group might contain and hold the therapist just as it does the members. The therapist might project these positive feelings onto the group members (T. Feldman, personal communication, December 13, 2000). Whereas Fenster, Phillips and Rapoport (1986) described the capacity of the pregnancy to nurture the real relationship in individual psychotherapy, this potential seems especially great in the psychotherapy group. Finally, our results suggest that women are somewhat more open to the therapeutic opportunities presented by their therapists' pregnancies than are men for both individual and group psychotherapy.

The Maternity Leave

Our pool of data concerning our participants' reactions was slender, but information on the incidence of acting out during the maternity leave was obtained. Therapists reported that acting out occurred in 63% of the groups (in contrast to 54% in the third trimester). The highest incident of acting out concerned attendance behaviors. In the seven groups where there was some acting out related to attendance, five involved premature termination from group. In contrast, in the third trimester, the attendance issue merely concerned members missing a session. A single incident of acting out and a single incident of suicidal behavior (an aspirin overdose) occurred. The maternity leave period is similar to the third trimester in that when acting out does occur, it tends to be consequential. One important question for future research is whether a thorough processing of members' reactions to the pregnancy diminishes the extent of acting out during these periods. In any case, the therapist must anticipate the potential for these untoward events in the clinical plan.

Therapist's Return to the Group

The therapist's return to the group signals a slight thematic shift. Although separation and abandonment themes commonly emerge, they are not nearly as dominating as they were in the second and third trimesters. Almost equivalent is the members' focus on sibling rivalry issues, and expressions of concern about the therapist's child, as well as the process of childbirth.

Relative to the second and third trimesters, the period of the therapist's return appears to be one of less engagement with the therapist's pregnancy. Therapists see this period as being a more tranquil one for members in contrast to the tumult of the last two trimesters. The lessened pre-occupation with abandonment and loss is likely due to the reassurance derived from the therapists' returns. At the same time, the therapist's baby—although no longer attending the group[3]—is more of a reality to members. Because all of our therapists provided basic information about the baby, such as the baby's gender, health condition and so on, sibling rivalry and curiosity about the baby was stimulated in some groups. Yet, a number of therapists spontaneously expressed surprise that members did not respond more strongly to their return. For many members, the relief at having the therapist back was accompanied by eagerness to have the therapist's pregnancy, absence and her baby put aside.

Therapist Reactions

Breen (1977) believed that the pregnant therapist's experience in the psychotherapy group would be different from her experience in the individual therapy situation. In the group, individuals other than the therapist fulfill members' needs. For this reason, using the therapist as a container for negative projections is perceived to be as risky as it is in individual therapy, where the patient is solely reliant upon the therapist. Furthermore, when the therapist is a member of a co-therapy team, the group can use splitting, assigning the roles of the all-good therapist and the all-bad therapist. Through the use of splitting, members are protected from the pain of integration, the pain that occurs when a basically good person engages in actions that are disappointing. These factors led Breen to see the group therapist as vulnerable to extreme negative feelings. As she noted about her own group, "I was rejected and *made to feel* the bad sexual mother" (italics added).

Other writers characterized their own reactions as they were leading groups during their pregnancies. Anderson (1994) talked about her discomfort with members' envy and their caretaking efforts vis-à-vis her. She indicated her dislike of having them acknowledge her vulnerability. Gavin (1994) discussed how her fear of members' envy and hostility led her to delay the announcement of the pregnancy. Rogers (1994) talked about how during the pregnancy, the therapist's boundaries between reality and fantasy are relaxed. Members' fantasies may be experienced as real to the therapist. Masochistic strivings on the part of the therapist may prevent her from placing appropriate limits on members' expressions of hostility toward her and her baby.

Generally, what has appeared in the literature is from the perspective of a therapist conducting a single group. The present authors believed that studying the reactions of group therapists across a large variety of groups might enable the identification of some common patterns of therapist response.

OUR FINDINGS ON THERAPIST REACTIONS

For each trimester and for the period following their return to the group, therapists were asked to describe (a) their pregnancy-related physical and emotional reactions while in the group, (b) alterations in their style of intervention relative to the pre-pregnancy period, and (c) their reactions to specific patient reactions (e.g., how the therapist responded to members' discovery of the pregnancy). Additionally, we presented the therapists with six possible patient reactions based upon reactions that had been identified in both the group and individual therapy literature. We asked the therapist to rate each in terms of how difficult each was for the therapist to receive. Therapists were able to indicate whether their group members did not exhibit any of the six reactions. They were also able to specify patient reactions beyond the six listed in the survey. Given that in Chapter 4, we provide an account of the therapist reactions, in this section we focus primarily on those responses distinguishing group psychotherapists from those using other modalities.

The Three Trimesters

Like individual therapists, group psychotherapists report their high level of self-focusing as being a major concern in their first trimester. The content of the self-focusing was variable. In some cases, a preoccupation with somatic symptoms (especially fatigue and nausea) emerged; in others, reflections on the pregnancy itself; and in still others, an overwhelming feeling of elation. Despite this self-focusing, most therapists did not perceive themselves as altering in any significant way their style of intervening (e.g., the use of here-and-now versus historical statements).

Another major theme for group psychotherapists during the first trimester is worry about the pregnancy being noticed. Our therapists reported expending considerable energy within the group, scrutinizing members for signs that the latter had indeed detected the pregnancy. In each instance, the therapist made it clear that such detection at the time would be an untoward event. Their apprehension appeared to be rooted in the reality that group has a multiplicity of observers; detection by any one might result in the entire group's learning about the pregnancy. In this sense, the group therapist has a lesser degree of control than does the individual therapist over the entrance of the pregnancy into the therapy. Unlike the individual therapist, the group therapist lacks the luxury of individualizing the date on which each patient learns about the pregnancy. On a personal level, the group aspect of patients' detection of the pregnancy is likely to intensify group therapists' sense of exposure.

Whereas in the first trimester group therapists worry about whether members will discover the pregnancy, in the second trimester their concern shifts to the optimal way in which to announce the pregnancy. Despite the anxiety over the moment in which the pregnancy was revealed, therapists described considerable relief once the announcement was made. As the comments of one therapist suggest, the secret of the pregnancy is experienced as a considerable burden.

Vignette 10.1
I was surprised they were surprised. I thought I was bulging, although I did wear clothes to cover it up. I was probably relieved. I really wanted to let [it]

out in December but I didn't. One colleague almost admonished me. She said that there is more information to gain if I would let members discover it on their own.

Group therapists often experience relief that members do not have a response to their pregnancies that is more sustained or negative. For example, one therapist said she was glad to have her expectation that members would "throw a fit" disconfirmed. Another therapist said she was pleased that the group returned to "business as usual" as quickly. However, as we will discuss, therapists have second thoughts about their eagerness to dispense so quickly with members' reactions to their pregnancies.

When group members do greet their therapists' news with signs of hostility, the former feel considerable distress, and especially so when the negative appears to be a whole group response. Specific responses to members' hostility are guilt over having abandoned members and irritation that members refused to share their happiness.

As noted previously, therapists frequently see group members as having very joyous and caregiving responses toward their therapists at this time. Group therapists have reactions to their group members in kind. One therapist leading an inpatient adolescent group expressed her pleasure in the following way, "I felt very warmed, loved by them." This therapist was similar to others in suggesting that the discovery of pregnancy provided an opportunity to be nurtured by the group members. Another therapist reflected the gratification possible in being a focus of the group, "I was fine. I felt special and a good part of that was the attention I received. I felt no discomfort or need to hide the pregnancy." Although our participants did not happen to express this sentiment, others such as DiPesa (2013) have noted that members' efforts to care for the group therapist can create challenges for the latter. DiPesa relates the anecdote of one group therapist who was interrupted in her effort to provide an educational lesson in a group psychotherapy session in Veterans' Hospital because one of the members was fearful that when the therapist stood at the blackboard, the boots she wore might destabilize her.

In the last trimester, group psychotherapists are both similar to and different from their individual psychotherapy counterparts. They are like individual psychotherapists in showing a return to the intense self-focusing that therapists observed in themselves in the first trimester. Multiple physical complaints, a felt inability to brook members' reactions to their pregnancies, and a yearning to be ensconced in the next phase of their lives led therapists to absent themselves from the group.

Group psychotherapists reported needing to make a variety of alterations in order to remain comfortable within the long therapy sessions. For example, one therapist needed to go to the bathroom during the group session. This behavior flew in the face of the group rule that once the session began, no member could leave. Another therapist put her feet up on another chair. Although individual therapists make many of these same accommodations, the clinical literature suggests that they are less fettered by worries of the appropriateness of these accommodations. These behaviors seemed to cause group therapists more consternation than they did their individual therapy counterparts because they are so thoroughly at odds with the group norms that the therapists had carefully cultivated.

The Maternity Leave

Our group psychotherapists were surprised at the extent to which they thought about the group members during their leaves. At times, the thoughts were of a positive nature. More typically, however, therapists worried about specific members or the group-as-a-whole, as seen in the next vignette:

> **Vignette 10.2**
> I was wondering if the group would keep going because it seemed attendance was dropping. I also wondered how they were connecting with the new co-leader. In retrospect, I think I would've tried to choose a person who is more compatible with me. I was concerned whether they would like it better without me or drop out. I was feeling insecure.

The therapist's apprehension about the survival of the group was common, as was her worry over her own survival as a leader (would they choose the other therapist over her?). Some therapists expressed a sense of urgency about getting back to the group lest it disintegrate altogether. This is a fear that seems to be greater for therapists with respect to their groups relative to their individual patients. Whereas a decision of an individual patient to end therapy affects only him or her, the decision of a group member affects the entire group and through a process of contagion can undermine the group's existence.

GROUP REFORMATION

During the early period of their return, group therapists suffered fatigue due to interrupted sleep and anxiety caused by the demand to juggle diverse responsibilities. Still, they saw themselves as having enhanced abilities to attend to and grasp their group members' reactions. For example, the leader of an outpatient group for incest survivors made the following comment: "I didn't feel anything special physically but emotionally I felt different. I was more open, less defended, more emotional, felt feelings more deeply." This heightened awareness is consistent with the observations of Fenster et al.'s (1986) individual therapists, who saw themselves as having a greater capacity for empathy due to their new maternal roles. Also, like Fenster et al.'s therapists, our interviewees saw themselves as having sensitivity to particular concerns that were directly relevant to their own life situation as new members. For example, one therapist said she was "more sensitive to the failures of the mother–child relationship."

Although our group psychotherapists took delight in the enhancement of their therapeutic skills, they also tended to feel vulnerable during the early portion of this new phase. Some therapists feel it is no longer their group; others observe that members look to them less for help. One of our therapists said, "My members were now used to the other leader. I felt that my role had been filled." To lessen feelings of insecurity and to re-assert their presence, some therapists become extremely active in the group. For example, one therapist remarked, "In the first session, I noticed myself being more active . . . It was my way of trying to re-integrate myself. I was trying too hard. I realized it and tried to lay back a little."

The Co-therapy Relationship

Unlike individual therapy, the group psychotherapist often functions as a member of a therapy team. To understand the group psychotherapist's experience of her pregnancy as it affects her work fully, it is necessary to examine both the therapist's relationship to her co-therapist during and after the pregnancy, and the vicissitudes in members' relationships to the co-therapist. For ease of exposition, the *therapist* is the pregnant member of the team whereas the *co-therapist* is the non-pregnant therapist. However, this terminology does not presume that the therapist was necessarily in the senior position.

Based on the interviewees' responses, the therapist's pregnancy appeared to affect positively the co-therapy relationship. Therapists felt nurtured by their co-therapists who, as the pregnancy progressed, took an increasingly active role in the group. Moreover, for the co-therapy team, an enhanced sense of effectiveness during the course of the pregnancy emerged as therapists saw that together, they were able to handle the challenges that the pregnancy posed. Along these lines, one therapist commented, "We are close and have had great success running groups. This just showed us how well we work together."

In contrast, the maternity leave seems to produce more complex changes. From the standpoint of the co-therapist, as perceived by the therapist, frustration and anger attend the extra work and burdens of managing the group alone. For instance, one therapist who was in a co-therapy team treating a very large group of severely disturbed members said, "By the time I returned, she was fried. She was a little angry but I understood. We both knew what was going on and it [her anger] was not the problem. That is why I came back early." At the same time, the co-therapist saw the opportunity to take a more active role as satisfying, particularly when that co-therapist was in the junior position. However, this greater satisfaction also led to disappointment on the return of the therapist.

The group's relationship with the co-therapist appears to change in ways that are less complex than their relationship with the therapist. Our interviewees observed that for the most part, the relationship with the co-therapist was strengthened as a function of the co-therapist's running the group during the therapist's absence. This enhanced relationship manifested itself in members' relying more on the co-therapist during crises and verbalizing a greater feeling of closeness to the co-therapist. The members and co-therapist became a subgroup, banding together perhaps in part to lessen feelings of sadness in relation to an abandoning and preoccupied therapist. Occasionally, the relationship with the co-therapist and the group moved in a negative direction. This less common effect occurred when the group had intense anger toward the therapist at the time she departed for her maternity leave. The co-therapist, in such a circumstance, seemed to be used as a displacement object.

Intervention Considerations

Many of the intervention issues that pregnant group therapists face are highlighted in the following vignette.

> **Vignette 10.3**
> Dr. Herbert, conducting a young adolescent group in a residential treatment center, told her group about her pregnancy in her fifth month. To her astonishment, she discovered that everyone knew about or suspected the pregnancy, except for two particularly isolated youths. One group member who had overheard staff talking had informed five of the other members. Another member said for some time, she thought the therapist looked pregnant, but recognized the therapist's altered appearance could be due to a mere weight gain. She did not want to risk mentioning her suspicion and potentially embarrassing the therapist.
>
> In the weeks that followed, group members focused on the pregnancy only occasionally. Members asked Dr. Herbert about the birth process and she shared information with them readily. Some of the members associated the pregnancy with recollections of their siblings' births. Dr. Herbert was gratified that the group members could talk about feelings of confusion and even hostility vis-à-vis their siblings, which they had not expressed earlier in the group. A month before she left on her maternity leave, members discussed the possibility of the co-therapist running the group. Dr. Herbert noticed the members' increased crankiness toward the co-therapist, but the manifestations of it were so subtle that the therapist commented on it neither to the group nor the co-therapist. Prior to her departure, members brought presents for the baby. She expressed gratitude, and a feeling of joy pervaded the group at the time of her departure.

Many of the therapists we interviewed would see this group as resembling ones they had led in several ways. The therapist engaged in minimal processing of the pregnancy with the group. Many therapists we interviewed also saw themselves as exploring their pregnancy with their group members only superficially, and they believed this neglect was to the detriment of their groups. Although like Dr. Herbert, our participants saw themselves as pursuing pregnancy-related themes, they did not feel they had attended sufficiently to the more subtle manifestations of reactions to the pregnancy, especially ones that could lead to the direct discussion of members' relationship with Dr. Herbert. In their retrospective evaluations of the pregnancy period, our participants felt that had they been more active in pursuing pregnancy-related material, especially members' more negatively tinged reactions, the members would have derived some unique benefit relating to this very special circumstance. Some therapists even felt that the acting out that occurred during their maternity leaves could have lessened had they been more encouraging of members' communication of negative reactions during their pregnancies. Our interviewees would have resonated with Dr. Herbert's failure to consider that any of the negative reactions being directed toward the co-therapist were in fact meant for her.

From an intervention standpoint, the task of the group therapist may be more difficult than that of the individual therapist. Our research shows that in a group, members are less likely than they are in individual therapy to come forth with negative reactions. They are also more likely to exhibit the pronatalist stance that is a reflection of the larger societal value of pregnancy. Therefore, the group therapist may need to exert herself considerably to see the indirect expressions of negative reactions and to respond to them with both alacrity and sensitivity.

A pregnant group therapist's decision making in the group might be beneficially influenced by a consideration of what actions on her part will promote the exploration of pregnancy-related member reactions. One major decision any pregnant group therapist must make is when to announce the pregnancy, and the considerations are somewhat different than in individual therapy. Dr. Herbert discovered that most of the members already knew she was pregnant. The fact that some members were privy to what other members were not created somewhat of an in-group versus out-group situation. Such a split, if unaddressed, can undermine a group's cohesion. Moreover, our research shows that it is not unusual, particularly when a group takes place in a larger treatment context, for members to hear about the pregnancy before the therapist announces it. Members' sensitivity to the possibility of embarrassing or invading the therapist's privacy leads them to suppress the communication of their knowledge. Therefore, once again, the therapist might need to assume a more active posture in seeking out hidden or indirect manifestations of members' detection of the therapist's pregnancy. The decision about the timing of the announcement should also take into account the other ways in which members could learn about the pregnancy. Generally, it is better for the therapist to apprise members of the pregnancy in a formal way than for them to hear of it informally from other staff, because such a formal announcement provides members the greatest latitude to explore their reactions.

Another therapist decision is when to announce the concrete plans for departure. Again, a number of our participants felt that they had not given group members sufficient notice of the particulars of their maternity leaves. Even if Dr. Herbert might have spurred more discussion by an earlier announcement, the more important element was the therapist's willingness to facilitate members in bringing to light the full range of their reactions. Nonetheless, had the therapist been more committed to processing these reactions, the 4-week period might have been constricting.

A third issue concerns the gifts given to the therapist by group members. Half of our therapists received baby gifts from members and among them, nearly half were presented with a gift by the entire group. Like Dr. Herbert, most of our participants accepted the gifts in an unquestioning way. Subsequently, none of our therapists expressed regret for accepting the presents. What several therapists questioned, however, was their abandonment of an exploratory attitude toward the gift. They felt that the presents did have unarticulated meanings to members and they could have assisted them in examining those meanings without diminishing the joy attached to their gift giving. Caught in the moment, the therapists seemed to see as their only alternatives exploration and rejection of the gift versus unexamined acceptance. Later, they realized that exploration could accompany the gift's acceptance.

The recommendation from our participants is clear. The pregnant therapist should foster within herself a willingness to help members reflect on all of their diverse reactions to her pregnancy. Although many factors may lead the therapist to shrink from responding in an exploratory rather than purely supportive way at this time, her adoption of a gently investigative posture will enable members to engage in valuable learning about themselves. In order to engage in such an exploration, members need time. Providing them with essential information about the unfolding of events well in advance of when they will occur supports members' exploratory efforts. For those groups in which a substitute therapist is used,[4] it is ideal if members can meet him or her well in advance of the therapist's departure. In this way, members have a fund of experience, albeit limited, to process their specific reactions to this individual.

Family and Couple Therapy

Although the birth process is a significant aspect of family and a cause of much joy, sorrow and conflict, surprisingly little has been written on the therapist's pregnancy and its impact on family and couple therapy. Perhaps the dearth of literature is related to the relatively brief nature of much of family and couple therapy. That is, the therapeutic relationship might in some cases lack the degree of depth that a longer-term relationship does. Or perhaps the therapist functions somewhat differently in a family system than with groups or individuals, so that the traditional transference/countertransference questions and problems are not as evidently present. The therapist as a figure might be less focal in family and couple therapy relative to other modalities. In much of family therapy, the family members' reactions to each other are more important than their reactions to the therapist. Because the therapist's pregnancy is not what precipitated anyone's entrance into treatment, it remains peripheral in a more focused treatment despite the appreciation that it could potentially make salient the hurts that brought the family into treatment.

Despite the lack of attention to the pregnant therapist in the family and couple therapy literature, we believe an examination of how the therapist's pregnancy affects family and couple therapists, and their clients, is important. We were able to garner some impressions from those individual and group therapists we interviewed who also do family and couple work, and commented upon it. In thinking both about their responses and about the distinctiveness of these two forms of multi-person treatment, we conclude that the work of the pregnant therapist might be abetted by an understanding of *multi-directed partiality*, a term coined by contextual family therapists (Boszormenyi-Nagy, Grunebaum, & Ulrich, 1991; Boszormenyi-Nagy & Spark, 1984), which has been applied in a variety of multi-person psychotherapies (Curtis & Dixon, 2005; Fullerton, 2014; Trotzer, 2004). Multi-directed partiality requires the therapist to take each member of the family's point of view, including, at times, those of deceased persons. It refers to the therapist's empathy, fairness, expectations for change, interaction with and professional commitment to helping each member of the family over the course of the therapeutic process. Although the therapeutic interaction involves each family member's secretly hoping that change and responsibility will be required for others and not necessarily for him or her, the therapist must apply even-handedness in her technique of engaging the family in the change process. Although the therapist may appear from time to time to "side" with a single member of the family, the overall plan involves a give-and-take for all family members. To accomplish this stance, the therapist must feel a connection to and empathy for each of the family members (or members of the couple) and they for her.

Broad Patterns in Family Therapy

Both therapist and clients have distinctive reactions as a consequence of the therapist's pregnancy.

THERAPIST REACTIONS

As we have stated previously in this book, pregnancy ushers in a new developmental phase for the therapist, which is accompanied by deepened empathy and possibly an altered pattern of identifications with family members. The specific profile of these identifications varies depending on her own intrapsychic constellations and those of her clients. Some therapists feel a new empathy for parents struggling with difficult children (e.g. hyperactivity, behavioral problems), whereas others feel might feel more judgmental of the parents' caregiving and disciplinary styles. As one therapist remarked, "I was in sheer disbelief that parents could be so uncaring. I felt much less empathic than before the pregnancy to their plight." However, this position is likely to change after the therapist returns to her practice, having now experienced the sleepless nights and unending anxieties of balancing indulgence with the development of healthy habits; an understanding of and empathy for the parents' plights and struggles grows. As one mother observed:

> Before I had my son, I not infrequently advised parents on limit-setting, time-outs and other childrearing and couples' problems. It was based on my training and what I read. Once I had my son, I realized how simplistic my understanding of family life was and how very unrealistic many of my suggestions were. Now I feel so much less certain about the "rights" and "wrongs" of childrearing. I appreciate how difficult it is to make decisions about some of the problems. In retrospect, I see that I was initially more blaming of them and now I feel more able to highlight and build on whatever strengths they have.

For children, especially those who are young, pregnant family therapists generally have increased empathy. One therapist told us,

> I became more maternal. I melted when those kids would come into the room. I had Erickson on my mind the whole time when I was pregnant, thinking of trust versus mistrust and the struggles these kids would have over that issue.

Adolescents, on the other hand, frequently provoked in the therapist negative reactions as the therapist found herself very firmly ensconcing herself in the parents' shoes.

Although pregnancy can be a catalyst for the therapist's deeper appreciation of difficult aspects of family life, it can also catch the therapist unaware of her own identifications with various family members and their roles. Consider, for example, a therapist who has recently returned from a maternity leave seeing a family related to a 6-year-old daughter's school phobia. If she is feeling acutely the pain of leaving her infant daily, she may be prone to identify too closely with the mother and fail to encourage parents to perform the parental task of letting go (Akhtar, 2016b) by helping the child to work through her separation anxieties. Likewise, a therapist who is disappointed with her husband's participation in childcare might feel a displaced irritation toward the father in a family therapy session. Thus, knowledge of these new "identifications" will help insulate the treatment from unhealthy multi-directed partiality.

FAMILY MEMBER REACTIONS

Members of a family will vary in their reaction and accommodation to the pregnancy, and this multiplicity is likely to pull the therapist in different directions in her exploratory efforts. Clients who themselves are mothers might make assumptions about the therapist's stance based on the latter's burgeoning maternity. For example, when one pregnant therapist recommended a change in level of care from partial to inpatient treatment for a child in the family, the mother became angry, saying, "How could you? You're going to be a mother. How would you feel when somebody does this to your child?" Children often have reactions suggesting the activation of distress over the entrance of new siblings into their families. For example, a young child in a family therapy session in which the pregnant therapist announces the pregnancy might show destructive behaviors toward toys in the room or engage in loud verbalizations that interfere with adult exchanges.

Like group members, family members might attempt to protect the therapist by minimizing their own difficulties, particularly as the pregnancy progresses. In some cases, the exploration of this caretaking of the therapist could be extremely helpful to one or more of the family members because such protective efforts could be in response to the activation of long-standing views of parental figures as being weak or needful.

Broad Patterns in Couple Therapy

Whether the therapist treats cohabitating or married individuals, or persons in a heterosexual or same-sex relationship, the goal is to help alleviate clients' relationship distress (Snyder, Castellani, & Whisman, 2006).[5] From an attachment theory perspective (Schachner, Shaver, & Mikulincer, 2003), couples' achievement of romantic love constitutes an activation of three behavioral systems: attachment, caregiving and sex. The therapist's capacity to support the couple in addressing these areas might be crucially affected, for good or ill, by her pregnant state, and may be mediated by the therapist experiencing the couple through the lens of her pregnancy or the couple's reaction to the pregnancy.

THERAPIST REACTIONS

A challenge to a couple's achieving a satisfying relationship is a lack of attachment security (Schachner, Shaver, & Mikulincer, 2003). One or both members of the couple might have come to adulthood with an insecure attachment style that hinders their ability to fully engage and find satisfaction in their most significant relationships. When couples enter treatment, even as members are feeling dissatisfied with one another, the presence of an attuned therapist enables them to feel that their needs are being met. The therapist's provision of warmth and safety allows the couple to be open with one another and communicative, thereby allowing for the repair of attachment difficulties and increasing attachment security. As has been noted in attachment research, when individuals are moved into a more secure mental space, they are more receptive to information about their partners that is discrepant with the model constructed of those partners (e.g., Mikulincer & Arad, 1999).

The therapist's pregnancy might induce in her feelings that facilitate or undermine the couple's feelings of security. For example, she may experience a greater awareness of her clients' need to be held in the therapeutic relationship. Her awareness of the fragility of her own fetus could heighten her attentiveness to each partner's hurts and vulnerabilities, as can be seen in this next vignette.

Vignette 10.4

Dr. Esters had seen a couple following her discovery of a favorable amniocentesis report. Her anxiety had been extremely heightened by the experience, but she greeted the couple, two prospective lesbian mothers, with a sense of relief. In past but recent sessions, Amy, the biological mother of their 8-month-old daughter, complained that Susanna, the non-biological mother, was unnecessarily fretting upon being shut out of their relationship. In turn, Susanna had expressed hurt that Amy was engaging in behaviors to marginalize Susanna's maternal role. In those past sessions, Dr. Esters had found herself feeling more fully aligned with Amy, and even caught herself thinking that Susanna's reaction was self-indulgent. The amniocentesis brought to the fore Dr. Esters's awareness of loss, as she feared receiving information about the child's viability and likely health. This trying circumstance helped her to achieve greater flexibility in her identifications and enabled her to realize the genuine pain Susanna was experiencing. When she communicated her empathy for Susanna in the session, Susanna visibly relaxed and went on to talk about the stress Amy must feel in needing to satisfy their daughter's physical and psychological needs. Amy then urged Susanna not to defer to her in making moment-to-moment caregiving decisions and invited her to take more initiative. In the session, Amy and Susanna went on to have some playful exchanges with one another. Dr. Esters noticed that her enriched awareness of loss not only enabled her to be more supportive of the couple but also of how she might have minimized some of her husband's anxieties vis-à-vis his role as caregiver and attachment object.

Dr. Esters's use of her pregnancy to gain insight into her clients redounded upon her own well-being as she achieved greater understanding of her own relationship. We explore this potential in our last chapter. For the present, our primary point is that each step of the pregnancy activates a host of feelings and thoughts, the awareness of which can be used to create a more secure environment for a couple to explore their dynamics. Indeed, Dr. Esters achieved multi-directed partiality, enabling her to repair injuries, thereby decreasing stress and enhancing each partner's ability to show love for the other. However, this treatment could have progressed otherwise had Dr. Esters's intense reactions to the unfolding events of the amniocentesis caused her to retreat from an immersion in her work with the couple. It stands to reason that such a withdrawal would have fostered insecurity in the couple leading to a strengthening of the negative features of their working models of one another and the therapist, and the dysfunctional behaviors associated with those models.

In some cases, a facet of the pregnancy can foster in the therapist an unexamined identification that diminishes one party's sense of security in the treatment, as is seen in this example provided by one couple therapist.

> **Vignette 10.5**
> Shortly before I became pregnant, a couple that was pregnant with their second child was referred to me by the wife's individual therapist. The wife had suffered from long-standing dysthymia. The wife complained about her husband's lack of support with their first child and his physical absence with his long hours at work. He complained that he needed her to help him with the family business and felt emotionally abandoned when they had their first child. They worked together with me for several months with some modest gains. The husband was more available and participatory in family life and the wife did some organizing of aspects of the family business.
>
> After I announced my pregnancy, I felt much more camaraderie with the woman as she shared some of her knowledge about parenting with me. It was subtle at first, but as I neared the end of my pregnancy, I became aware that her husband had withdrawn from his participation in family life and in the session as well. His wife reported that she enjoyed coming to the sessions and seemed to have little awareness of her husband's absence at home. It was not until my pregnancy leave that this pattern became apparent when her individual therapist later told me that she had relapsed into a moderate depression.

Here, the therapist's unexplored identification with the woman hindered her from seeing how the current situation constituted a re-enactment of an old injury for the husband, leading him to engage in his customary withdrawal. Were the therapist to recognize her pregnancy as a potentially significant event for him, she might have helped him to plumb his own reactions in a way that might have catalyzed considerable psychological growth for him and for them as a couple.

CLIENT REACTIONS

For couples, the customary reaction to the therapist's pregnancy is likely to rest upon their own developmental stage as a couple. Young couples who are anticipating building a family may greet the therapist's pregnancy with particular excitement borne out of their identification with her. However, if the couple has been struggling to conceive or experienced multiple miscarriages (Gerber, 2016)—if indeed, conflicts related to fertility issues have brought them into therapy—then, the therapist's pregnancy is likely to induce pain. As noted previously, many clients will shrink from the expression of any negativity because of a fear that the therapist in her fragile state will be unable to bear it. Therefore, the therapist must be actively reassuring that she welcomes the exploration of the significance of her pregnancy for the couple and that she is sufficiently robust to participate in it.

For couples in the active phase of parenting, the pregnancy of the therapist sensitizes them to the common ground they have with her. However, as our preceding example suggests, the pattern of identifications can shift based upon this new information. The therapist must be sensitive to whether she is now being perceived as the demanding, preoccupied or fretful partner, and how she can helpfully contain these projections, and create an environment in which they can be re-owned by one or both of the parties. As in the case of group members, members of the couple may see in the therapist's pregnancy the opportunity to bestow upon her their own wisdom and practical suggestions, a sharing that frequently has an esteem-boosting effect on clients.

For elderly couples, the therapist's pregnancy could provide an opportunity to reminisce about their own parenting experiences. In some cases, regrets might surface over their own parenting shortcomings. The therapist would do well to be attuned to parents' comparing—to their detriment—an idealized view of the therapist-as-parent with their own real-life experiences. However, in general, elderly individuals tend to have a positive response to the therapist's pregnancy (Herrin, 2001) and, as in the case of middle-aged couples, this response often takes the form of nurturing efforts vis-à-vis the therapist. Moreover, the therapist's slower pace as the pregnancy advances may lead the couple to feel more in synchrony with her from a kinesthetic standpoint (Herrin, 2001).

Couples who have chosen to be childless, regardless of their age, might see the therapist's pregnancy through the lens of the stigma commonly associated with their life choice. Commonly, individuals who elect not to procreate and rear children are subjected to negative judgments by pronatalist societies that see parenting as an imperative for married individuals. The therapist's pregnancy can easily be construed as a reproach of their decision. As the pregnancy progresses, the couple may progressively see the therapist as not being in their camp. For older couples that are involuntarily childless, the therapist's pregnancy might activate particular regrets such as the woman's putting off childrearing to pursue a career. Indeed, Sives's (2014) research shows that involuntary childlessness presents a set of losses to a couple, and the pain associated with them has great staying power due, in part, to its hidden character. A therapist's sensitivity to this source of suffering could provide the couple a unique opportunity to explore it, thereby potentially lessening its hold.

Adoptive Parents and Biological Fathers in Multi-person Therapies

We classify adoptive parents and non-adoptive fathers together in this section because of one feature that they share: the child does not physically enter the treatment room as does the child of a pregnant therapist. Consequently, during the expectancy period, these parents-to-be have much greater discretion concerning whether and what to disclose about the entrance of the child into the family. However, some differences are present among them. Particularly for those expectant parents who pursue international adoption, typically a hiatus from the group is necessary as the adopting parents emigrate the child and install him or her in the family. The therapist faces the task of what to tell either group members or participants in family or couples therapy as to why the therapist's extended absence is occurring. In a setting in which members have been encouraged to share their thoughts, feelings and fantasies about the therapist, speculation about the reasons for the absence are likely to be shared. For example, some patients will wonder whether the therapist is confronting a health issue. Without being apprised of the reality of the therapist's situation, patients may enter the period of separation from the therapist with a high level of anxiety. Such a prospect is likely to compel the therapist in the direction of disclosure. Still, the issues of when to disclose and how much to disclose remain.

Both authors of this text had the experience of disclosing an adoption plan to a group. In consistency with the literature on group members' reactions to the therapists' pregnancies, group members had reactions that were far less intense than those of individual therapy clients. Any expression of the typical themes of abandonment, envy, and competition were muted. Their reactions often seemed to be informed by stereotypic notions concerning adoption. For example, members construed the therapists' pursuing adoption as motivated by altruism, an interpretation that was proffered by no individual therapy patient. It was as if in the group, broad societal notions about biological versus adoptive families shaped the interactions, whereas in the individual situation, the specific dynamics of the therapist–patient relationship held sway. Indeed, group members may articulate notions about adoption that the therapist experiences as manifestations of *adoptism* (Steinberg & Hall, 2000), the notion that non-biological family connections are somehow less valuable than biological connections. Such occurrences might evoke in the therapist a range of negative emotions. The group members may also embrace the notion of the virtuousness of the therapist as a means of avoiding the possibility that the therapist is infertile (of course, it might also be the case that her partner is infertile). The virtuous therapist could extend her giving spirit to the group members, whereas the infertile therapist might not have the necessary resources—that is, be enough of a woman in their eyes—to mother the group properly.

Three of the fathers in our sample conducted psychotherapy groups. They indicated that they did not share news about their partners' pregnancies. Nonetheless, one therapist felt that the members sensed that the father was awaiting a baby. For example, he reported that the members seemed more disposed to look at the male–female co-therapy team as a parental dyad. At the most pragmatic level, men tend not to announce the arrival of the child because it is not demanded by the situation. Looking a little more deeply, however, we might consider the possibility that for the father, the introduction of this personal element may seem gratuitous, that is, sharing an aspect of one's life that ostensibly has nothing to do with the group. It is perhaps out of this sense that many male therapists recoil from doing so. Worry about overstimulating members with evocative personal information might be particularly great when the therapist is working with group members functioning at the borderline level who easily become dysregulated (Karterud, 2015). An alternative explanation, however, emerges from the observation that male therapists respond somewhat similarly to male patients to the imminent arrival of the child. Although research (Lecours, Bouchard, & Normandin, 1995) has pointed to stylistic differences between male and female therapists, whether they are operative in this circumstance is yet to be determined. Guy, Guy and Liaboe (1986) share their important observation that frequently, patients have multiple routes to finding out that the therapist is expecting a child. For example, one patient was able to make this discernment merely on changes she discerned in the therapist's interventions. By not inviting patients' reactions, the male therapist may be consigning patients to bear their burden silently.

Two of the three fathers did not take off any sessions after the baby was born; one was absent for two sessions. In terms of how the fathers felt after the baby was born, one father observed, "Initially, I was very tired—up a lot. Tended to be a little less crisp because of fatigue . . . There were times I would've rather been at home. The fatigue lasted over a year." The other two fathers noticed no particular reaction in their work life. In addressing what was most difficult, one father said that he ran a men's group and felt disappointment that the members seemed unresponsive to his changed status. In particular, he thought it would be a stimulus for them to talk about unresolved conflicts about having children, but this did not occur. Another interesting circumstance was a man who was leading a group of gay men with a gay co-therapist. He, however, was heterosexual. After his return, the other therapist announced to the group that he was a new father. In that discussion, it came out that he was straight. This therapist felt the announcement should have been collaboratively and carefully arranged given that the revelation of his sexual orientation had very significant implications for his work in the group.

Practical Implications

- The modality makes a difference: the therapist should not expect the same responses from clients in multi-person therapy as in individual therapy.
- Although in group psychotherapy as in individual therapy, the therapist might be tempted to avoid particular boundary crossings such as gift giving, patients may be deprived an opportunity to engage in important discoveries if the therapist takes a completely non-interpretive stance.
- To maximize learning and minimize acting out, members should be given as much time as possible to adapt to changes that the therapist anticipates.

- If a substitute therapist is engaged, the group should have an opportunity to meet that individual well before the therapist's departure.
- The therapist's pregnancy is especially evocative in couple and family therapy given that the therapist is in the process of building a family. Hence, it should serve as a potent stimulus for deeper and broader work.
- Adoptive parents and biological fathers may see a more muted response from groups, couples and families relative to the reactions to pregnant therapists. This does not mean that palpable reactions that have significance for the client are not present.

Notes

1. Freud wrote about acting out in 1914 with respect to repeating versus remembering. He defined acting out as the expression of affect or conflict entailing a motor discharge that serves the individual defensively, in that he or she remains unaware of the unconscious conflictual material. Contemporary use has widened "motoric discharge" to include more complex social interactions.
2. This latter finding was included in our study because of Breen's (1997) observation that a distinctive feature of male participation in the group at this time is their production of considerable content related to same-sex attraction. Later accounts emphasized men's production of increased sexual content in general. Our questionnaire did not encompass this possibility, but we hope those developed for future studies do.
3. Some therapists did, indeed, bring their babies to the group, but this was generally in the case of adolescent groups.
4. One advantage of using a substitute therapist is that it provides an opportunity for a consultation on the group. Each therapist has a unique perspective on and reactions to group members and the group process. The long-term therapist can learn from the substitute therapist's observations. For this advantage to be maximally realized, the leave-taking therapist should think about it in this way.
5. We do not deal in this section with types of couple therapy other than romantic adult relationships.

CHAPTER 11

Expectant Parents' Relationships With Peers, Supervisors and the Workplace

All mental health professionals operate within a network or community of professionals. In some instances, this network is well defined, as in the case of a therapist who does her work in a residential treatment center in collaboration with other members of the treatment team. In other instances, the network is more amorphous, as in the circumstance of the private practitioner who may depend on other professionals for referrals and collaboration on specific cases. Regardless of the nature of the network, we argue that to fully grasp the dynamics of the psychotherapeutic process between patient and expectant parent during and following the arrival of the child, one must understand the therapist's relationship with her professional context during this period.

A Theoretical Framework

General systems theory (GST) (von Bertalanffy, 1966) provides a useful framework for understanding the relationships between the pregnant therapist and her professional network. According to GST, any social system can be described as existing within a series of infinitely larger supersystems, and having embedded within it a series of infinitely small subsystems. Hence, the therapist–patient unit would be embedded in a larger social system such as the patient and staff community on a particular hospital unit, which is in turn embedded in the larger unit of the hospital. Both the therapist—in our case, the expectant therapist—and the patients themselves constitute social systems whose members might be considered to be the various psychological forces that operate within each.

A fundamental tenet of systems theory is that the nested systems within any hierarchy have boundaries that are permeable to one another, leading to a constant ingress and egress of information from one system to another. A change in one system will then reverberate to the other systems within a series of systems. Consequently, dynamics related to the therapist's expectant status that enter the therapist's and patient's intrapsychic also permeate the patient–therapist relationship, and ultimately, the treatment system in which the relationship exists.

Likewise, dynamics within the treatment system seep into the patient–therapist relationship. Hence, any adequate analysis of the effects of the therapist's status as a prospective parent must be bidirectional, looking at how broader system dynamics affect those of the patient and therapist and vice versa.

The literature has focused almost exclusively on the pregnant therapist in her workplace, to the neglect of other expectancy conditions. Within the literature on the pregnant therapist, different writers on this topic have emphasized one system or another as having a causal role in how other systems in the hierarchy handle the therapist's status. For example, Baum and Herring (1975) described the power of the pregnant therapist's own dynamics in influencing how the broader treatment environment regarded the pregnancy. Butts and Cavenar (1979) provided a counterpoint to the Baum and Herring analysis:

> We do not believe that the interpersonal conflicts are, in most cases, the result of the manner in which the pregnant resident reacts to her colleagues and supervisors; rather, we suggest that intrapsychic conflicts may be generated in the pregnant resident as a result of peer reactions to her.
>
> (p. 1587)

From a general systems theory perspective, one would expect to see each level of the hierarchy as affecting other levels. Certainly the broader system's stance toward accommodating those needs rooted in staff members' personal lives is going to affect stress, vulnerability to developing an array of symptoms, physical and psychological, and interpersonal behaviors at work. By the same token, however, a therapist who manifests great trepidation about the viability of balancing and integrating the professional and personal aspects of her life probably will shape the setting's reaction to her pregnancy. Suppose a staff member is frequently late for work because of morning sickness but has a personal motto of keeping "private things private." Other staff then might question her commitment. The ultimate discovery of her pregnancy may do little to alleviate their irritation. This reciprocal relationship undoubtedly exists not only for pregnancy but also for all forms of expectant parenting. In the sections that follow, we attempt to understand better this reciprocal relationship and focus on a relationship of particular importance: the supervisory relationship.

The Dynamics of the Setting

Settings in which mental health professionals work vary greatly in their ways of responding to individuals who are expecting to introduce a child into their lives. Although we characterize responses as adaptive and maladaptive, we do not assume that a particular setting easily falls into one category or another. The setting in which an expectant parent is showered with well wishes might be the same setting in which expectant parents are reprimanded for making adjustments to their schedule to fulfill family needs. Nonetheless, in a broad way, organizations can be characterized as having a fundamentally supportive or adaptive stance versus an undermining or maladaptive stance to this life transition.

Adaptive Institutional Responses

When an organization's response is fundamentally adaptive, four features characterize it. First, the transition to parenthood is broadly perceived as an event of major significance in the life of the mental health professional, an event having major ramifications for the therapist's work prior to and following the arrival of the child.

Second, the climate of the organization is such that different feelings toward the expectant parent can be safely expressed and that a balance in the expression of both positive and negative feelings is achieved. Typically, people will express joyful feelings. Staff who already have children may take delight in the happiness that awaits the expectant parent. Staff members who yearn for children might identify with the expectant parent's success and feel greater hopefulness about their own circumstances. One of our psychologist interviewees told us how she had often felt that prior to her pregnancy, she was met with aloofness by the psychiatrists within her institution. Then, during her pregnancy, many of these same individuals took initiative in speaking with her with surprising cordiality. For example, they shared stories about their own children. Generally, negative reactions will also be present. For some co-workers, seeing another's success in building a family might beget sorrow and envy, especially for those who have suffered long-standing deprivation in this area. Worries about how work relationships will change, based on the expectant parent's new status, might be stimulated. Fears about what slack co-workers will need to pick up for the expectant parent could be engendered.

Third, the expectant parent's work responsibilities during the period leading up to the arrival of the child are modified appropriately. Such modifications are often necessitated by pregnancy, but also by other expectancy conditions. The prospective father may have to devote more time to care for his firstborn as his wife is placed on bedrest during her second pregnancy. Prospective parents who are adopting internationally might need to spend considerable time abroad. The flexibility the work site demonstrates at this time might be reflective of the same quality once the parent returns from parental leave and has the ongoing responsibility of juggling work and home. Research has shown that this organizational flexibility is a major contributor to such important factors as marital satisfaction after the birth of a child (e.g., Tomlinson & Irwin, 1993) and the woman's balanced sense of herself as both an employee and a mother (Fursman, 2002). Fourth, preparations are made for the prospective parent's leave well in advance of parental leave. When these four features are present, the organization can both fulfill its goal of providing services and safeguard the well-being of the expectant parent and the other employees with whom he or she works.

Common Maladaptive Institutional Patterns

Yet, many organizations do not achieve this gold standard. From the literature and from our own data, we delineate four institutional response patterns, all having in common the creation of a stressful and even toxic environment for the expectant parent. These features are not ones that are not unique to therapeutic contexts; rather, they have been observed in a great range of work environments (Gross & Pattison, 2007). What we point out are some common ways these trends manifest in the settings in which therapists commonly work.

Denial and Minimization

Within the workplace, a particularly common response pattern is denial and minimization (Hennekam, 2016). These processes operate on a general level when those in the setting act as if transitions to parenthood, most especially pregnancies, do not occur. This phenomenon is especially prominent when the setting is dependent for service delivery on psychology interns, psychiatric residents and other therapists in training. Often in interviews for training programs, the notion is advanced that the trainee's personal life should recede during the training period. Reciprocally, some prospective trainees are reluctant to inquire at the interview about the policies an organization has regarding parental leave out of fear that such queries may lessen their desirability to the setting.

Attempts to discourage new parenting responsibilities do not seem especially successful. For example, in Auchincloss' (1982) second postgraduate year, 3 of the 12 residents (half of the women) became pregnant. Baum and Herring (1975) reported that at their institution, out of 20 female residents, 35% became pregnant over the course of their residency. Moreover, we have noted large number of pregnancies among the psychology interns and psychiatric residents whom we have supervised. We have also seen a high percentage of male trainees transition to fatherhood. Therefore, it would seem that the transition to parenthood is *de rigueur* for trainees.

The neglect of sites to do any planning in relation to this likely occurrence (such as identifying additional personnel who can be tapped during the therapist's maternity leave) represents a form of institutional denial that sets the stage for innumerable difficulties. Among these difficulties is the great likelihood that additional work demands will befall the existing staff, leading to greater internecine tensions (Hilty et al., 2005; Tinsley, 2000). In some instances, the burden on other staff can be sufficiently great to compromise their satisfaction with their work. Also, such institutional denial creates a context in which staff fail to recognize when patients are reacting, implicitly or explicitly, to the therapist's life transition. In being unassisted with their responses, patients are deprived of the opportunity to learn from them and are vulnerable to enacting them within the treatment. Benedek (1973) describe the case of staff being surprised and confused at reactions of an adolescent girl who began to speak about "wild sexual exploits, missed menstrual periods and breast engorgement" (p. 367) following her recognition of the pregnancy of her therapist. Rather than making the connection between the therapist's pregnancy and the patient's thought content, the staff initially and incorrectly conjectured that the patient herself must be pregnant.

Denial occurs on a more individual level when, following the announcement of the imminent arrival of a child, staff act as if nothing of significance has happened. Denial can be particular dramatic in relation to the pregnant therapist. Even as staff offer warm congratulations, they might proceed to make no modifications in her work expectations. For example, Branchey (1983) described the following behavior of hospital administrators during her pregnancy, "Their reaction was to schedule me to be on night call and to take me to give a grand rounds presentation a few days before the expected delivery date" (pp. 135–136). One manifestation of denial is staff members' ignoring the work hazards present for the pregnant therapist, requiring a protective response on her part. One of the authors encountered denial when she found that in her seventh month of pregnancy, staff had difficulty fathoming why she would be reluctant to work with a newly admitted inpatient who had a history of assaulting staff. For expectant fathers, the absence of the kind of physical stimulus that pregnancy provides allows denial to exert itself more tenaciously, particularly if the father himself makes little of the impending event. Moreover, gender-based assumptions about childcare, and by extension, preparation for childcare might be seen as exclusively the expectant mother's province. Adoptive parents are also especially likely to encounter a work setting's blindness to their transitional needs.

Therapists are not alone in obtaining this type of response to their life transition. In fact, in other types of practice, staff denial can be even greater. Matozzo (1999) interviewed 10 psychologists, all of whom were therapists, and 9 physicians, none of whom was a psychiatrist. Most of the psychologists saw the first trimester as being the most difficult, whereas physicians experienced the third trimester as the most demanding. Perhaps physicians have greater physical demands than psychologists, thereby making the third trimester more arduous for the former. The physicians noted that a primary stressor during the third trimester was the response of administration and colleagues toward their advanced pregnancies. The expectation of other professionals, they noted, was that their work be minimally affected by their pregnancies. In fact, one physician reported that when she was 7 months pregnant, she continued to work although her amniotic fluid was low. She acted against the medical advice she received because of her conviction that not to do so would jeopardize her standing in the work environment. The literature (e.g., Bergström et al., 2009; Hemp, 2004) has coined this phenomenon *presenteeism*, the behavior of being in the workplace when common sense would dictate otherwise. It is the opposite of absenteeism. Although presenteeism can be rooted in the dynamics of the present person, it can also be attached to the dynamics of the settings, as in this case.

A final manifestation of denial is when the staff within the site urge the therapist to promote denial in her dealings with her patients. For example, Grossman (1990) reported how one pregnant therapist was instructed by her boss not to reveal her pregnancy to her patients until she was "beginning to show." The therapist said, "to have to keep it sort of secret until this other person felt it was okay was very unnatural" (p. 66).

Hostility and Sadism

A second pattern is related to the first and is suggested by the prior examples: the direct or indirect expression of hostile or sadistic impulses toward the expectant therapist. These trends are related in that when the social environment denies or minimizes the impact of the expectancy, it fails to accommodate itself to the special needs of this individual and thereby imposes undue hardship on him or her. Therefore, denial might sometimes work in the service of hostility. However, despite efforts to mask it, hostility might appear quite clearly. For example, Butts and Cavenar (1979) described the reactions to an obviously pregnant resident's oral presentation of her work with a psychotic adolescent in an intensive psychotherapy. Members of the group were in agreement that the case should be transferred immediately because the pregnancy would "drive him crazy" (p. 1588). The pregnancy was likened to the stimulus of a therapist "who might have his right arm missing; it can't be missed" (p. 1588). Notably, the supervisor who had been working on this case did not share this view. Unsurprisingly, the therapist felt considerable distress following the conference as well as confusion about whether to work with the patient. Her relationships with the other conference attendees were strained for some time thereafter. While Butts and Cavenar focused on other aspects of the group's response, we were struck by the group's effort to inflict hurt by making the therapist feel damaged by virtue of her pregnancy. However, in other cases, the hostility will be more modulated as when residents of a training program complain that the pregnant therapist is obtaining too much special consideration (McLaren, 2008).

Sometimes, the hostility is rooted in a view that the therapist is not entitled to have a child. This is particularly true for trainees who might be expected to devote all of their attention to training (Finch, 2003; Walsh, Gold, Jensen, & Jedrzkiewicz, 2005). Baum and Itzhaky (2006) interviewed five social work supervisors in five different Israeli social welfare agencies. The supervisors expressed a great deal of negative affect toward their pregnant supervisees. A common theme in the supervisors' narrative material was that the supervisee had misplaced priorities—she was building a family at a time when she should have been focusing on learning to become a social worker. This view also extends to new hires, who can be seen as having put into the organization an insufficient amount of time to warrant any special consideration. As Gross and Pattison (2010) point out, hostility from older co-workers can be rooted in envy related to accommodations that may be available to prospective parents in today's work culture that were unavailable to them.

In Baum and Itzhaky's (2006) previously mentioned study, supervisor hostility was also based on the supervisors' perceptions that the supervisee had waited too long to share the fact of the pregnancy with the supervisor. These investigators suggest that because the supervisee ordinarily shares material of a private nature with the supervisor in order to better accomplish her clinical work, the withholding of the news of the pregnancy violates the supervisor's expectations of closeness in the relationship.

Over-Solicitude

A third pattern of response, over-solicitude, occurs oftentimes in reaction to the aforementioned hostility and sadism and is seen most conspicuously in response to pregnancy relative to other pre-parenting conditions. As we have previously noted, within Euro-American cultures, the manifestation of positive responses toward a woman's pregnancy is strongly expected. Staff members are often placed in a conflictual situation between the urge to express a feeling and to avoid the reprobation that violating a cultural norm brings. They may also be inclined to defend against hostility because often, pregnant women are perceived as warmer than others in the workplace (Masser, Grass & Nesic, 2007), and this benevolent persona might make these especially objectionable as targets for hostility. Along the same lines, the pregnant staff member may be a symbol for staff members' early caregivers, figures toward whom the expression of hostility might also have been unacceptable. Finally, the therapist herself may discourage expressions of hostility, thereby placing a demand on the patient to adopt a defensive strategy in relation to it.

The compromise formation solution is often the expression of exaggerated solicitude toward the pregnant woman, a defensive maneuver that expresses both sides of the conflict. On the one hand, positive sentiment is expressed; on the other, discomfort is generated in the recipient. Butts and Cavenar (1979) described an example of this interactional pattern in a supervisor's behavior toward a supervisee:

> When the resident became pregnant, the supervisor experienced a flood of feelings and many dreams about the pregnancy. He felt angry and betrayed, yet patronizing and protective toward her. He was aware of his special efforts to make everything easier for the resident: this was a reaction formation against underlying hostile impulses. The supervisor's patronizing attitude was to the resident's detriment: as he regressed because of his own conflicts and expected less performance from the resident, she regressed and performed less well.
>
> (p. 1588)

Another form this over-solicitude faces is unwanted advice from others who describe normative ways of balancing home and work while being insensitive to the pregnant woman's desire to find balance in her own way (Hennekam, 2016).

Pregnancy Preoccupation

A fourth pattern contrasts strikingly with the prior three, but can sometimes coexist with the others. Often, the pregnancy generates an excitement that is quite intense but without the forced quality of the enthusiasm based on reaction formation. Gross and Pattison (2007) write about how the intense focus of many upon individual women's pregnancies might be due, in part, to the fact that pregnancies are no longer commonplace. With the falling birthrate, individuals encounter fewer and fewer people in their environments who are in this state. Consequently, it truly is something special.

In some instances, this response may reveal what Bion (1959) identified as a *basic assumption pairing group*. It occurs when a group (in this case, the staff) has an unconscious fantasy that a Messiah, in this case, the therapist's baby, will rescue it from its difficulties and woes. Auchincloss (1982) reported a possible activation of such a basic assumption group in her residency training group. The members of the group were excited about one resident's pregnancy but implicitly refused to address the practical difficulties it created. Auchincloss (1982) hypothesized that the "Messianic fantasy protected the group members from the dangerous competitive feelings, dependency needs and repression that threaten all beginning psychiatric trainees" (p. 820). One common manifestation of an activated pairing basic assumption group is that staff appear to think of nothing other than the pregnancy and relate to the therapist almost exclusively in her role as expectant parent. The accompanying collective mood state is one of giddiness and festivity. We have heard nothing similar to this reaction in the accounts of expectant biological fathers or adoptive parents. It appears that a pregnancy is needed to induce this reaction.

Although in our discussion we have contrasted organizations in terms of those showing adaptive versus maladaptive responses to the therapist's pregnancies, certainly most organizations will show a combination of such features. Furthermore, as the following vignette provided by one of our interviewees suggests, any given response may have both elements.

Vignette 11.1

During my pregnancy, I received an unusually high number of referrals, mostly from colleagues who knew that I was pregnant and knew that I would be taking some time for maternity leave. The closer I got to my due date, the more referrals I received. This phenomenon struck me as strange, as on the one hand, it felt like a loving, generous gesture . . . that my friends and colleagues perhaps wanted to give something to me in support of the pregnancy. On the other hand, I felt as though I was being offered something that people knew I would obviously have to refuse. In that sense, it was as though I was being teased: I have something that I know you want but can't have now . . . I also felt: many of these people referred to me are women who know what it is like to have a new child, who understand the demands.

Why aren't they being more supportive in the direction of encouraging me to take time off from work? I felt as though there were some abandonment fears on others' part and anger, as well, that I was planning to exit the work scene for a brief period of time. Perhaps there was envy, as well, toward the notion of my having a baby.

The reader will notice that this therapist detected in the responses of her work associates many of the themes that were discussed in Chapter 2 as transferential responses patients have toward people in their lives, including their therapists.

Effects of Institutional Responses

The responses of the institution induce a host of reactions in expectant therapists. One reaction is surprise that peers responded in a way so at odds with the therapist's expectations of them. Disappointment is an aspect of this surprise: our interviewees reported having hoped for more empathy and consideration than they actually received. Part of the reason for this surprise and disappointment might have been that these therapists placed their energy into the correct anticipation of *patient* reactions. With colleagues, perhaps they expected responses that were positive rather than ambivalent or negative. Such off-the-mark expectations result when expectant therapists neglect to appreciate the complex reactions that their status begets in others.

Frequently, expectant therapists mirror their colleagues' responses to them. For example, the sense of abandonment that staff and colleagues sometimes feel vis-à-vis the pregnant therapist is reciprocally evoked in the therapist as she witnesses her needs being ignored. The setting's denial can easily lead the therapist to deny the enormity of the changes occurring in her life, changes requiring a multitude of accommodations (Fenster et al., 1986). A setting can induce a therapist who is already uncomfortable with her vulnerability to "blame herself for what she sees as self-indulgence" (Fenster et al., 1986, p. 67).

Although the aforementioned changes represent concordant responses (Racker, 2012) between the setting and the therapist, the therapist, based upon a variety of factors including her personality dynamics, may exhibit complementary responses (see Chapter 3 for a discussion of concordant and complementary reactions). For example, a therapist who finds herself in an environment that ignores her needs may become extremely demanding and convey a sense of entitlement. A person who finds herself the object of envy might flaunt her pregnancy triumphantly. Of course, while most therapists have an affinity for a particular type of response, by no means is the therapist compelled to act out any given reaction. Rather, each nascent reaction provides the basis for a more thorough understanding of the workplace dynamics—be it a treatment team, a hospital administration or one's network of referral sources—with the potential for more sensitive relating to others within the setting.

What can make staff responses perplexing to the expectant therapist is that negatively toned and positive-toned responses can exist alongside one another. The staff members who complain bitterly about any extra work they are asked to absorb are the same staff who plan a lavish baby shower for the expectant therapist. The societal pronatalism that dictates the expression of positive feeling for pregnant women leads to overt expressions of enthusiasm and more covert expressions of hostility and disapproval. The pregnant therapist is readily led to mistrust her perceptions of the negatively rooted behaviors in the midst of positive gestures. The ambiguity hinders the pregnant therapist from clearly seeing what problem is at hand and what might be done about it.

We have concerned ourselves primarily with the emotional effects of these institutional responses. However, physical responses can occur as well. For example, Schneider-Braus and Goodwin (1985) noticed that their sample of six pregnant therapists, all residents in psychiatry, had an unusual number of third-trimester complications (preeclampsia, premature labor in a twin gestation, fetal growth retardation and cesarean sections). Phelan (1988) found that psychiatric residents (along with residents in obstetrics-gynecology and surgery) had higher hypertension rates during pregnancy than the population of pregnant women at large. It stands to reason that these difficulties are in part attributable to institutional policies that discourage women from making appropriate allowances for their pregnancies.

Recommendations for the Workplace

Institutions would benefit themselves and their employees by accepting that employees will become expectant parents. Like any regular occurrence affecting all stakeholders in the settings—therapists, staff, patients, patients' families—a plan should be developed to address the complexities created by this transition. We recommend that any comprehensive plan have five components.

Workplace Policies for Expectant Parents

First, if it is not already present, a policy regarding all expectancy conditions should be established. The policy should include benefits available for the to-be mother or father—whether it includes paid or unpaid leave, the amount of time available, options for extension, possible provisions for the new mother or father such as time available for sick children and so on. The United States is one of the few countries to offer fewer than 6 months' leave to care for a young child, and so the expectant or new parent will be dependent upon the generosity of the workplace to have time beyond this limit (Ray, Gornick, & Schmitt, 2010). Around the world, guaranteed parental leave for fathers is far less common than for mothers, a policy that reinforces gender inequalities (Ray et al., 2010) and is particularly disadvantageous for fathers in same-sex relationships. This is true despite the evidence that paternal leave is associated with multiple positive outcomes for the child. For example, Flacking, Dykes and Ewald (2010) found, perhaps paradoxically, that infants whose fathers did not take a paternity leave were much less likely to be breastfed during the first year of life. Stated differently, the father's participation in the infant's life is an important support to breastfeeding. Fortunately, in some countries such as Sweden, Norway and Greece, fathers are treated much more favorably. For example, in Sweden, a couple receives a total amount of parental leave time with 48% being reserved for the father. During the leave, the father receives 51% of his salary (Ray et al., 2010). For those countries with either no or minimal paternity leave, greater stress will be placed upon the mother to remove herself from the workplace extendedly.

Reading Resources

Second, expectant parents, who are also mental health professionals, as well as their co-workers, benefit from the presence of resources to use during the pregnancy and re-entry periods. The compilation of readings related to the pregnant therapist is particularly feasible given the fairly substantial corpus of writings in this area. The literature is now extensive enough that in selecting relevant readings, one can achieve a fair degree of specificity in terms of the population of the patients treated, the setting, and the characteristics of the therapist. Less is available on mental health professionals who are expectant adoptive parents or biological fathers. Hopefully, this literature will expand and deepen in the decades to come.

Staff Support

Third, a staff person who could cultivate this topic as an area of specialty could be of immense benefit to the workplace. The person who ideally had experienced this life transition could serve as a consultant not only to the expectant employee but also to supervisors and other staff working with him or her (Baum & Herring, 1975). Hennekam (2016) found that when pregnant women have access to role models who have experienced this life transition while working have far better transitional experiences than those who do not. This individual, having a special sensitivity to the individual and group issues that arise when a staff member is awaiting a child, can assist staff in achieving awareness of the possible indirect reactions to conflicts evoked by the expectancy in all social strata of the workplace. The resource person could become knowledgeable about ways of ameliorating the risk of particular activities. For example, therapists typically have the demand to sit for long periods of time. Potentially, the resource person could offer tips concerning different postures that might relieve the stress on the body from this particular physical demand or suggest supports such as a lumbar roll to ease postural strain.

A primary function of both the readings and the onsite specialist is that they might assist pregnant and other expectant therapists in forming more accurate anticipations of what they are likely to experience. For example, according to the literature (e.g., Schneider-Braus & Goodwin, 1985), pregnant women frequently underestimate the severity of physical symptoms in their first trimester, symptoms often necessitating considerable adjustment in workload and schedule. The results of our study and those of Bashe (1989) suggest that female therapists often fail to realize that at the end of their pregnancies, prior to delivery, they will long for a respite from work. Many regret forming a plan to work until their due dates. Most mothers and fathers underestimate the demands that will be made on them on their return, such as the problems arising when their children are ill (Auchincloss, 1982; Schneider-Braus & Goodman, 1985). Prospective fathers often misgauge the strength of patient reactions to their transition (Guy, Guy, & Liaboe, 1986). The formation of more accurate expectations enables more effective planning and diminishes the stress when inevitable problems arise.

Academic programs that are sending students to clinical sites might supplement the supervisory resources present within the clinical sites. For example, developing a network of graduates who have gone through the transition to parenthood and who are willing to mentor current trainees could be of great benefit. These mentors would also have had experience in negotiating the transition to parenthood while satisfying requirements as a trainee and also as a student (e.g., the dissertation).

Staffing Guidelines

A fourth component is the existence of guidelines and policies in relation to the practical issues that arise pertaining to expectant staff (Finch, 2003). For example, if a pregnant therapist needs to take time off from work to attend to health needs, are there certain activities that must be made up at some point, such as evenings on call? Will additional personnel be hired, or will the current staff be expected to absorb the load of the pregnant therapist? How will the extra work be distributed? These guidelines should include all categories of expectancy. Formally adopted guidelines embraced after a period of deliberation and discussion are likely to take into account a greater variety of perspectives and needs of all parties than the impromptu, hasty decision making that occurs in relation to individual staff members' pregnancies. As such, a course of action that results from the application of these guidelines is less likely to produce acrimony and dissension (Shreier & Mahmood, 1988) than ad hoc decision making. Also, these guidelines are a savings for the expectant therapist who is spared from having to duplicate the problem-solving efforts of past pregnant therapists in the setting during a period when time and energy may be limited.

Staff Support Groups

Fifth, just as all-important staff transitions and issues are discussed at staff meetings, so too should the circumstance of a staff member expecting a child in all its implications for the workplace. When there are several expectant therapists within the same setting, the institution of a support group should be considered. It might include individuals who have already transitioned through this process who are able to share their insights as well as those who are aspiring to build a family (Schneider-Braus & Goodwin, 1985). Such a group could cover a range of issues. The group's collective problem-solving resources might be used in relation to the practical issues that arise. Members' discussions could culminate in recommendations to the setting about the guidelines mentioned earlier. It could also be used to address psychological conflicts related to this area, such as the conflict between the wish to be perfect and all-capable as a professional and the desire to withdraw from the professional realm and attend fully to the child's imminent arrival.

Provisions for Parents Upon Return to the Workplace

What the employee needs from a workplace will differ once that employee has become a parent. Return to the workplace will be expedited immeasurably if a setting demonstrates the willingness to accommodate those needs. For example, parents will need flexibility to accommodate problems in childcare and sickness of children. Women who are breastfeeding will require quiet, private places to pump breast milk, a sufficient break to engage in this activity, refrigeration to store breast milk, and workplace cribs for those who are able to breastfeed on site (Rojjanasrirat, 2004; Suyes, Abrahams, & Labbok, 2008). The Affordable Care Act mandates many of these requirements (United States Department of Labor, 2010). Summarizing existing research, Haviland, James, Killman and Trbovich (2015) note that workplaces that facilitate breastfeeding enjoy decreased healthcare costs, lessened employee absenteeism, more robust employee retention, better employee morale and more favorable public relations. To the extent that parents know prior to their leave what resources are in place for their return, to that same extent, these parents will be able to return to the workplace with less regret and more enthusiasm.

Responses of the Therapist

The expectant therapist's behavior makes a difference in how the system responds to his or her expectant state. Stated in the language of general systems theory, the therapist is a subsystem of the broader system of treatment in which that therapist functions. Information constantly flows from the parent-to-be to the broader system, a flow that inevitably alters the system receiving it. In this section, we note several patterns of response that have been observed to undermine the therapist's maintenance of a constructive working relationship with those in the workplace, prior to the arrival of the child and following the return to work. This presentation is followed by recommendations in the form of a description of modes of response on the part of both parties—the therapist and the broader environment—that maximize the therapeutic and relationship-building potential of the therapist's transition to parenthood.

Common Therapist Reactions

Our own research and the literature suggest that three generally maladaptive stances on the part of the expectant therapist are particularly common.

Denial and Minimization

Like staff within the setting, the therapist might engage in denial about many aspects and consequences of the pregnancy or other expectant state (Wiesenthal, 2008). The denial can take a variety of forms. The therapist might deny that the expectant state is affecting his or her work; that preparations need to be made for a period of absence, however long; and that the therapist's professional life might be altered to some degree upon his or her return following the arrival of the child. On a behavioral level, this denial might manifest itself as an unwillingness to talk about the transition to parenthood particularly as it affects his or her current work. When this reticence occurs in the supervisory relationship, it denies the supervisor the opportunity to help the supervisee gain understanding of how the feelings, thoughts and impulses stimulated by the transition shape that supervisee's clinical work. The denial might also show itself in a tendency to take on additional responsibilities (Schneider-Braus & Goodwin, 1985). For example, a pregnant woman might sign up to be on committees despite the fact that her upcoming leave would challenge her ability to participate on the committee meaningfully. In some cases, the operative factor is fear of loss of control. Being away from the workplace stimulates anticipatory anxiety, which a heightened involvement in activities prior to the maternity leave may lessen. Also palpable might be doubts about one's success in fulfilling a new, parental role, doubts that might be allayed in seeing oneself function in a conspicuously competent way in one's current role. Also operative might be a fear that others in the workplace will have an altered perception of the expectant co-worker. Indeed, studies (Greenberg & Ladge, 2009; Pattison, Gross, & Cast, 1997) have demonstrated that pregnant women tend to be seen as less capable and invested in their professional lives. Such responses constitute stigma in that they entail seeing an individual through the lens of a negative stereotype (Fox & Quinn, 2015). Anticipating stigma, women who work in a strongly male culture may fear being seen as weak or soft because of their burgeoning maternity. Again, a high level of work activity might be expected to counter this perception. The therapist might also practice denial and minimization by failing to plan for the maternity leave. Perhaps, in addition to other previously mentioned factors, the therapist has a sense of loss connected to leaving work and the specter of scaling back work responsibilities in the future or giving up work altogether. By not acknowledging his or her impending departure, the therapist can avoid recognizing all of the losses that may attend that departure.

By failing to recognize and address the professional–personal tensions that inevitably exist in a transition of this enormity, a therapist's planning is likely to be inadequate to serve his or her needs. Moreover, that expectant therapist is likely creating a circumstance where he or she will experience as intrusions commitments that were agreed upon during the period in which the therapist was minimizing or denying the transitional realities of new parenthood. An academic psychologist in the following vignette provides a clear illustration of the consequences of a pregnancy governed in the workplace by minimizing and denying.

Vignette 11.2

There I was, 24 hours after I delivered my baby cesarean section, holding this incredible little baby. Any pain I felt was masked by this indescribable, exhilarating experience. In what I discovered later to be a rare moment, he was sleeping next to me after I had tried to breastfeed him. I was jilted out of my reverie by the harsh sound of the telephone. A woman at the other end said, "Dr. X, this is Y (book editor). I just have a couple of questions on your manuscript." I became momentarily disoriented, having no memory for the final version of a chapter that I had sent to the publisher only days ago. Because my chapter had been one of the last to be completed, in a moment of psychotic denial, I had readily agreed to have this editor call me at the hospital as if it were a motel room of a conference I was attending that week. I don't even remember if I acknowledged that this "conference" would center around my first child's birth. I felt more than a small annoyance at her at that time, that my limited maternity leave was eroded by these demanding editors who did not have the decency to preserve the sanctity of my hospital stay. Yet, I had taken on this project knowing that it would be a horse race as to whether the chapter or the delivery would finish first. I did not want colleagues to think that my pregnancy would interfere with my academic commitments.

Although this illustration is dramatic, the tendency to feel regret over commitments made during the expectancy period is extremely common.

Withdrawal

The next two patterns we consider, withdrawal and entitlement, contrast greatly with the first. Withdrawal occurs when the therapist expresses a lessened level of interest and involvement in work activities. To some extent, the phenomenon is natural: a child's entering a family is an event of such enormous proportions that it is natural for other aspects of a person's life to recede in importance. One of the authors remembers attending a workshop during her pregnancy and finding the presenter's remarks far less compelling than her baby's kicks. When the pregnancy or adoption is complicated, such a withdrawal is likely to be even more extended and pronounced.

In the absence of such complications, prolonged disengagement from the everyday world might have other meanings. It could reveal an effort to separate the self from others' troubling reactions toward the expectancy. For example, were the therapist to sense others' hostility toward her, a flight response would be natural. However, the therapist might also recoil from positively toned responses, such as when a therapist might be uncomfortable with other staff members' attempts to nurture her. One of our interviewees told us of her extreme discomfort when the staff had a surprise shower for her on the unit and how she felt like shrinking from that event. The pregnant therapist might also wish to withdraw from others who feel comfort in connecting with her pregnancy in tactile ways. Another interviewee talked about how odd it seemed to her that other staff who barely knew her would walk up to her and pat her stomach. She found herself attempting to avoid such interactions. Alternatively, the withdrawal might be a defense against long-standing, pre-expectancy issues associated with work; that is, the expectancy, like any other consuming personal life event, might provide a sanctuary from work-related tensions.

Entitlement

A sense of entitlement entails an abrogation of other's needs, feelings, capabilities or any combination thereof. It might appear as an expectation on the part of the expectant therapist to be liberated from having to articulate her needs (e.g., "Isn't it obvious I can't do that?"). Entitlement is seen in the therapist who becomes highly disappointed or aggravated that others (unknowingly) schedule a meeting at a time when she is beset by fatigue or morning sickness. This posture might also show itself in the failure to assist others whose professional activities are affected by the expectancy, for example, neglecting to provide a substitute therapist with critical information about a patient to enable effective treatment during the maternity or paternity leave. It also reveals itself in an unwillingness to tolerate the diverse feelings others have about the consequences of the pregnancy for them. An example would be a pregnant therapist who has no empathy with others' irritation at having to work longer hours, cover more patients, or be on call more frequently (e.g., "I can't believe they just wouldn't be happy for me and would want to help out.").

Like the aforementioned patterns, the intrapsychic reasons for this pattern are complex and, in part, stem from the long-standing interpersonal style of the therapist. That is, a therapist who customarily responds with a sense of entitlement to an array of life events is prone to do so as well in regard to his or her status of being an expectant parent. Relative to other expectancy conditions (e.g., adoption), the physical and physiological alterations of pregnancy might lead to its evocation in this circumstance and not others. The emergence of a sense of entitlement could represent a backing away from the complexity created by the pregnancy in a professional woman's life. By declaring, implicitly, others' needs and reactions less important than her own, she protects herself from having to reckon with them. For both biological and adoptive mothers, a sense of entitlement might be a reaction to a perception, based in reality or not, that the setting devalues women's family pursuits. The entitlement could be an attempt to desensitize herself to the negativity while asserting her needs in an environment that is assumed to be unreceptive to them.

What are the consequences within the setting of the therapist showing these patterns? The therapist's denial or withdrawal can collude with a system seeking to do the same in relation to the therapist's expectancy. At worse, particularly in the case of the pregnant woman, such collusion can endanger her well-being. For example, tasks might be given and accepted that pose a health risk to the therapist and her baby. For example, some research literature (see Salihu, Myers, & August, 2012, for a review) suggests a relationship between long work hours and low birth weight. Among the various professional groups, psychiatric residents are perhaps most likely to encounter demands to serve back-to-back shifts or have an excessively long work day. For all expectancy conditions, these maladaptive modes of dealing with the expectancy hinder the development of good strategies for (a) addressing any patient reactions to the expectancy, (b) obtaining coverage as the expectant therapist attends to medical and other needs, and (c) ensuring that all workplace responsibilities are covered during parental leave. Even if no real problems emerge in connection with the use of denial and minimization, these defenses ensure that the stimulus the expectant state might provide for therapists' and patients' psychological growth is unlikely to be realized.

Recommendations for Therapists

For the mental health professional who is awaiting the arrival of a child—be it through pregnancy or adoption—we would recommend that he or she approach other staff with all of the relevant issues associated with this status in a thoughtful rather than off-handed way. Just as it is important to consider the characteristics of the patient in making such decisions as when to announce that one is an expectant parent, so too is it helpful to assess the organization and its likely stance toward this development. For example, in an organization in which the therapist's absence for maternity leave creates a variety of staffing challenges, plenty of time should be allowed for working through the various difficulties.

The pregnant professional, Benedek (1973) noted, might find it helpful to share with staff bits of information about her plans on an ongoing basis so as to challenge tendencies toward denial and minimization. She suggested further that the pregnant professional help staff to anticipate how each patient is likely to react to the pregnancy. Benedek raised the intriguing notion that by considering patients' likely reactions, staff members have an outlet, albeit a relatively non-threatening disguised one, for their own varied responses. We think prospective fathers and adoptive parents could also beneficially employ these strategies. The difference, however, is that whereas staff are compelled to recognize that revelation of the pregnancy is inevitable, they might question whether the expectant father or adoptive parents needs to disclose that he or she is awaiting a child.

On the one hand, this questioning could foster very interesting and worthwhile discussion on therapist self-disclosure. On the other, such a position on the part of staff could evoke a variety of reactions on the part of the other-than-pregnant expectant therapist who might interpret that position as a devaluation of his or her status (see Brabender and Whitmore, 2014, for further discussion).

The Supervisor–Supervisee Relationship

Because family building occurs earlier than later in a clinician's career, frequently expectant professionals are in supervision. The tenor of this relationship is key to the supervisee's ability to provide competent services to clients. Given the intensity of therapist and client reactions during and following the expectancy period, the supervisee is in a position to benefit greatly from the supervisor's clarifications and insights. The critical nature of supervision during the therapist's pregnancy is expressed well in the following quote:

> The supervisor's challenge is to help the analyst avoid converting this important milestone in her life [the pregnancy] into a millstone or stumbling block in the analysis of her patient. The supervisor can help the analyst turn the evocative nature of the pregnancy into a positive force for the analysis.
>
> (Goldberger et al., 2003, p. 442)

What is true for analysis is also true for psychotherapy. The therapists we interviewed indicated that the supervisor was all-important in helping the pregnant therapist to recognize what technical modifications were necessary during the pregnancy. For example, one of our interviewees mentioned how difficult it was for her during her pregnancy when her patients expressed concern for her. She stated, "I wanted to be the caretaker, not be taken care of by others." Her supervisor had had two pregnancies of her own while functioning as a therapist. It was only through her supervisor's input, she felt, that she was able to receive rather than spurn patients' nurturing and not respond to them in an overly analytical, detached and defensive way. Her supervisor was also instrumental in encouraging her to be active in bringing up the pregnancy and making it clear to patients that it was fair material for their reactions. She said that if left to her own inclinations, she would have proceeded as if the pregnancy were irrelevant to her work with the patients and was off-limits for their commentary.

The supervisor can be enormously helpful as the supervisee contends with the patient's acting out in relation to the therapist's expectant state. Wiesenthal (2008) provides an illustration of her own work during her residency involving a patient who had an abortion and subsequently learned of her therapist's pregnancy. The patient, after expressing a range of negative feelings, began to miss sessions. It was the supervisor who helped this therapist to see the importance of phoning the patient and encouraging further exploration of the patient's feelings. The patient returned to treatment and engaged in productive work.

The supervisor can be a powerful advocate for the supervisee within the broader setting. For example, in the Butts and Cavenar case (1979) described earlier, the supervisor having a perspective that was independent of the other staff was critical to the therapist's capacity to remain responsive and helpful to a patient following the staff's expression of skepticism about her likely effectiveness. In fact, the supervisor's distance enabled him to assist the supervisee in recognizing the group dynamic responses to the pregnancy that underlay their skepticism. Earlier it was suggested that an expectant therapist could encourage the staff to grapple with the implications of his or her new status by sharing details of it on an ongoing basis during the staff meetings (e.g., "I think I'm getting clearer on how long I'll be staying out for my paternity leave"). In fact, if the expectant therapist is a trainee, it might be essential that he or she receive public support from a supervisor in doing so. Otherwise, it could be easy for staff to misconstrue such sharing in negative terms by, for example, viewing it as a manifestation of the therapist's self-indulgence and self-absorption.

Supervisory Difficulties

Despite the potential usefulness of the supervisory relationship to the pregnant therapist, numerous examples appear in the literature of supervisors not only failing to be supportive but actually undermining their supervisees' work during this time. For example, Butts and Cavenar (1979) described a case in which a resident, 7 months pregnant, was treating an obsessive-compulsive man in intensive psychotherapy. When the patient neglected to give any mention of the pregnancy, the therapist wondered in supervision whether she should introduce the topic. According to Butts and Cavenar,

> The supervisor responded that the resident perceived the lack of attention to her pregnancy as a narcissistic injury and that the patient should pay no more attention to the pregnancy than he might new shoes or glasses that the resident might have.
>
> (p. 1588)

Butts and Cavenar explained the supervisor's response in terms of his history: he, an only child, had had great ambivalence over the arrival of his second child and now the supervisee was having a second child. Like the patient, the supervisor might have wanted to sidestep the feelings aroused by this circumstance. Goldberger et al. (2003) document other supervisory obstacles that can arise:

> These [reactions] can range from annoyed distancing from the pregnant analyst to overinvolved counter-identification. Supervisors may get vicarious pleasure from the candidate's pregnancy; they may project from their own experiences of pregnancy. Supervisors who have themselves had

difficulty with pregnancy (either their own or that of a spouse) may assume that the candidate will have similar difficulties.

(p. 459)

Our own participants attested to the importance of the intrapsychic life of the supervisor in that supervisor's capacity to be helpful during a supervisee's pregnancy. One of our participants described how her supervisor had urged her to attend a symposium that was on the topic of the pregnant therapist. She explained that traveling to the conference at that advanced point in her pregnancy would be too arduous for her and that she needed the time to prepare for the baby's coming. Despite her explanation, the supervisor did not relent. The therapist observed:

> I felt as though the supervisor was endeavoring to be helpful to me, to offer me something useful. However, I was extremely put out by his constant reminding me of the conference and asking me if I had made arrangements, if I was intending to go. It felt extremely unempathic. I thought: He's looking at me like I am the mother and he wants for some reason to make me work and work for him.

The supervisee tried to understand the supervisor's insensitivity—a departure from his usual behavior—in terms of his dynamics. She speculated that the supervisor, being a middle child in a large family, had resented his mother for the deprivations he experienced due to the births of the later children. At the same time, he wanted to find ways to be helpful to her.

Whether this dynamic speculation had any accuracy, it is certainly the case that supervisors, like patients and other staff, find their supervisees' pregnancies to be emotionally evocative based on their own dynamic histories. Supervisors are immune to none of the transferential responses outlined in Chapter 2. Yet, the structure of the supervisory relationship might make these natural reactions at once more painful and impermissible to the supervisor himself or herself. For example, it might be disturbing to feel both nurturing toward and envious of the supervisee.

Another factor leading supervisors to avoid assisting the supervisee with the effects the pregnancy has on the treatment process is the worry that such aid might turn the supervision into therapy (Imber, 1995). However, what distinguishes such assistance from therapy is the goal of the intervention. In supervision, the attempt is to enable the supervisee to treat her patient more effectively; in therapy, the goal is to advance the well-being of the patient. Finally, although the literature has described resources for the pregnant therapists to help them address pregnancy-related reactions, the literature for supervisors is just emerging and non-existent for other expectancy conditions.

Although supervisors might have similar reactions to the supervisor's other colleagues, particular reactions might be distinctive. For example, it is not unusual for a supervisor to identify with the supervisee, regarding that supervisee to be an idealized version of self. Such idealization can satisfy the supervisor's impulse toward generativity (Erikson, 1950) and can compensate for perceived deficiencies in his or her professional self. As part of this idealization, the supervisor takes narcissistic satisfaction in the supervisee's progress and accomplishments. The supervisee's expectancy might be perceived as a fundamental shift in the supervisee's priorities from career to domestic life. When supervisors attempt to deny the expectancy or place even greater demands on the supervisee, it might be an effort to preserve the gratifications attached to the idealization. In the prior example of the conference-promoting supervisor, this wish might have given rise to a compromise formation. On the one hand, the supervisor might have been trying to maintain connection to the supervisor's professional self by urging her to exert herself to attend a career-related event. On the other hand, the fact of the event's connection to the pregnancy might signify a conscious or unconscious attempt by the supervisor to see the supervisee's identity in broader terms.

The extent to which the supervisor constructs a complex image of the supervisee that comprehends parenthood is likely to be affected by the supervisor's own history in this regard. If the supervisor has had children and has experienced the complications arising from the simultaneous pursuit of career and parenthood, a potential exists for the supervisor's conveyance of a very special sort of empathy to the supervisee. However, this potential might not be realized by the professional who is also a parent if that individual is actively involved in fending off painful affects associated with past or current decisions. For example, one supervisor expressed shock and dismay that a pregnant resident did not call her unit immediately the day that she had been rushed to the hospital for the treatment of an ectopic pregnancy and kept the treatment team guessing on her whereabouts. This supervisor was one who continually lamented that the sociocultural climate gave women fewer options when she had her children 25 years ago. It seemed she felt she was forced to compromise her children's well-being significantly to maintain her career. In some sense, she was envious of this resident who, despite her misfortune, could simply give way to her personal life.

Just as the supervisor might have distinctive reactions to the supervisee, so might the latter have unique reactions to the former. The supervisor might be seen as having a special capacity to provide the supervisee with essential emotional nutrients during this period. As has been pointed out repeatedly in the literature, it is common for expectant parents to need considerable emotional support during the period of awaiting a child. The combination of the supervisor's authority over, and close contact with, the supervisee might lead the supervisee to harbor an expectation of receiving such support from the supervisor. If the supervisor fails to do so, the supervisee's disappointment might be quite acute and could even compromise the working relationship that the parties had forged, as we see in the next vignette.

Vignette 11.3

A new supervisor who had herself never experienced pregnancy was confused when her supervisee began to withdraw progressively over the course of her pregnancy. One manifestation of the withdrawal was that the supervisee was less forthcoming about details of her cases. At some point, the supervisor confronted the supervisee about the change. The supervisee said she was "turned off" by the indifference of the supervisor who had not once inquired as to how her pregnancy was going. The supervisor was in turn hurt because she claimed that although she was very curious about the pregnancy, she felt she had taken particular pains to preserve a boundary between the personal and the professional. She experienced learning about the details of the pregnancy as forbidden voyeuristic gratification. Her own inexperience as a supervisor led her to attempt to compartmentalize spheres of experience that are necessarily related in a way that produced an intense sense of deprivation in her supervisee.

Another determinant of the reactions of supervisors and supervisees to one another during the supervisee's expectancy is a phenomenon known as *parallel process* (Searles, 1955; Morrissey & Tribe, 2001; Mothersole, 1999). Parallel process occurs when a structural or dynamic feature appearing in one subsystem of a system replicates itself in another subsystem of that same system. Fenster et al. (1986) provide numerous examples of how the dynamic existing between supervisor and supervisee replicates that between the patient and the pregnant therapist. The existence of parallel processes is readily understood within a systems theory perspective in terms of the permeability of boundaries between subsystems within a system (von Bertalanffy, 1966). The constant flow of information leads the dynamic elements present in one subsystem to enter another, thereby creating isomorphies. These isomorphies can have varying effects, positive and negative. For the expectant therapist, if the repetition simply means that a regressive solution to expectancy-related conflicts reverberates through many or all of the subsystems in which the therapist is involved, this reverberation is likely to intensify any distressing aspects of the therapist's experience. The following vignette illustrates such a phenomenon.

Vignette 11.4

A hospital administrator felt that the psychology interns were excessive in their requests for time off due to various personal situations. In one intern's case, the request for time off was for a maternity leave. The administrator levied a criticism at the internship director, who reported to the administrator, that she had not made wise choices in the selection of interns. She had picked individuals who were in some fashion fettered rather than free to pursue their work responsibilities. The director received this criticism with silent hostility. With the pregnant intern she supervised, she found herself being harshly critical of the intern's work. The intern became more and more withdrawn and essentially deprived the director-supervisor of material available for critique.

In this example, the structure of the relationship between the supervisor and the administrator to whom she reported repeated itself in the supervisor–supervisee relationship. The players acted out negatively toned feelings such as hostility. They might have used these feelings as a point of departure for exploring how the institution could adapt to the inevitable changes in the lives of staff and how the staff could accommodate the needs of the institution in the midst of these changes. The analyzed reverberation of the top-level administrator's non-support of the interns in the supervisor–supervisee relationship undermined the quality of the supervision, thereby hindering the supervisee's work.

In the case highlighted in the following vignette, however, the repetition of the dynamics in subsystems of a system enriched in favorable ways the interactions of staff members.

Vignette 11.5

Dr. Moritz, a supervisor of a pregnant therapist, Perry, noticed that during the latter's mid-trimester, her interpretations were "off" relative to her usual level of attunement. Perry herself complained of having a sense of ineffectuality with many of her patients and did not seem to benefit from the supervision sessions. Neither party, independently or collaboratively, could put an interpretive finger on the problem. Dr. Moritz also observed that a number of the supervisee's patients had a reaction to her pregnancy that took the form of demands such as the rescheduling of appointment times; the demands appeared to escalate as the pregnancy progressed. The supervisee's effort seemed to be the accommodation of these demands with minimal effort at the analysis of their motivational base. Again, this was unusual for Perry. One reason Dr. Moritz became aware of these demands was because it affected her: in order to accommodate her patients, the supervisee requested that her supervisor modify their schedule of appointments. Although the supervisor had some misgivings about making the requested changes and felt some irritation at having to do so, she found herself complying with Perry's wishes. Not to do so, she felt, seemed unkind and ungenerous.

Dr. Moritz's reflections on the changes with Perry's pregnancy led her to notice that a parallel process had developed between the therapist and her patients, and the supervisor and the supervisee. Like Perry, Dr. Moritz was unwilling to be a frustrating agent because of the guilt connected to that role. Perry's guilt was related to her belief that the effects of her pregnancy would be more negative than neutral or positive for her severely disturbed patients. Relatedly, Dr. Moritz's guilt was connected to her fear of failing to be the all-giving nurturer. In both supervisor and supervisee, the acts of over-accommodation to avoid guilt led to irritation and disattunement. Dr. Moritz achieved greater insight into the dynamics between Perry and her patients through her recognition of the parallel dynamics. As Perry was helped to identify and actively evaluate her notion that she was damaging her patients through her pregnancy, she was able to direct her energy to understanding patients rather than managing her guilt and the therapies moved forward. Dr. Moritz, too, was better able to distinguish between reasonable accommodations and ones that would unduly disrupt her own professional functioning. Plumbing the parallel process led to a strengthening of the alliance between Dr. Moritz and Perry. Of course, parallel process is observed in expectant conditions other than pregnancy, as the following vignette illustrates.

Vignette 11.6

An expectant father-supervisee, Nigel, told his supervisor, Dr. Tomkins, that his wife was having a baby in 3 months but he didn't anticipate needing to take more than a day off. Dr. Tomkins was a relatively new supervisor and had yet to encounter a wide range of situations in the course of providing supervision. Dr. Tomkins warmly congratulated the intern and internally registered that he was glad it would create no disruption vis-à-vis Nigel's responsibilities. Nigel mentioned that he was planning on apprising neither other patients nor other staff members. He asked Dr. Tomkins to keep the information confidential, and Dr. Tomkins agreed. Nothing out of the ordinary occurred for the next 2 months. One month prior to Nigel's date of delivery, Nigel's wife needed to be hospitalized. For a week, Nigel needed to take off considerable blocks of work to take care of his 8-year-old daughter while his mother-in-law made arrangements to absorb childcare responsibilities. Other staff had to pick up the slack, and were irritated by it. Nigel was surprised at their irritation because he had expected them to be joyful for him. A few of Nigel's patients were angry as well. While the patient irritation was expressed to Nigel, the staff annoyance was directed toward Dr. Tomkins, who recognized that he and Nigel had been unified in their avoidance of an event that held promise of affecting Nigel's workplace far more than they were willing to acknowledge. Dr. Tomkins and Nigel both acknowledged their responsibility for the untoward developments and established for themselves the goal of repairing relationships.

In this example, the developmental status of the supervisor might have made him particularly vulnerable to entering into a parallel process with Nigel and his patients. As Falender and Shafranske (2004) note, the new supervisor can exhibit rigidity in interpreting roles, and consistent with this inconsistency is a failure to integrate personal and professional facets of self.

Practical Implications for the Supervisory Relationship

As has been discussed throughout this book, the expectancy of the therapist is evocative of certain thematic material and provides a host of special issues in terms of intervention. Stated simply, this period is, and should be, a departure from business as usual. Consequently, it is a time in which the therapist does well to take advantage of all resources available, and one of those resources is supervision. Ideally, the supervisor is someone who has familiarity with the clinical phenomena associated with pregnancy and other expectancy states. The supervisor should be someone who has forged or can forge a strong supervisory alliance with the trainee, a bond that has been demonstrated to be associated with an array of positive outcomes (Watkins, 2012). The supervisor should also have the knowledge and skills to help the supervisee cope with the powerful institutional dynamics that can be stimulated by the therapist's disclosure that he or she is expecting a child. The supervisor should also have a deep knowledge of ethical issues and skill in helping the therapist to navigate the complex boundary issues that can emerge at this time.

From the standpoint of the supervisor, our recommendation is that he or she strive to be aware of the complexity of forces bearing on the therapist and the supervisory relationship. Supervision is also made more effective by the supervisor's mindfulness and tolerance of the strong affects and impulses that the expectancy is likely to evoke from him or her. Although some supervisors might choose to share these responses directly with the supervisee as a way of fostering openness, others may use them for understanding the supervisory relationship better and to identify parallel processes between the supervisory and therapy relationships that will further the latter. The supervisor should see as part of the supervisory process the natural human response of inquiring into the well-being of the therapist. This demonstration of the supervisor's caring can reduce stress and invite self-disclosures that might be germane to the therapist's work. The supervisor should also attend to all aspects of the supervisee's identity in arriving at an understanding of those supervisee responses in the treatment situation. For example, the supervisee's own cultural background may predispose him or her to have a relatively open versus closed stance in regard to sharing with others a personal transition. For example, Baum and Itzhaky (2006) noted that supervisees who come from orthodox religious background might have inhibitions about sharing the news of the pregnancy because such communications entail acknowledging their own sexuality. The supervisor aware of this cultural bias can assist the supervisee in developing creative compromises that will give his or her background, the needs of the setting, and the supervisees' clients their due. Finally, given the strong (and often negative) effects that institutional dynamics may have on the expectant therapist, an appropriate role for the supervisor might be that of advocate, so that the expectant therapist enjoys an environment conducive to growth in realms both professional and personal.

Recommendations

- Work sites and supervisors should recognize that pregnancy and other expectancy conditions are natural phenomena in the lives of trainees and early career professionals. Organizations and supervisors should develop resources to accommodate the needs of both the workplace, the supervisee, and the expectant parent/therapist. Where possible, academic training programs should supplement these resources.

- Although work settings frequently have positive reactions to the therapist's expectancy of a child, negative reactions also occur based upon unconscious impulses and feelings stimulated by the expectancy and the practical difficulties created by the therapist's transition. The therapist should be ready for the full range of staff reactions, with positive and negative reactions often occurring alongside one another. The therapist might find it reassuring to know that many others have encountered the same reactions.
- Therapists who are expectant parents also have reactions within the work setting that can hinder their adjustment in the setting during this period. A response that recognizes the momentousness of the transition as well as the way it impinges on others enables the therapist to engage in constructive problem-solving.
- To deal with the workplace challenges of this transition, the expectant therapist should tap all available resources including supervision, reading, workplace guidelines, and if available, participation in a workplace conversation group for expectant parents.

CHAPTER 12

Conclusions and Future Directions

When either the therapist or the patient is making the transition to parent, the effects of the process on therapy are potentially incalculable. This book has dealt with the therapist's expectancy. We leave it to others to focus on the equally important topic of the client's expectancy. At times, the physical, psychological and social transformation of the therapist can overwhelm and consume him or her with a kaleidoscope of personal feelings. In response to the intrusion in the case of pregnancy and the therapist's preoccupations in all expectant conditions, patients also have varied and intense feelings—joy, envy, anger, apprehension and so on. Such reactions require acknowledgment and exploration by the therapist, often aided by a supervisor. The therapist's feelings, urges, fantasies and cognitions, conscious and unconscious, have the power to disrupt treatment. At the same time, they offer the therapist the occasion for personal and professional growth and the possibility of exploring with patients areas made salient by this special life passage, ones that possibly were not available for scrutiny earlier in the treatment.

In this final chapter, we sum up what we know about the pregnant therapist, parents in non-traditional families, and the expectant father. We highlight the major patient and therapist reactions that have been described in the literature, including research conducted since our last edition, and that have been suggested by the responses of our interviewees. Fourteen years after we wrote our first edition of this book, it is still true that we know more about the pregnant therapist, particularly a heterosexual woman parenting within the context of a traditional marriage, than any other configuration. Therefore, our conclusions about her situation will be more detailed than those concerning the circumstances of other expectant parents. Following our review, we revisit some of the major decisions the expectant therapist must make. We then identify directions for future research.

Major Points

1. Although all expectancy states could instigate strong responses on the part of the patient, the pregnancy of the therapist is a particularly potent stimulus

because the baby enters the physical space of the therapy. The pregnancy stimulates a number of themes that either might not have emerged previously or not with the same intensity. The most common themes are separation and loss, competition, sexuality, envy and jealousy, and anger. The exploration of these themes constitutes opportunities in the treatment, but with many patients, therapists must actively foster it. The pregnancy also underscores facets of the real relationship, the acknowledgment of which also has therapeutic potential. For example, the patient might experience a realistic concern for or nurturance in relation to the therapist. For the therapist, these moments might be novel and esteem building, and they could further enhance the therapeutic relationship. Some evidence suggests that for adoptive therapists and expectant fathers, the same core issues are at play and in fact, can emerge with greater suddenness given that these therapists are not presenting patients with progressively discernible evidence of a life transition.

2. A number of factors, many of which are characteristics of the patient, influence the patient's response to the therapist's pregnancy. Age and gender emerge as particular important factors. In general, men are less overtly responsive to the pregnancy than women, a difference that is especially pronounced in adolescence. Whereas female patients frequently exhibit excitement and curiosity, males tend to show withdrawal and constriction.

One variable that has been almost entirely neglected is the sexual orientation of the patient. Whether the gender differences observed in a heterosexual population exist in gay, lesbian and bisexual individuals is unknown and an important area for future study. For example, one could imagine a lesbian patient feels some envy of the heterosexual pregnant therapist for the relatively easier situation she has to negotiate with medical personnel, family, and important others on the way to becoming a parent. Gender identity is another unexplored variable: do transgender men and women show different behaviors and identifications with the pregnant therapist than cisgender individuals? As McCluskey (2016) stated, this area of future research is important. The diagnostic status of the patient is also important both from the standpoint of level of ego function and personality style. For example, individuals who function at a borderline level are likely to show a greater disposition toward acting out than individuals organized at either the psychotic or neurotic levels, and this disposition is likely to be more pronounced if the person has a histrionic rather than obsessive-compulsive style. With respect to other expectant conditions, the work has not yet been done to know how individual factors affect patient reactions. For these conditions, different patient variables might be of importance other than those affecting the pregnant therapist–patient dyad. For example, it stands to reason that in the case of the adopting therapist, the adoptive versus nonadoptive status of the patient is of relevance to patient reaction.

3. Events related to the pregnancy, such as miscarriage or infertility, take an inestimable toll on the therapist and often require the introduction of special resources such as extra supervision or therapy to be manageable both in terms of therapist and patient well-being.

4. Modalities of treatment vary in the extent to which they are conducive to the emergence of different themes related to the pregnancy. For example, individual therapy appears to facilitate the emergence of issues of competition and sharing more readily than does group psychotherapy. The group situation, on the other hand, seems to stimulate caretaking responses toward the therapist. At the same time, considerable commonalities exist among the modalities in terms of emerging themes. For example, in both group and individual therapy, themes connected to abandonment, separation and loss are particularly prominent. Family and couple therapies are modalities in need of much further study. What we also do not know is how therapist characteristics interact with type of modality in their effects on the patient–therapist dyad. For example, to what extent does the expectant therapist's status of being a member of a sexual minority affect individuals in group versus individual therapy? We might suppose that because in group psychotherapy, members are less dependent upon the therapist, perhaps the therapist's characteristics are less important. However, like all suppositions, this one must be confirmed (or disconfirmed) by research. Some clinical observations have accrued about fathers in group psychotherapy, and they suggest that relative to expectant mothers, expectant fathers receive far less attention. The confirmation and elucidation of such a difference might tell us something broader about how group members perceive male versus female therapists.

5. During the therapist's pregnancy, and upon her return to work following her maternity leave, the therapist's emotional and cognitive experience as a therapist is likely to be affected by the event of pregnancy itself and, in the case of the primiparous therapist, her new role of mother. Throughout the book, but particularly in Chapters 3 and 4, we described how the shifting physical and psychological events resonate in the treatment situation. For example, we discussed how in the first and third trimesters the therapist's absorption with the pregnancy makes the achievement of a continuous attunement to the patients and the material he or she presents more difficult. We have also pointed out that the therapist's sensitivity to certain issues, such as the struggles some patients experience in being good parents, is enhanced as the woman becomes a parent. In the cases of adoption and expectant fatherhood, the psychological changes are also very significant and have potential to influence the therapist's work. Although adoptive parents, expectant fathers and lesbian non-biological mothers do not have the direct experience of physical changes themselves, they too are affected emotionally by the physical status of the child and the biological mother.

6. From moment to moment, how the therapist reacts to the patient, during her pregnancy and upon her return to work, is shaped by how the patient responds to her, her pregnancy and her status as a new parent. The therapist's ability to take stock of these reactions will enhance or limit her ability to be helpful to the patient through all of the life changes the therapist is experiencing.

7. The workplace also influences the therapist's responses. Despite the pronatalist value of society, it appears from our survey of the literature that many work settings in practice fail to support the needs of the pregnant employee and her family and subtly discourage time and emotional space for parenting. In fact, some settings create impediments to her responding in a therapeutically optimal way to her patients both before and after childbirth. Many workplaces fail to provide even the basic resources to safeguard the mother and child's well-being, such as a private spot where the mother can pump her milk so that she can continue to breastfeed. Fathers and adopting parents, whose expectancies are less perceptible, are treated with even less sensitivity. However, workplace culture is rooted in societal culture. Many countries such as the United States fail to have policies such as paid parental leave that support the building of a family.

8. Prospective parents from non-traditional families have special challenges from those in traditional families but also have resources to offer that emanate from their structure. For example, LGBT parents might have to cope with client responses rooted in heterosexism or transphobia. However, these families tend to offer their children the value of tolerance in a more consistent way than other types of families. Single parents must bear a greater amount of stress in parenting but provide a model for their child of how to develop a network of support.

9. Further research is needed on expectant therapists building non-traditional families, including those not covered in this text (e.g., multi-racial families, families in which parents are cohabitating).

10. The therapist who is an expecting and new parent undergoes an irreversible transformational change that reverberates through her personal and professional life. In order to accommodate to life with this new being, the therapist must revisit his or her ideas about work and family balance. A reallocation of energies is often needed. Typically, change occurs in a stepwise fashion in the patient–therapist interaction, colleague interchange and supervisor-supervisee exchanges. These shifts are presented throughout the book but particularly in Chapters 2, 3, 4, 6 and 11. These changes are most difficult when the therapist is struggling with his or her competence in each of these domains. Chapters 4 and 11 suggest that personal therapy, supervision or a senior colleague who can serve an advisory function can help greatly in enabling the therapist to come to some point of contentment with a revised professional identity and an augmented parental identity.

Decision Making

Throughout this text, we have made numerous suggestions about how the therapist might handle the series of decisions he or she must make while anticipating the arrival of a child into the therapist's family. In this section, we integrate information from prior chapters by discussing and, in some cases, contrasting the approaches of therapists in different treatment situations at varying stages of the transition to parenthood.

The Therapist's Disclosure of the Expectancy of a Child

When, what and how to disclose that the therapist is expecting a baby are issues with which therapists in this life must grapple. The variation in how therapists do so is highlighted by the contrasts between the following vignettes.

Vignette 12.1
For much of her 2-year treatment, Madison, 16, had been prone to extreme negative feelings toward the therapist. In expressing these feelings, she alternated between rageful explosions in the sessions and acting-out incidents consisting primarily in missing sessions. A year ago, one instance of possible suicidal activity occurred involving an overdose of over-the-counter medication. Madison claimed it was inadvertent, but the therapist saw it as a reaction to the therapist's announcement that she (the therapist) would be away for 2 weeks. Madison proceeded through a 4-month period in which she showed much greater containment of negative feelings. During this period, when the therapist disappointed her by announcing that she was taking another vacation, Madison expressed her feelings verbally to the therapist. It was during this vacation that the therapist discovered she was pregnant. The therapist knew that she wanted to take a 3-month maternity leave. She dreaded giving Madison the news; she worried it would usher in a new period of acting out. Over the first 3 months of the pregnancy, Madison gave no sign either directly or derivatively of recognizing a change in the therapist.

Vignette 12.2
Alex, a mildly depressed but highly functioning young woman in her mid-twenties, had been in treatment for 2 months. She was an extremely harsh critic of herself and used the treatment as an opportunity to identify faults and castigate herself. The therapist considered herself somewhat eclectic and used both psychodynamic and cognitive-behavioral components in conducting the treatment. Over the brief course of treatment, Alex had shown some amelioration of her mood as well as a lessening of her harsh self-criticism. Recently, she had been preoccupied with her friends' being married and having babies while she remained, so it seemed to her, frozen

in time. The therapist noted that on an occasion when she needed to cancel a session at the last minute, Alex was able to take this interruption in stride.

The patients in these vignettes differ in their ages and levels of ego functioning. The treatment circumstances also vary, particularly in terms of treatment tenure and the therapists' theoretical orientations. In Chapter 8 on the developmental status of the patient, we discuss some of the intense reactions of adolescent girls in responding to their therapists' pregnancies. That Madison has tended to react to disappointments in her relationship with the therapist with acting out, even self-destructive acting out, naturally leads the therapist to be concerned about how she might respond to the discovery of the pregnancy. Although Madison has shown some improvement in her ability to experience and express her feelings, the great potential for the therapist's pregnancy to be felt as a keen disappointment might compel her to respond in her former way, which would reduce her sense of vulnerability vis-à-vis the therapist. Based on these factors, the therapist might consider informing Madison at a relatively early point in the pregnancy so that the dyad has a full opportunity to explore the conflicts activated by the revelation.

In contrast, Alex's relationship with the therapist is a fledgling one. She has not yet come to trust the therapist sufficiently to be bothered greatly by her absence. As was discussed in Chapter 3, it is important for the therapist to have an open stance concerning the patient's reactions. Although the pregnancy of the therapist is potentially a significant one for the patient, it is not necessarily an evocative event. One factor affecting the degree of importance this event holds for the patient is the degree of development of the relationship, a variable that itself is influenced by the amount of time that patients and therapists have been together.

Another distinguishing factor between the two patients is level of functioning. Because Alex is more mature than Madison, she is likely to deal with any frustrations she might feel in relationship to the pregnancy with containment. In the therapy process, Alex is giving evidence of having registered some information about the therapist's pregnancy. Her comments about her friends might be a derivative expression of a possible comparison between the therapist and herself. In view of all of these factors, the therapist can have a somewhat more relaxed posture with Alex than can Madison's therapist. Alex's therapist can wait and see if Alex's reactions to the pregnancy become more direct and in this way, provide the therapy with the greatest amount of information concerning not only her conscious but also, unconscious reactions to the pregnancy.

The general principle to be extracted from this comparison is that the discussion about when to announce the pregnancy should be an individual one predicated on a consideration of a variety of patient characteristics. Among these characteristics are developmental status and level of psychological (ego) functioning. The more information about the patient the therapist considers, the more sensitively timed any communication about the pregnancy are likely to be. Unfortunately, in some settings such as a residential treatment center, the therapist cannot customize the communication because patients share information with one another.

For some therapists, the announcement of the pregnancy might bring other revelations such as the therapist's sexual orientation, or married versus single status. Patients might have responses to these aspects in ways that pose challenges to the therapeutic alliance. For example, the patient might exhibit disapproval of a single woman's choice to assume the role of solo parent. Transgender therapists might encounter the patient's cisgenderism just as gay and lesbian therapists might be confronted with heterosexism. For these more complicated situations, therapists can benefit from additional supports such as individual or group supervision, which is likely to be especially effective when those providing supervision have personal understanding of the therapist's circumstance.

For adopting therapists and prospective fathers, the decision of whether and when to announce that a baby is expected is a more active one given that the patient might not otherwise learn of this life change prior to its happening. This difference can make the decision a somewhat more difficult one. We have found that therapists in these situations are more likely to worry that their own conflictual concerns are driving their decisions. We would argue that, just as in the case of the pregnant therapist, a careful reflection on all of the characteristics of the patient is extremely useful in addition to considering one's own motives for the possible disclosure. The therapist in making the decision should also keep in mind that such information is in the public domain. The therapist must weigh the effects on the real relationship and the therapeutic alliance of obtaining this news from the therapist versus other channels.

Planning the Leave

Following the disclosure of the expectancy, the next major decision the therapist must make is when to schedule the leave and what supports should be provided for the patient during the therapist's absence, however long or short. Some of the factors bearing on this decision will be highlighted in the following vignette, featuring a therapist who was adopting a child.

Vignette 12.3

Sheldon is a 30-year-old man with paranoid symptoms. He had been seeing his therapist for only 3 months following a stay in a residential treatment center. At the time he began with the therapist, she was expecting to adopt a baby domestically within 4 months. During their initial meeting, she had alluded to her impending adoption of a baby and noted that if they continued to work together, a 1-month disruption in the treatment would occur.

Sheldon's relatives, who had been contacted by his neighbors, had pressured him to admit himself to a residential treatment center. The neighbors were troubled by several angry outbursts that followed his interpretation of minor events as actions against him. While in the residential treatment center, Sheldon had been placed on a small dose of antipsychotic medication and his anxiety diminished considerably. He had had a successful experience in a problem-solving group and this success led to his referral to a similar but somewhat less structured outpatient group. In the outpatient group, Sheldon was voluble, speaking out frequently in an effort to provide advice or comfort to another member. Although he did share information about himself, it was mainly to give inspirational talks about problems he had solved rather than current struggles. He took delight in a member's comment that he seemed like one of the therapists. He harkened back to the comment frequently in sessions. Sheldon continued to be seen on an outpatient basis by his medicating psychiatrist who maintained a collegial relationship with him, often soliciting from Sheldon during their monthly sessions his abundant views on current political situations.

In addition to being referred for psychiatric monitoring and outpatient group therapy, Sheldon was also referred for supportive individual therapy. His behavior in individual treatment was in stark contrast with his behavior in the group. He repeatedly claimed he had nothing to say. Occasionally, he would embark on a diatribe against the leader of the country. When the therapist suggested that perhaps he was worrying about her ability to conduct the therapy, he became outraged and made insinuations about the intactness of her thought processes. However, gradually, he appeared to be more forthcoming about his frustrations with his neighbors and his conviction about their malevolence toward him.

As the birth of the baby approached, she increasingly worried about what to do about Sheldon. She felt that Sheldon's connection with the group was firm and his connection with her was tenuous. At the same time, she suspected that the lack of trust he felt in their relationship was part and parcel of his personality organization: given their amount of time together, the relationship might be as good as it could be. She wondered whether she should arrange for a substitute therapist. She also contemplated transferring him to another therapist altogether. She considered encouraging him to continue with his group and his medicating psychiatrist during her absence while possible seeing the latter more frequently.

The planning of the therapist's leave requires a comprehensive case review as well as an assessment of the resources available to the patient. When the patient is relatively high functioning and the maternity or paternity leave is brief, the therapist need not introduce the complication of a substitute therapist. In fact, some patients might see such a suggestion as condescending on the part of the departing therapist. However, for patients who are lower functioning and at risk for behaving in ways that are highly detrimental to themselves and others, further support is in order. Yet, whether a substitute therapist is an appropriate support must be evaluated on a case-by-case basis: use of a substitute therapist requires the patient's capacity to form relatively quickly a tie with a caretaking person. Patients such as Sheldon with profound mistrust need a lengthy period of relationship building. As therapists are making their decisions, they should exercise care not to unduly weight their own interests. Departing therapists frequently worry that substitute therapists might become permanent therapists. However, ethical practice demands that the well-being of the patient be given priority over the therapist's needs.

In the instance of Sheldon, the therapist had three other resources to deploy during her leave: the psychiatrist, the group therapist and herself. The medicating psychiatrist could perform some monitoring function. However, to do this adequately, monthly meetings might be insufficient. A major challenge for the psychiatrist would be to obtain the necessary information while maintaining rapport. Any obvious shift in the relationship in the direction of greater exploration or any behaviors on the part of the psychiatrist that would alter the power differential in the patient's perception might jeopardize the psychiatrist's status as a resource during the individual therapist's parental leave. The second resource is the group therapist. One possibility would be for the group therapist to function also as an individual therapist during the parental leave. The advantage of this arrangement is that Sheldon already had some measure of trust in the group therapist. The disadvantage is essentially the same as that with the psychiatrist, namely, the potential for introducing a threatening element in the relationship that would place it in jeopardy. The third resource is the departing therapist herself. Although the therapist planned to suspend sessions for a certain period, she might be able and willing to have some phone contact with the patient. For example, she could check in with the patient at several points during her absence.

Ultimately, the plan that could support the patient's well-being and safeguard the therapeutic relationship during the leave is one that entails the orchestration of all of these resources. Doing so would require a high level of communication among all persons providing Sheldon treatment. Oftentimes, the development of a plan for patients during a therapist's parental leave, especially when patients are vulnerable in some way (as in the case of children or lower functioning adults), involves a high level of coordination among the providers of mental health services. A group of professionals who might not have functioned as a true treatment team might be required to become such a unit in order to serve the patient's needs adequately during the period of the therapist's departure.

The Gift Dilemma

In many cases, the therapist will be the recipient of presents, typically for the baby, but in some cases for himself or herself. The therapist would do well to assume he or she is going to receive presents and develop a particular plan for dealing with such an occurrence. The first question the therapist must pose to himself or herself is whether or not to accept the present. Our research and that of others suggests that a therapist almost always accepts gifts for the baby. The only instance in which therapists choose not to accept a gift is when the gift is inappropriate (i.e., crosses a boundary the therapist wishes to maintain). Where therapists depart from one another is in the extent to which the meaning of the present is explored with the patient. Whereas some merely express gratitude, others engage the patient in an investigation of the significance of the gift. In developing an approach to the gift dilemma, the therapist must weigh the objectives of safeguarding the therapeutic alliance, ensuring the patient's stability during the leave, and taking advantage of opportunities for therapeutic growth. These objectives should be considered in the light of the specific factors of the case, factors related to the modality, the patient and other variables suggested in the following vignettes. This one highlights the modality factor.

Vignette 12.4

In an outpatient group of male and female adults organized primarily at the upper borderline level, a surprise shower was given for the therapist 3 weeks before her maternity leave. Throughout her pregnancy, members had been extremely reticent to express any sort of negative reactions to the pregnancy. Yet members exhibited contentiousness toward the student co-therapist (the supervisee of the pregnant therapist). During the surprise shower, members presented the therapist with a painting for the baby's room, a picture of a beatific mother cuddling her slumbering child. "To the best therapist and mother in the world" was written on the card that was signed by each group member. The members appeared eager for the co-therapist to see the inscription.

In Chapter 10, we describe how the members of a psychotherapy group are less likely than individual therapy patients to express negative feelings in relation to the therapist's pregnancy. This group is true to form. Yet, glimmerings of negativity could be detected in members' responses to the co-therapist. In responding to the group gift, the therapist should keep in mind the objective of ensuring the group's stability during her leave. In addition to missing an opportunity for learning, lack of processing of members' negatively toned feelings, especially their anger, might result in acting out during the maternity leave. This worry is particularly realistic given members' developmental status (i.e., being organized at the borderline rather than neurotic level). Such acting out, particularly if taking the form of absence and precipitous terminations, could undermine the integrity of the entire group. Alternatively, members might show extreme expressions of anger that the co-therapist might have difficulty addressing productively. Such difficulty might be compounded by the supervisor's failure to model how to work with the group's anger.

In this situation, then, the therapist might use her remaining time in the group to identify the group's use of splitting to manage members' anger in relation to the therapist. Members could be helped to see that the Madonna in the picture was actually the therapist for whom they wished rather than the therapist that they had. Members' failure to express anger in relation to the therapist was likely due, in part, to their fear of its destructive value: the anger might destroy the therapist, her baby or themselves. In fact, more potentially destructive are the alternate indirect means the members might find to give these feelings expression. Therefore, the detoxification of members' anger is an important task (Kibel, 1981). Detoxifying anger entails helping members to see that their anger is a reasonable response to the situation and that their catastrophic fantasies about the possible consequences of the direct verbalization of anger toward the person evoking the anger are not likely to be realized.

The therapist seeking to explore the connection between a gift and negative feelings about the pregnancy has an advantage in the group situation relative to the individual situation. In the group, the potential of interpreting warded-off, unacceptable feelings or impulses as shared psychological elements lessens the narcissistic sting attached to them (Kibel, 1981). Although members on an individual level might resist giving expression to negative feelings because of their shame and humiliation about these feelings, in a group setting, the recognition that others, too, have these reactions makes them far more tolerable. Moreover, the group, in the language of attachment theory, provides a secure base for members to explore any attachment anxiety stimulated by the upcoming departure of the therapist (Marmarosh & Tasca, 2013), anxiety that is laced with anger toward the therapist for having created this separation crisis.

The therapist's response to a gift should take into account the patient's developmental level and narcissistic tie to the gift. These features figure prominently in the next vignette.

Vignette 12.5

John, an 8-year-old boy, had been placed in a residential treatment center because of extreme acting-out behavior in his school setting. Not only had he engaged in behavior threatening to other children (e.g., throwing another child off a school bus), but also had engaged in some self-destructive behaviors, such as eating glue during an art project. On admission to the residential treatment center, he was assigned to a psychology intern in her fourth month of pregnancy for play therapy. Because of the supervisor's concern that the child's unacknowledged awareness of the pregnancy might precipitate episodes of acting out, he was told very early on about the pregnancy (although it was unlikely that he would still be at the center when she took her maternity leave). In his play, he expressed anger toward the mother doll and the baby doll, frequently pounding the latter on the floor yelling, "Bad, bad!" At the same time, he expressed curiosity about the pregnancy and continually asked the therapist if the baby was a boy. When the therapist said she didn't know, John said he hoped it was. Gradually, his level of aggression, although never disappearing altogether, diminished in intensity.

A month prior to the therapist's departure for her leave and 3 weeks prior to John's commencement of his summer leave, he brought her a sculpture he had made in art class of a puppy. He said it was a present for the baby boy. The art therapist later shared with his individual therapist the fact that he took great satisfaction in making the puppy for the therapist and was very excited about giving it to her. He said, "The baby is really going to love this little guy."

The therapist had acted consistent with the thinking in much of the child literature (e.g., Callahan, 1985), that children should be given maximal time to react to the pregnancy separately from the maternity leave itself. The therapist's apprising the child of the pregnancy at a relatively early point enabled the child to delve into competition-related issues in his play therapy. The child's spontaneous expression of warmth toward the therapist's baby seemed to be a consequence of his having reckoned with the intensity of his anger. Although the gift might have some elements of an effort to defend against negative feelings, it was also a genuine expression of his positive feelings.

The child often experiences a gift that he or she has made as an extension of self. For this reason, the rejection of the gift (an unlikely act by any pregnant therapist) or even its exploration, would most likely lead the child to experience narcissistic hurt. The long-term impact of the hurt, particularly in view of the therapist's upcoming departure, might not justify any surfeit meaning that can be extracted through the gift's exploration.

The case of John illustrate an important connection between the therapist's announcement of the pregnancy, the processing of the pregnancy, and the therapist's stance toward a gift. To the extent that the therapist ensures that the patient (a) knows about the pregnancy for a sufficient period before the leave and (b) is given encouragement and opportunity to explore pregnancy-related reactions, the burden is lifted from the interpretation of the gift to discover important dimensions of the patient's response to the pregnancy. The therapist is thereby liberated to respond to the real relationship aspect of the gift.

Announcement of the Arrival of the Child in the Family

Once the birth has occurred, or in the case of adoption, the arrival of the child in the family, the therapist must decide whether and how to communicate this event to patients and what details to share. Again, the decision should be predicated on knowledge of the patient's characteristics and dynamics. The following vignette illustrates the concerns of a therapist in such a circumstance.

Vignette 12.6
Reba was a therapist with a large practice. Her high-risk pregnancy was a difficult one, with frequent bleeding. Reba continually feared the loss of the pregnancy. Nonetheless, she was able to carry the baby full-term. Moreover,

because of the sedentary nature of her work, she found she had little disruption in her sessions and patients were not aware of the problems she was experiencing. When the baby was born, he was admitted to the NICU for 2 months. During the first few weeks of this period, on several occasions, the infant ceased to breathe and needed to be resuscitated. However, the infant survived these episodes, left the hospital, and thrived.

Shortly after birth, Reba wondered what to do about each of her patients. She knew that many of them were waiting with excitement to learn the news of the birth. She also needed to inform patients that the dates of their treatment resumption were uncertain. Yet, she felt that her son's ability to survive was in question. She was distraught and felt she had few emotional resources to deal with their reactions to specific features of the situation. As she contemplated her predicament, she realized that there were two subgroups of patients. One subgroup, she anticipated, would be able to be given relatively minimal information about her difficulties and withstand the ambiguities. She thought she might write a short note indicating that the baby was a boy and was born with some health problems. She would also indicate that she would be back in touch when she was able to schedule an appointment. She would remind them of the name and number of the person providing coverage for her if the patient had any additional concerns.

She puzzled over another subgroup of patients, one of whom was Holly. Holly was a 22-year-old woman who had a histrionic personality style and was organized at the borderline level. Her late adolescent and young adult life was scattered with self-injurious acting out. The therapy had had a stormy course, with transferences to the therapist rapidly swinging from negative to positive. The therapist's pregnancy had seen the relationship's more consistent residency in a negative transference pattern. Holly's expression of death wishes toward the baby had been frequent, as had periods of self-condemnation for these expressions. In fact, Reba had gone into supervision to help herself manage her reactions to the patient's hostility toward the baby so that she would not join with the patient's self-rejection. Now that the baby's life was in jeopardy, she feared that Holly would believe she had caused the infant's difficulties and that this inference would instigate a new series of acting-out incidents. Holly had begun to be seen during the therapist's absence by a substitute therapist. Reba began to form a plan wherein the substitute therapist would give her the information about the birth complications. She planned to apprise the therapist of her concerns over the link Holly might draw between the child's problems and her murderous wishes.

Reba had a clear recognition of the importance of tailoring her communications to the individual needs of her patients. For some patients, the provision of information beyond a few basic facts might have been emotionally burdensome. For others, the anxiety-arousing potential of the information required that patients be given a forum to address their fears, fantasies, associations and other emotional reactions.

With patients such as Holly, Reba recognized the need to institute a higher level of support than with others. In fact, this vignette highlights an advantage of using a substitute therapist. Because of the uncertainties associated with pregnancy and delivery, the substitute therapist provides a safety net should either the time frame change (e.g., the maternity leave begins earlier or lasts longer) or untoward events occur (e.g., a death of the child or a decision by the therapist not to return to work). Whereas higher functioning patients might be able to brook these uncertainties and difficulties, lower functioning patients are likely to benefit from protections against more self-detrimental means of independently managing unforeseen events. In this instance, then, Reba had an excellent resource available to help her to assist this patient from afar.

Another important dimension of this case is Reba's recognition of what she could manage during her crisis with her child. Attending to her own needs as well as those of her child and her patients was too demanding to permit her to do justice to all parties. Therefore, she appropriately relegated responsibility to the substitute therapist to both convey the information about the therapist and to explore the Holly's reactions to it. The new parent's recognition of his or her limitations is critical to serving everyone's well-being before, during and after the child's entrance into the family.

For therapists who are new fathers, new adoptive parents or non-biological gay and lesbian expectant parents, the announcement is likely to be a difficult decision when the therapist has not forecasted that such an event was to take place. For gay and lesbian individuals, the disclosure of sexual orientation might also come with the parenting disclosure making the decision of sharing information more complicated. What poses a special burden for patients is when an extended leave of the therapist coincides with the news of the arrival of the child. A strong recommendation is that therapists in all expectancy conditions will develop a plan about what information is to be shared before a child's arrival so that the patient has adequate time to explore each piece of information with a still-available therapist.

In all of the treatment situations that arise related to the therapist's expectant parenthood, the development of an appropriate intervention strategy requires weighing a variety of factors including characteristics of the patient (including diagnosis, level of functioning, background of trauma, childbearing history, etc.), the modality of treatment and type of therapeutic work being done and the treatment setting, as well as the specifics of the therapist's personality and situation. Therefore, the formulation of a uniform policy that is not subject to re-evaluating as events unfold is unlikely to be the optimal strategy for the expectant therapist. Flexible, individualized approaches with vigilance for possible countertransferential motives are what will benefit both the patient and therapist during the latter's life changes.

Final Note

The event of a therapist becoming a parent is profound and requires all of the knowledge we can amass. We believe that the study of therapists anticipating the entrance of a child into the family will advance only through substantial changes in how this topic is addressed (i.e., what methodologies are employed and what facets of the transition are addressed). Significant limitations exist in the methodologies employed in the exploration of early parenting situations. For the most part, this circumstance has been investigated from the vantage point of the therapist. What is the therapist experiencing? What does the therapist *see* the patient experiencing? Certain, the perspective of the therapist is essential. However, a comprehensive understanding of the phenomena associated with these life changes demands other viewpoints as well.

A rich source of information is that provided by patients themselves. A few of the therapists we interviewed also had the perspective of being the patient of a pregnant therapist at a previous point in their lives. They observed that their therapy technique was informed by their experiences of being on "the other side of the couch." From those few studies that have been done using patient perspectives, it is evident that they offer a distinctive point of view. For example, in the Katzman (1993) study of eating-disordered patients, the investigators discovered that the patients had a conscious realization of the pregnancy considerably before their articulation of it. This finding could have implications for the timing of the therapist's announcement. More recently, McCluskey (2016), who interviewed eight clients who had experienced their therapists' pregnancies for their duration, found that therapists' announcements of their pregnancies did not automatically lead clients to recognize the inevitability of a break in treatment. This finding makes clear the importance of the therapist actively alerting patients to this aspect. McCluskey also found that the patients who are covered by substitute therapists often experience loyalty conflicts, and consider staying with the substitute therapist. This is the kind of reaction that could easily be hidden from the therapist. Vandereycken and DeKerf (2010) presented 69 eating-disordered patients with a questionnaire in which they compared their reactions to the therapist's pregnancy in comparison with the pregnancies of other significant individuals in their lives. They found that these patients perceived the therapists' pregnancies as more consequential for how they regarded themselves. Such a finding is consistent with the theme of this book, that the expectancy of the therapist is a matter of some moment. However, obtaining these insights requires that the clients themselves are asked about their experiences.

Other perspectives are available. For example, systematic observations might be collected from other professionals who work with the therapist, in the capacities as co-therapist, treatment team member, administrative supervisor, staff support person and so on. Professionals in these roles can make an important contribution not only because they provide another set of eyes to witness clinical phenomena, but also because they, too, in their work as clinicians, might be affected by the therapist's imminent parenthood. To know fully the clinical effects of this life change, it would be essential to assess its influence on each member of a treatment community. Furthermore, each perspective—that of the therapist, patient and the other professionals in the treatment environment— has validity in its own right and adds to the complex clinical picture that any significant life transition produces.

Another methodological point concerns when the data is collected. Much of the study data available—including our own—is retrospective. This is an unsurprising finding given the challenges of collecting current data. For example, how can the interviewer collect data from the therapists in their first trimester, given that many are unwilling to reveal their pregnancies (or other expectant states) to their professional communities? Yet, memory can distort the therapist's experience of many aspects of his or her experience. On the other hand, the therapist might recognize aspects of his or her experience that were less accessible during the pregnancy. Therefore, the literature benefits from both current and retrospective observations. Each provides us with distinctive information; each informs us of the limits of the other.

Therapists building families use a multiplicity of routes and come to parenting with a kaleidoscope of identities. The literature has barely begun to explore these varied routes and identities and their significance for clinical practice. In the past 15 years, greater attention has been given to gender identity and sexual orientation in the professional literature, but that interest has not extended to the topic of the therapist's building a family. From an even superficial contemplation of the situation of the gay or lesbian therapist, for instance, it is apparent that complexities are present in such matters as announcing the upcoming birth of a child that are not present for heterosexual individuals. The neglect within the literature means that individuals so circumstanced will be on their own in navigating their course. Expectant fathers and adoptive parents are also deserving of more careful attention, including the kinds of systematic efforts that have taken place for pregnant therapists that have occurred across nearly four decades.

Another area of needed inquiry concerns therapist decision making. We have discussed throughout this book that the therapist's expectancy ushers in a host of important clinical decisions. Therapists must decide when to announce the expectancy, how to handle gifts, whether to use alternate therapists, and other considerations. Although much has been written about these decision-making points, virtually no research has been done looking at the effects of particular types of decisions with patients of different characteristics.

Finally, an area in need of further investigation concerns the influence of the therapist's theoretical orientation. In our investigation of group therapists, we discovered that the same set of themes emerges in the treatment across therapists using different theoretical orientations. For example, our small sample of therapists using cognitive-behavioral and interpersonal orientations recognized the abandonment and sibling rivalry themes that psychodynamic therapists have long observed in the material of their patients. Would our finding of common themes be replicated in other studies? We also found that some thematic specificity exists in group versus individual psychotherapies. This finding, too, bears replication and expanded study. Once there is some clarity concerning the effects of the therapist's expectancy within differential theoretical orientations and modalities, then the pressing issue will become how these thematic elements can be tapped to maximal therapeutic advantage.

Building a family is one of the most basic of human activities. Becoming a parent is one of the most profound transitions a human being could undergo. Although the study of the therapist's expectancy has occurred over four decades, we are still in the very beginning stage of understanding the ways in which it shapes and is shaped by work as a therapist. Through our fledgling efforts, we have hoped to inspire others to pursue this area of study further. We look forward to learning of others' contributions.

Bibliography

Abbasi, A. (2014). *The rupture of serenity: External intrusions and psychoanalytic technique*. London: Karnac Books.

Abend, S. M. (1982). Serious illness in the analyst: Countertransference considerations. *Journal of the American Psychoanalytical Association, 30*, 365–379.

Addati, L., Cassirer, N., & Gilchrist, K. (2014). *Maternity and paternity at work: Law and practice across the world*. Geneva: International Labour Office.

Adelson, M. (1995). Effect of therapist's pregnancies on transference and countertransference: A case history. *Journal of Clinical Psychoanalysis, 4*(3), 383–404.

Aizley, H. (2006). Introduction: Mommy delirious. In H. Aizley (Ed.), *Confessions of the other mother: Nonbiological lesbian moms tell all* (pp. ix–xiii). Boston, MA: Beacon Press.

Akhtar, S. (2016a). Guilt: An introductory overview. In S. Akhtar (ed.) *Guilt: Origins, manifestations, and management* (pp. 1–15). Lanham, MD: Jacob Aronson.

Akhtar, S. (2016b). The impact of contemporary culture on maternal functions: An overview. In S. Akhtar (Ed.), *The new motherhoods: Patterns of early child care in contemporary culture* (pp. 81–106). Lanham, MD: Rowman & Littlefield.

Albertini, M., & Kohli, M. (2009). What childless older people give: Is the generational link broken? *Ageing and Society, 29*(8), 1261–1274. https://doi.org/10.1017/S0144686X0999033X

Alio, A. P., Salihu, H. M., Kornosky, J. L., Richman, A. M., & Marty, P. J. (2010). Feto-infant health and survival: Does paternal involvement matter? *Maternal and Child Health Journal, 14*(6), 931–937. https://doi.org/10.1007/s10995-009-0531-9

Allen, D. W. (1977). Basic treatment issues. In M. J. Horowitz (Ed.), *Hysterical Personality* (pp. 283–328). New York: Jason Aronson.

Allison, J. (2011). Conceiving silence: Infertility as discursive contradiction in Ireland. *Medical Anthropology Quarterly, 25*(1), 1–21.

Allison, K. C., & Sarwer, D. B. (2016). Body image disturbance during pregnancy and the postpartum period. In A. Wenzel (Ed.), *The Oxford handbook of perinatal psychology* (pp. 231–251). New York: Oxford University Press.

Al-Mateen, C. S. (1991). Simultaneous pregnancy in the therapist and the patient. *American Journal of Psychotherapy, 45*(3), 432–444.

Almeida, C. P. de Sá, E., Cunha, F. F., & Pires, E. P. (2012). Common mental disorders during pregnancy and baby's development in the first year of life. *Journal of Reproductive and Infant Psychology, 30*(4), 341–351. https://doi.org/10.1080/02646838.201 2.736689

Almond, R. (2015). Patients' pregnancies during treatment: The influence of the analyst's psychology. *Psychoanalytic Dialogues, 25*(3), 344–358. https://doi.org/10.1080/104818 85.2015.1034560

Alperin, R. M. (2001). Barriers to intimacy: An object relations perspective. *Psychoanalytic Psychology, 18*(1), 137–156.

Amato, P. R. (2001). Children and divorce in the 1990s: An update of the Amato and Keith (1991) meta-analysis. *Journal of Family Psychology, 15*, 355–370.

American Pregnancy Association. (2016, August). *Miscarriage: Signs, symptoms, treatment and prevention.* Retrieved October 3, 2016, from http://americanpregnancy.org/ pregnancy-complications/miscarriage/

American Psychological Association. (2002). Ethical principles of psychologists and code of conduct. *American Psychologist, 57*(12), 1060–1073. https://doi.org/10.1037/ 0003-066X.57.12.1060

American Society for Reproductive Medicine. (2012). *Age and fertility: A guide for patients.* American Society for Reproductive Medicine. Retrieved from www.asrm. org/uploadedFiles/ASRM_Content/Resources/Patient_Resources/Fact_Sheets_and_ Info_Booklets/agefertility.pdf

An, Z. (2014). The dilemma of receiving support from in-laws: A study of the discourse of online pregnancy and childbirth support groups. *China Media Research, 10*(3), 32–43.

Anderson, L. (1994). The experience of being a pregnant group therapist. *Group Analysis, 27*(1), 75–85.

Anderson, M. V., & Rutherford, M. D. (2013). Evidence of a nesting psychology during human pregnancy. *Evolution and Human Behavior, 34*(6), 390–397. https://doi. org/10.1016/j.evolhumbehav.2013.07.002

Anderson, N., Fallon, A., Brabender, V., & Maier, L. (2000, April 28). *Emerging themes in group versus individual psychotherapy during the therapist§s pregnancy* (Poster session). Philadelphia, PA: Philadelphia Area Group Psychotherapy Society Annual Conference, Widener University.

Anderson, V. N., Fleming, A. S., & Steiner, M. (1994). Mood and the transition to motherhood. *Journal of Reproductive and Infant Psychology, 12*(2), 69–77. https://doi.org/10. 1080/02646839408408870

Apfel, R. J., & Keylor, R. G. (2002). Psychoanalysis and infertility myths and realities. *The International Journal of Psychoanalysis, 83*(1), 85–104.

Arrighi, B. A., & Maume, D. J. (2000). Workplace subordination and men's avoidance of housework. *Journal of Family Issues, 21*(4), 464–487. https://doi.org/10.11 77/019251300021004003

Asher, W. J., Vogler, T. C., Bovee, K. C., Holtzapple, P. G., & Hamilton, R. W. (1976). In vivo performance of liquid membrane capsules. *Transactions—American Society for Artificial Internal Organs, 22*, 605–611.

Ashway, J. A. (1984). A therapist§s pregnancy: An opportunity for conflict resolution and growth in the treatment of children. *Clinical Social Work Journal, 121*(3), 3–17.

Atkinson, D. R., Brady, S., & Casas, J. M. (1981). Sexual preference similarity, attitude similarity, and perceived counseling credibility and attractiveness. *Journal of Counseling Psychology, 28*(6), 504–509. https://doi.org/10.1037/0022-0167.28.6.504

Atlas-Koch, G. (2008). Three pregnancies and psychoanalysis: A thin line between fusion and separateness. *The Psychoanalytic Review, 95*(2), 259–283. https://doi.org/10.1521/prev.2008.95.2.259

Auchincloss, E. L. (1982). Conflict among psychiatric residents in response to pregnancy. *American Journal of Psychiatry, 139*(6), 818–820.

Aumann, K., Galinsky, E., & Matos, K. (2011). *The new male mystique*. New York: Families and Work Institute.

Babb, P. L., McIntosh, A. M., Fernandez-Duque, E., & Schurr, T. G. (2014). Prolactin receptor gene diversity in Azara's owl monkeys (Aotus azarai) and humans (Homo sapiens) suggests a non-neutral evolutionary history among primates. *International Journal of Primatology, 35*(1), 129–155. https://doi.org/10.1007/s10764-013-9721-9

Bach, P., & Hayes, S. C. (2002). The use of acceptance and commitment therapy to prevent the rehospitalization of psychotic patients: A randomized controlled trial. *Journal of Consulting and Clinical Psychology, 70*(5), 1129–1139. https://doi.org/10.1037//0022-006X.70.5.1129

Bales, K. L., Maninger, N., & Hinde, K. (2012). New directions in the neurobiology and physiology of paternal care. In O. Gillath, G. Adams, & A. Kunkel (Eds.), *Relationship science: Integrating evolutionary, neuroscience, and sociocultural approaches* (pp. 91–111). Washington, DC: American Psychological Association. Retrieved from http://content.apa.org/books/13489-005

Ballou, J. (1978). The significance of reconcilative themes in the psychology of pregnancy. *Bulletin of the Menninger Clinic, 42*, 383–413.

Balsam, R. (1974). The pregnant therapist. In R. Balsam & A. Balsam (Eds.), *Becoming a psychotherapist* (pp. 265–288). Boston: Little Brown.

Balsam, R. H. (2012). The pregnant mother and the body image of the daughter. In P. Mariotti (Ed.), *The maternal lineage: Identification, desire, and transgenerational issues* (pp. 113–138). New York: Routledge.

Barbanel, L. (1980). The therapist's pregnancy. In B. L. Blum (Ed.), *Psychological aspects of pregnancy, birthing, and bonding* (pp. 232–246). New York: Human Sciences Press.

Bar-Tura, N. B. (2012, April 23). *Impact of patient pregnancy on psychodynamic psychotherapy* (Doctoral Dissertation). The Chicago School of Professional Psychology, Chicago, IL. Retrieved from UMI Dissertation Publishing. (UMI No. 3536307)

Bartlett, E. E. (2004). The effects of fatherhood on the health of men: A review of the literature. *The Journal of Men's Health & Gender, 1*(2–3), 159–169. https://doi.org/10.1016/j.jmhg.2004.06.004

Bashe, E. (1989). *The therapist's pregnancy: The experience of patient and therapist in psychoanalytic psychotherapy* (Doctoral Dissertation). Rutgers University, New Brunswick, NJ.

Bassen, C. R. (1988). The impact of the therapist's pregnancy on the course of analysis. *Psychoanalytic Inquiry, 8*(2), 280–298.

Bateman, A., & Fonagy, P. (2004). *Psychotherapy for borderline personality disorder: Mentalization-based treatment.* Oxford: Oxford University Press. Retrieved from www.oxfordclinicalpsych.com/view/10.1093/med:psych/9780198527664.001.0001/med-9780198527664

Baum, D. (2009, April 21). *Brown anthropologist examines stigma of infertility in Nigeria | News from Brown.* Retrieved August 7, 2016, from https://news.brown.edu/articles/2009/04/infertility

Baum, N. (2010). Dual role transition among first time pregnant social work student trainees. *Social Work Education, 29*(7), 718–728. https://doi.org/10.1080/02615471003599335

Baum, N., & Itzhaky, H. (2006). Pregnancy as a secret in supervision. *Arete, 29*(2), 33–43.

Baum, O. E., & Herring, C. (1975). The pregnant psychotherapist in training: Some preliminary findings and impressions. *American Journal of Psychiatry, 132*(4), 419–422.

Becker, G. (1994). Metaphors in disrupted lives: Infertility and cultural constructions of continuity. *Medical Anthropology Quarterly, 8*(4), 383–410.

Beebe, B., Jaffe, J., & Lachmann, F. (1992). A dyadic systems view of communication. In N. J. Skolnick & S. C. Warshaw (Eds.), *Relational perspectives in psychoanalysis* (pp. 61–81). El Dorado Hills, CA: Analytic Press.

Benedek, E. P. (1973). The fourth world of the pregnant therapist. *Journal of American Medical Women§s Association, 28,* 365–368.

Benedek, T. (1959). Parenthood as a developmental phase; a contribution to the libido theory. *Journal of the American Psychoanalytic Association, 7*(3), 389–417.

Bennett, S. M., Litz, B. T., Lee, B. S., et al. (2005). The scope and impact of perinatal loss: current status and future directions. *Professional Psychology, Research and Practice, 36,* 180–187.

Bergström, G., Bodin, L., Hagberg, J., Lindh, T., Aronsson, G., & Josephson, M. (2009). Does sickness presenteeism have an impact on future general health? *International Archives of Occupational and Environmental Health, 82*(10), 1179–1190. https://doi.org/10.1007/s00420-009-0433-6

Berkman, C. S., & Zinberg, G. (1997). Homophobia and heterosexism in social workers. *Social Work, 42*(4), 319–332. https://doi.org/10.1093/sw/42.4.319

Berkson, M. (n.d.). *Exploring religious aspects of infertility treatments by Mindy Berkson.* Retrieved August 7, 2016, from www.articlecity.com/articles/religion/article_946.shtml

Berman, E. (1975). Acting out as a response to the psychiatrist§s pregnancy. *Journal of the American Medical Women's Association, 30*(11), 456–458.

Bernica, N. (2001). *Attitudes of social workers toward gay and lesbian adoption* (1405848 M.S.W.). California State University, Long Beach, Ann Arbor, MI. Retrieved from http://proxy.lib.utk.edu:90/login?url=http://search.proquest.com/docview/194107525?account id=14766

Bhar, S. S., & Kyrios, M. (2007). An investigation of self-ambivalence in obsessive-compulsive disorder. *Behaviour Research and Therapy, 45*(8), 1845–1857. https://doi.org/10.1016/j.brat.2007.02.005

Bianchi, S. M., Sayer, L. C., Milkie, M. A., & Robinson, J. P. (2012). Housework: Who did, does or will do it, and how much does it matter? *Social Forces, 91*(1), 55–63. https://doi.org/10.1093/sf/sos120

Bibring, G. L. (1959). Some Considerations of the psychological processes in pregnancy. *The Psychoanalytic Study of the Child, 14*(1), 113–121. https://doi.org/10.1080/00797308.1959.11822824

Bibring, G. L., Dwyer, T. F., Huntington, D. S., & Valenstein, A. (1961). A study of the psychological processes in pregnancy and of the earliest mother-child relationship: II methodological considerations. *The Psychoanalytic Study of the Child, 16*, 9–73.

Bienen, M. (1990). The pregnant therapist: Countertransference dilemmas and willingness to explore transference material. *Psychotherapy: Theory, Research, Practice, Training, 27*(4), 607–612. https://doi.org/10.1037/0033-3204.27.4.607

Bion, W. (1959). *Experiences in groups*. London: Tavistock.

Bjørnholt, M. (2014). Changing men, changing times—fathers and sons from an experimental gender equality study. *The Sociological Review, 62*(2), 295–315. https://doi.org/10.1111/1467-954X.12156

Blankenhorn, D. (1995). *Fatherless America: Confronting our most urgent social problem*. New York: Basic Books.

Blencowe, H., Cousens, S., Oestergaard, M. Z., Chou, D., Moller, A.-B., Narwal, R., . . . Lawn, J. E. (2012). National, regional, and worldwide estimates of preterm birth rates in the year 2010 with time trends since 1990 for selected countries: A systematic analysis and implications. *The Lancet, 379*(9832), 2162–2172. https://doi.org/10.1016/S0140-6736(12)60820-4

Bliss, C. (1999). *The social construction of infertility by minority women*. Doctoral Dissertation. Retrieved from www.gerrystahl.net/personal/family/dissertation.pdf

Blos, P. (1980). Modifications in the traditional psychoanalytic theory of female adolescent development. *Adolescent Psychiatry, 8*, 8–24.

Blos, P. (1985). *Son and father: Before and beyond the oedipus complex*. New York: Collier MacMillan.

Blumberg, R. L., & Coleman, M. T. (1989). A theoretical look at the gender balance of power in the american couple. *Journal of Family Issues, 10*(2), 225–250.

Bolognini, S. (2006). The profession of ferryman: Considerations on the analyst's internal attitude in consultation and in referral. *The International Journal of Psychoanalysis, 87*(1), 25–42.

Borders, L. D., Penny, J. M., & Portnoy, F. (2000). Adult adoptees and their friends: Current functioning and psychosocial well-being. *Family Relations, 49*(4), 407–418.

Boszormenyi-Nagy, I., Grunebaum, J., & Ulrich, D. (1991). Contextual therapy. In A. S. Gurman & D. P. Kniskern (Eds.), *Handbook of Family Therapy* (pp. 200–238). New York: Brunner/Mazel.

Boszormenyi-Nagy, I., & Spark, G. (1984). *Invisible loyalties: Reciprocity in intergeneration family therapy*. New York: Brunner/Mazel.

Botsford Morgan, W., & King, E. B. (2012). Mothers' psychological contracts: Does supervisor breach explain intention to leave the organization? *Human Resource Management, 51*(5), 629–649. https://doi.org/10.1002/hrm.21492

Boyce, P., Condon, J., Barton, J., & Corkindale, C. (2007). First-time fathers' study: Psychological distress in expectant fathers during pregnancy. *Australian and New Zealand Journal of Psychiatry, 41*(9), 718–725. https://doi.org/10.1080/00048670701517959

Brabender, V. M., & Fallon, A. E. (2013). Setting the stage: The adoptive parent in context. In V. M. Brabender & A. E. Fallon (Eds.), *Working with adoptive parents: Research, theory, and therapeutic interventions* (pp. 1–22). New York: Wiley.

Brabender, V. M., & Mihura, J. (2016). The construction of gender and sex, and their implications for psychological assessment. In V. Brabender & J. Mihura (Eds.), *Handbook of gender and sexuality in psychological assessment* (pp. 3–43). New York: Routledge.

Brabender, V. M., Swartz, S., Winzinger, M., & Fallon, A. E. (2013). The adoptive mother. In V. M. Brabender & A. E. Fallon (Eds.), *Working with adoptive parents: Research, theory, and therapeutic interventions* (pp. 61–104). Hoboken, NJ: Wiley.

Brabender, V. M., & Whitmore, A. E. (2013). *Working with adoptive parents: Research, theory, and therapeutic interventions* (V. Brabender & A. Fallon, Eds.). Hoboken, NJ: Wiley.

Branchey, Z. (1983). Letters to the editor: Pregnant residents in the 1960s. *American Journal of Psychiatry, 140*, 135–136.

Braun, K., & Champagne, F. A. (2014). Paternal influences on offspring development: Behavioural and epigenetic pathways. *Journal of Neuroendocrinology, 26*(10), 697–706. https://doi.org/10.1111/jne.12174

Breen, D. (1977). Some differences between group and individual therapy in connection with the therapist's pregnancy. *International Journal of Group Psychotherapy, 27*(4), 499–506.

Bretherton, I. (2010). Fathers in attachment theory and research: A review. *Early Child Development and Care, 180*(1–2), 9–23. https://doi.org/10.1080/03004430903414661

Breuer, J., Freud, S., & Brill, A. A. (1895). *Studies in hysteria* (Standard ed., 2). London, England: Hogarth. Retrieved from www.myilibrary.com?id=892237

Bridges, N. A., & Smith, J. M. (1988). Viewpoint: The pregnant therapist and the seriously disturbed patient: Managing long-term psychotherapeutic treatment. *Psychiatry, 51*(1), 104–109. https://doi.org/10.1080/00332747.1988.11024384

Brier, N. (2008). Grief following miscarriage: A comprehensive review of the literature. *Journal of Women's Health, 17*(3), 451–464. https://doi.org/10.1089/jwh.2007.0505

Brodzinsky, D. M. (2011). Children's understanding of adoption: Developmental and clinical implications. *Professional Psychology: Research and Practice, 42*(2), 200–207. https://doi.org/10.1037/a0022415

Brooks, G. R., & Gilbert, L. A. (1995). Men in families: Old constraints, new possibilities. In R. F. Levant and W. F. Pollack (Eds.), *A new psychology of men*. New York: Basic Books.

Brouwers, M. (1989). The pregnant therapist at the university counseling center. *Journal of College Student Psychotherapy, 4*(1), 3–15.

Browning, D. H. (1974). Patients' reactions to their therapist's pregnancies. *Journal of the Academy of Child Psychiatry, 13*, 468–482.

Butts, N. T., & Cavenar, J. O. (1979). Colleagues' responses to the pregnant psychiatric resident. *American Journal of Psychiatry, 136*(12), 1587–1589.

Byrnes, M. J. (2000, June). *The impact of therapist pregnancy on the process of child psychotherapy* (Doctoral Dissertation). DePaul University, Chicago, IL. Retrieved from UMI Dissertation Publishing. (UMI No. 9982603)

Cacciatore, J. (2013). Psychological effects of stillbirth. *Seminars in Fetal and Neonatal Medicine, 18*(2), 76–82. https://doi.org/10.1016/j.siny.2012.09.001

Cacciatore, J., DeFrain, J., & Jones, K.L.C. (2008). When a baby dies: Ambiguity and stillbirth. *Marriage & Family Review, 44*(4), 439–454. https://doi.org/10.1080/01494 920802454017

Cacciatore, J., Frøen, J. F., & Killian, M. (2013). Condemning self, condemning other: Blame and mental health in women suffering stillbirth. *Journal of Mental Health Counseling, 35*(4), 342.

Cacciatore, J., Schnebly, S., & Froen, J. F. (2009). The effects of social support on maternal anxiety and depression after stillbirth. *Health & Social Care in the Community, 17*(2), 167–176. https://doi.org/10.1111/j.1365-2524.2008.00814.x

Cairney, J., Boyle, M., Offord, D. R., & Racine, Y. (2003). Stress, social support and depression in single and married mothers. *Social Psychiatry and Psychiatric Epidemiology, 38*(8), 442–449. https://doi.org/10.1007/s00127-003-0661-0

Callanan, D. L. (1985). Children's reactions to their therapist's pregnancy. *Child Psychiatry and Human Development, 16*(2), 113–119.

Camilleri, P., & Ryan, M. (2006). Social work students' attitudes toward homosexuality and their knowledge and attitudes toward homosexual parenting as an alternative family unit: An Australian study. *Social Work Education, 25*(3), 288–304.

Campbell, I. E. (1989). Common psychological concerns experienced by parents during pregnancy. *Canada's Mental Health*, March, 2–5.

Cassidy, J., & Shaver, P. R. (Eds.). (2016). *Handbook of attachment: theory, research, and clinical applications* (Third edition). New York: Guilford Press.

Ceballo, R., Lansford, J. E., Abbey, A., & Stewart, A. J. (2004). Gaining a child: Comparing the experiences of biological parents, adoptive parents, and stepparents. *Family Relations, 53*(1), 38–48. https://doi.org/10.1111/j.1741-3729.2004.00007.x

Census Bureau. (2015). *Quick facts: United States*. Retrieved from https://www.census.gov/quickfacts/table/PST045215/00

Chandler, N. B. (1998). *Stress and marital satisfaction among first time expectant fathers* (Doctoral Dissertation). California School of Professional Psychology, Los Angeles, CA. Retrieved from UMI Dissertation Publishing. (UMI No. 9831015)

Chandra, A., Copen, C. E., & Stephen, E. H. (2013). Infertility and impaired fecundity in the United States, 1982–2010: Data from the National Survey of Family Growth. *Natl Health Stat Report, 67*(67), 1–19.

Chang, S.-R., Chao, Y.-M., & Kenney, N. J. (2006). I am a woman and I'm pregnant: Body image of women in Taiwan during the third trimester of pregnancy. *Birth, 33*(2), 147–153. https://doi.org/10.1111/j.0730-7659.2006.00087.x

Chasseguet-Smirgel, J. (1984). The femininity of the analyst in professional practice. *International Journal of Psycho-Analysis, 65*, 169–178.

Chiaramont, J. (1986). Therapist pregnancy and maternity leave: Maintaining and furthering therapeutic gains in the interim. *Clinical Social Work Journal, 14*, 335–348.

Child Welfare Information Gateway (2016). *Adoption statistics*. Retrieved from https://www.childwelfare.gov/topics/systemwide/statistics/adoption/

Chodorow, N. (1999). *The reproduction of mothering: Psychoanalysis and the sociology of gender* (2nd ed.). Berkeley, CA: University of California Press.

Chong, A., & Mickelson, K. D. (2016). Perceived fairness and relationship satisfaction during the transition to parenthood: The mediating role of spousal support. *Journal of Family Issues, 37*(1), 3–28. https://doi.org/10.1177/0192513X13516764

Civin, M. A., & Lombardi, K. L. (1996). Chloe by the afternoon: Relational configurations, identificatory processes, and the organization of clinical experiences in unusual circumstances. In B. Gerson (Ed.), *The therapist as a person: Life crisis, life choices, life experiences, and their effects on treatment*. Hillsdale, NJ: Analytic Press.

Clark, A., Skouteris, H., Wertheim, E. H., Paxton, S. J., & Milgrom, J. (2009). My baby body: A qualitative insight into women's body-related experiences and mood during pregnancy and the postpartum. *Journal of Reproductive and Infant Psychology, 27*(4), 330–345. https://doi.org/10.1080/02646830903190904

Clark, M., & Ogden, J. (1999). The impact of pregnancy on eating behaviour and aspects of weight concern. *International Journal of Obesity, 23*(1), 18–24.

Clarkson, S. E. (1980). Pregnancy as a stimulus. *British Journal of Medical Psychology, 53*, 313–317.

Clay, R. A. (2006). Battling the self-blame of infertility for women and men facing infertility, the challenge to stop faulting themselves and start managing stress and making choices. *American Psychological Association, 37*(8), 44–45.

Cohn, D., Livingston, G., & Wang, W. (2014). *After decades of decline, a rise in stay-at-home mothers.* Pew Research Center. Retrieved from www.pewsocialtrends. org/2014/04/08/after-decades-of-decline-a-rise-in-stay-at-home-mothers/

Cole, D. S. (1980). Therapeutic issues arising from the pregnancy of the therapist. *Psychotherapy: Theory, Research, and Practice, 17*(2), 210–213.

Coleman, (1969). Psychological state during first pregnancy. *American Journal of Orthopsychiatry, 39*, 788–797.

Coley, R. L., Votruba-Drzal, E., & Schindler, H. S. (2009). Fathers' and mothers' parenting predicting and responding to adolescent sexual risk behaviors. *Child Development, 80*(3), 808–827. https://doi.org/10.1111/j.1467-8624.2009.01299.x

Comeau, K. M. (1987). When the nurse psychotherapist is pregnant (Implications for transference-countertransference). *Perspectives in Psychiatric Care, 3*(4), 127–131.

Condon, J. T., & Corkindale, C. J. (1998). The assessment of parent-to-infant attachment: Development of a self-report questionnaire instrument. *Journal of Reproductive and Infant Psychology, 16*(1), 57–76. https://doi.org/10.1080/02646839808404558

Condon, J. T., & Dunn, D. J. (1988). Nature and determinants of parent-to-infant attachment in the early postnatal period. *Journal of the American Academy of Child Adolescent Psychiatry, 27*(3), 293–299.

Cook, E. P. (1987). Characteristics of the biopsychosocial crisis of infertility. *Journal of Counseling & Development, 65*(9), 465–470. https://doi.org/10.1002/j.1556-6676.1987. tb00756.x

Cosgrove, L. (2004). The aftermath of pregnancy loss: A feminist critique of the literature and implications for treatment. *Women & Therapy, 27*(3–4), 107–122. https://doi. org/10.1300/J015v27n03_08

Côté-Arsenault, D. (2003). Weaving babies lost in pregnancy into the fabric of the family. *Journal of Family Nursing, 9*(1), 23–37. https://doi.org/10.1177/1074840702239489

Counselman, E. F., & Alonso, A. (1993). The ill therapist: therapists' reactions to personal illness and its impact on psychotherapy. *American Journal of Psychotherapy, 47*(4), 591–602.

Cousineau, T. M., & Domar, A. D. (2007). Psychological impact of infertility. *Best Practice & Research Clinical Obstetrics & Gynaecology, 21*(2), 293–308. https://doi.org/10. 1016/j.bpobgyn.2006.12.003

Cowan, C. P., & Cowan, P. A. (1988). Who does what when partners become parents: Implications for men, women, and marriage. *Marriage & Family Review, 12*(3–4), 105–131. https://doi.org/10.1300/J002v12n03_07

Crawford, I., McLeod, A., Zamboni, B. D., & Jordan, M. B. (1999). Psychologists' attitudes toward gay and lesbian parenting. *Professional Psychology: Research and Practice, 30*(4), 394–401. https://doi.org/10.1037//0735-7028.30.4.394

Crawley, R., Lomax, S., & Ayers, S. (2013). Recovering from stillbirth: The effects of making and sharing memories on maternal mental health. *Journal of Reproductive and Infant Psychology, 31*(2), 195–207. https://doi.org/10.1080/02646838.2013.79 5216

Crowl, A., Ahn, S., & Baker, J. (2008). A meta-analysis of developmental outcomes for children of same-sex and heterosexual parents. *Journal of GLBT Family Studies, 4*(3), 385–407. https://doi.org/10.1080/15504280802177615

Crowley, J. E., & Kolenikov, S. (2014). Flexible work options and mothers' perceptions of career harm: Mothers' perceptions of career harm. *The Sociological Quarterly, 55*(1), 168–195. https://doi.org/10.1111/tsq.12050

Cui, W. (2010). Mother of nothing: The agony of infertility. *Bulletin of the World Health Organization, 88*(12), 881–882. https://doi.org/10.2471/BLT.10.011210

Cullen-Drill, M. (1994). The pregnant therapist. *Perspectives in Psychiatric Care, 30*(4), 7–13.

Cullington-Roberts, D. (1994). The absent psychotherapist. *Psychoanalytic Psychotherapy, 8*(1), 63–76. https://doi.org/10.1080/02668739400700061

Cullington-Roberts, D. (2004). The psychotherapist's miscarriage and pregnancy as an obstacle to containment. *Psychoanalytic Psychotherapy, 18*(1), 99–110. https://doi.org/10.1080/14749730410001656543

Curtis, E. A., & Dixon, M. S. (2005). Family therapy and systemic practice with older people: Where are we now? *Journal of Family Therapy, 27*(1), 43–64. https://doi.org/10.1111/j.1467-6427.2005.00298.x

Dagan, Y., Lapidot, A., & Eisenstein, M. (2001). Women's dreams reported during first pregnancy. *Psychiatry and Clinical Neurosciences, 55*(1), 13–20.

Daugirdaite, V., Akker, O. van den, & Purewal, S. (2015). Posttraumatic stress and post-traumatic stress disorder after termination of pregnancy and reproductive loss: A systematic review. *Journal of Pregnancy, 2015*, 1–14. https://doi.org/10.1155/2015/646345

Davidson, M. J. (2011). The dark side of the rainbow: A research model of occupational stress in lesbian, gay, and bisexuals (LGBs) in the workplace. In S. Groschl (Ed.), *Diversity in the workplace: Multi-disciplinary and international perspectives* (pp. 169–184). New York: Routledge.

Davis, R. D., & Millon, T. (1999). Models of personality and its disorders. In T. Millon, P. H. Blaney, & R. D. Davis (Eds.), *Oxford textbook of psychopathology* (pp. 485–522). New York: Oxford Press.

Deben-Mager, M. (1993). Acting out and transference themes induced by successive pregnancies of the analyst. *The International Journal of Psychoanalysis, 74*, 129–139.

De Frain, J., Martens, L., Stork, J., & Stork, W. (1990). The psychological effects of a stillbirth on surviving family members. *OMEGA—Journal of Death and Dying, 22*(2), 81–108. https://doi.org/10.2190/A8VB-08XR-ACGH-2GYG

Deka, P. K., & Sarma, S. (2010). Psychological aspects of infertility. *BJMP, 3*(3), 336.

Dell'Antonia, K. (2012, June 20). *Pregnancy rates rise for women over 40*. Retrieved October 3, 2016, from http://parenting.blogs.nytimes.com/2012/06/20/pregnancy-rates-rise-for-women-over-40/?_r=0

Delmore-Ko, P., Pancer, S. M., Hunsberger, B., & Pratt, M. (2000). Becoming a parent: The relation between prenatal expectations and postnatal experience. *Journal of Family Psychology, 14*(4), 625–640. https://doi.org/10.1037/0893-3200.14.4.625

DelPriore, D. J., & Hill, S. E. (2013). The effects of paternal disengagement on women's sexual decision making: An experimental approach. *Journal of Personality and Social Psychology, 105*(2), 234–246. https://doi.org/10.1037/a0032784

Demos, J. (1994). The changing faces of fatherhood: A new exploration in american family history. In S. H. Cath, A. R. Gurwitt, & J. M. Ross (Eds.), *Father and child: developmental and clinical perspectives* (pp. 425–445). Hillsdale, NJ: Analytic Press.

Deutsch, F. M. (2001). Equally shared parenting. *Current Directions In Psychological Science, 10*(1), 25–28.

Deutsch, H. (1944). *The psychology of women: A psychoanalytic interpretation*. New York: Grune and Stratton.

Deutsch, H. (1945). *The Psychology of women, Vol. II: Motherhood*. New York: Grune & Stratton.

Devi, A. M., & Chanu, M. P. (2015). Couvade syndrome. *International Journal of Nursing Education and Research, 3*(3), 330. https://doi.org/10.5958/2454-2660.2015.00017.4

Dewald, P. A. (1982). The clinical importance of the termination phase. *Psychoanalytic Inquiry, 2*, 441–461.

Dewald, P. A. (1994). Countertransference issues when the therapist is ill or disabled. *American Journal of Psychotherapy, 48* (2), 221–230.

Diamond, D. (1992). Gender-specific transference reactions of male and female patients to the therapist's pregnancy. *Psychoanalytic Psychology, 9*(3), 319–345. https://doi.org/10.1037/h0079379

DiPesa, A. C. (2013). *Beyond the office doors: The relationship between psychotherapists' disclosures of personal life events and their professional identity* (Master's Thesis). Smith College School for Social Work.

Domash, L. (1984). The preoedipal patient and the pregnancy of the therapist. *Journal of Contemporary Psychotherapy, 14*(2), 109–119.

Donkor, E. S. (2008). *Socio-cultural perceptions of infertility in Ghana*. Retrieved from http://umkn-dsp01.unisa.ac.za/handle/10500/9829

Doss, B. D., Rhoades, G. K., Stanley, S. M., & Markman, H. J. (2009). The effect of the transition to parenthood on relationship quality: An 8-year prospective study. *Journal of Personality and Social Psychology, 96*(3), 601–619. https://doi.org/10.1037/a0013969

Downey, D. B. (1994). The school performance of children from single-mother and single-father families: Economic or interpersonal deprivation? *Journal of Family Issues, 15*(1), 129–147. https://doi.org/10.1177/019251394015001006

Dufton, K. (2004). Somebody else's baby: Evidence of broken rules and broken promises? *Psychoanalytic Psychotherapy, 18*(1), 111–124. https://doi.org/10.1080/14749730410001656552

Dunkel Schetter, C., Saxbe, D. E., Cheadle, A. C. D., & Guardino, C. M. (2016). Postpartum depressive symptoms following consecutive pregnancies: Stability, change, and mechanisms. *Clinical Psychological Science, 4*(5), 909–918. https://doi.org/10.1177/2167702616644894

Dyrdal, G. M., & Lucas, R. E. (2013). Reaction and adaptation to the birth of a child: A couple-level analysis. *Developmental Psychology, 49*(4), 749–761. https://doi.org/10.1037/a0028335

Dyson, E., & King, G. (2008). The pregnant therapist. *Psychodynamic Practice, 14*(1), 27–42. https://doi.org/10.1080/14753630701768958

Earle, S. (2003). "Bumps and boobs": Fatness and women's experiences of pregnancy. *Women's Studies International Forum, 26*(3), 245–252. https://doi.org/10.1016/S0277-5395(03)00054-2

Ellman, C. S. (2000). The empty mother: Women's fear of their destructive envy. *The Psychoanalytic Quarterly, 69*(4), 633–657. https://doi.org/10.1002/j.2167-4086.2000.tb00579.x

Ellman, C. S. (2011). Anonymity: Blank screen or black hole. In A. B. Druck (Ed.), *A new Freudian synthesis: Clinical process in the next generation* (pp. 157–172). London, England: Karnac Books.

Ellwood, D. T., & Jencks, C. (2001). *The growing differences in family structure: What do we know? Where do we look for answers?* Cambridge, MA: Harvard University. Retrieved from www.russellsage.org/sites/all/files/u4/Ellwood%26Jencks.pdf

Elsevier. (2010, August 22). *Oxytocin: It's a mom and pop thing—ScienceDaily.* Retrieved February 27, 2016, from www.sciencedaily.com/releases/2010/08/100820101207.htm

Elster, A. B., & Panzarine, S. (1983). Teenage fathers: Stresses during gestation and early parenthood. *Clinical Pediatrics, 22*(10), 700–703. https://doi.org/10.1177/000992288 302201005

Erbil, N., Şenkul, A., Başara, G. F., Sağlam, Y., & Gezer, M. (2012). Body image among Turkish women during the first year postpartum. *Health Care for Women International, 33*(2), 125–137. https://doi.org/10.1080/07399332.2011.603977

Erickson, R. J. (2005). Why emotion work matters: Sex, gender, and the division of household labor. *Journal of Marriage and Family, 67*(2), 337–351.

Erikson, E. H. (1950). *Childhood and society.* New York: W. W. Norton.

Erikson, E. H. (1994). *Identity, youth and crisis.* New York: Norton.

Erikson, E. H., & Erikson, J. M. (1998). *The life cycle completed* (Extended version). New York: W. W. Norton.

Etchegoyen, A. (1993). The analyst's pregnancy and its consequences on her work. *International Journal of Psychoanalysis, 74*(1), 141–149.

Evan B. Donaldson Adoption Institute. (1997). *"Benchmark adoption survey: Report on findings."* New York: Princeton Survey Research Associates. Retrieved from htta://www.adoptioninstitute.org/survey/Benchmark_Survey_1997.pdf.

Evan B. Donaldson Adoption Institute. (2002). *National adoption attitudes survey.* Harris Interactive, Inc. Retrieved from www.adoptioninstitute.org/old/survey/Adoption_Attitudes_Survey.pdf

Fagan, J., & Barnett, M. (2003). The relationship between maternal gatekeeping, paternal competence, mothers' attitudes about the father role, and father involvement. *Journal of Family Issues, 24*(8), 1020–1043. https://doi.org/10.1177/0192513X03256397

Falender, C. A., & Shafranske, E. P. (2004). *Clinical supervision: A competency-based approach.* Washington, DC: American Psychological Association.

Fallon, T. (2013). Therapeutic interventions with adopted children and adoptive parents: A psychoanalytic developmental approach. In V. M. Brabender and A. E. Fallon (Eds.), *Working with adoptive parents: Research, theory, and therapeutic interventions* (pp. 181–194). Hoboken, NJ: Wiley.

Fallon, A., Brabender, V., Anderson, N., & Maier, L. (1995, March 1). *Survey of pregnant group therapists.* Philadelphia Area Group Psychotherapy Society Lecture Series. Friends Hospital, Philadelphia, PA.

Fallon, A., Brabender, V., Anderson, N., & Maier, L. (1998). Therapist's perceptions of differences in the responses of group and individual psychotherapy patients to the therapist's pregnancy. *Focus,* November, 3–5.

Farr, R. H., Forssell, S. L., & Patterson, C. J. (2010). Parenting and child development in adoptive families: Does parental sexual orientation matter? *Applied Developmental Science, 14*(3), 164–178. https://doi.org/10.1080/10888691.2010.500958

Farr, R. H., & Patterson, C. J. (2013). Coparenting among lesbian, gay, and heterosexual couples: Associations with adopted children's outcomes. *Child Development, 84*(4), 1226–1240. https://doi.org/10.1111/cdev.12046

fatherhood. (n.d.). *Collins English dictionary—Complete and unabridged, 12th edition 2014.* Retrieved from www.thefreedictionary.com/fatherhood

Fatoye, F., Adeyemi, A., & Oladimeji, B. (2004). Emotional distress and its correlates among Nigerian women in late pregnancy. *Journal of Obstetrics and Gynaecology*, *24*(5), 504–509. https://doi.org/10.1080/01443610410001722518

Fedewa, A. L., Black, W. W., & Ahn, S. (2015). Children and adolescents with same-gender parents: A meta-analytic approach in assessing outcomes. *Journal of GLBT Family Studies*, *11*(1), 1–34. https://doi.org/10.1080/1550428X.2013.869486

Feldman, R., Gordon, I., Schneiderman, I., Weisman, O., & Zagoory-Sharon, O. (2010). Natural variations in maternal and paternal care are associated with systematic changes in oxytocin following parent—infant contact. *Psychoneuroendocrinology*, *35*(8), 1133–1141. https://doi.org/10.1016/j.psyneuen.2010.01.013

Fenster, S. L. (1983). Intrusion in the analytic space: The pregnancy of the psychoanalytic therapist (Doctoral dissertation, Adelphi University). *Dissertation Abstracts International*, *44*(3-B), 909.

Fenster, S. L., Phillips, S. B., & Rappaport, E. R. G. (1986). *The therapist's pregnancy: Intrusion in the analytic space*. New Jersey: The Analytic Press.

Fernandez-Duque, E., Valeggia, C. R., & Mendoza, S. P. (2009). The biology of paternal care in human and nonhuman primates. *Annual Review of Anthropology*, *38*(1), 115–130. https://doi.org/10.1146/annurev-anthro-091908-164334

Ferree, M. M. (2010). Filling the glass: Gender perspectives on families. *Journal of Marriage and Family*, *72*(3), 420–439. https://doi.org/10.1111/j.1741-3737.2010.00711.x

Finch, S. J. (2003). Pregnancy during residency: A literature review. *Academic Medicine*, *78*(4), 418–428. https://doi.org/10.1097/00001888-200304000-00021

Finnbogadóttir, H., Crang Svalenius, E., & K Persson, E. (2003). Expectant first-time fathers' experiences of pregnancy. *Midwifery*, *19*(2), 96–105. https://doi.org/10.1016/S0266-6138(03)00003-2

Flacking, R., Dykes, F., & Ewald, U. (2010). The influence of fathers' socioeconomic status and paternity leave on breastfeeding duration: A population-based cohort study. *Scandinavian Journal of Public Health*, *38*(4), 337–343. https://doi.org/10.1177/1403494810362002

Foli, K. J. (2010). Depression in adoptive parents: A model of understanding through grounded theory. *Western Journal of Nursing Research*, *32*(3), 379–400. https://doi.org/10.1177/0193945909351299

Foulkes, S. H. (1975). *Group analytic psychotherapy: Methods and principles*. London, England: G. Kamos.

Fox, A. B., & Quinn, D. M. (2015). Pregnant women at work: The role of stigma in predicting women's intended exist from the workforce. *Psychology of Women Quarterly*, *39*(2), 226–242. Doi: 10.1177/0361684314552653.

Franche, R.-L., & Bulow, C. (1999). The impact of a subsequent pregnancy on grief and emotional adjustment following a perinatal loss. *Infant Mental Health Journal*, *20*(2), 175–187. https://doi.org/10.1002/(SICI)1097-0355(199922)20:2<175::AID-IMHJ5>3.0.CO;2-Q

Franche, R. L., & Mikail, S. F. (1999). The impact of perinatal loss on adjustment to subsequent pregnancy. *Social Science & Medicine (1982)*, *48*(11), 1613–1623.

Franklin, A. J., & Davis, T. (2000). Therapeutic support groups as primary intervention for issues of fatherhood with African American men. In *Interventions for fathers*. Binghamton, NY: Haworth Press.

Freeman, N. (2005). When the therapist is infertile. In A. Rosen & J. Rosen (Eds.), *Frozen dreams: Psychodynamic dimensions of infertility and assisted reproduction* (pp. 50–68). New York, NY: Analytic Press/Taylor & Francis Group.

Freud, S. (1905). *Fragment of an analysis of a case of hysteria* (Standard ed., Vol. 7, pp. 1–122). London, England: Hogarth.

Freud, S., & Breuer, J. (1895). Studies on hysteria (Second edition). London: Hogarth.

Friedman, M. E. (1993). When the analyst becomes pregnant—twice. *Psychoanalytic Inquiry, 13*(2), 226–239. https://doi.org/10.1080/07351699309533935

Friedewald, M. E., Fletcher, R., & Fairbairn, H. (2005). All-male discussion forums for expectant fathers: Evaluation of a model. *Journal of Perinatal Education, 14*(2), 8–18. https://doi.org/10.1624/105812405X44673

Frøen, J. F., Cacciatore, J., McClure, E. M., Kuti, O., Jokhio, A. H., Islam, M., & Shiffman, J. (2011). Stillbirths: Why they matter. *The Lancet, 377*(9774), 1353–1366. https://doi.org/10.1016/S0140-6736(10)62232-5

Frosch, A. (2002). Transference: Psychic reality and material reality. *Psychoanalytic Psychology, 19*(4), 603–633. https://doi.org/10.1037/0736-9735.19.4.603

Frost, J., Bradley, H., Levitas, R., Smith, L., & Garcia, J. (2007). The loss of possibility: Scientisation of death and the special case of early miscarriage: The scientisation of death and early miscarriage. *Sociology of Health & Illness, 29*(7), 1003–1022. https://doi.org/10.1111/j.1467-9566.2007.01019.x

Fulcher, M., Sutfin, E. L., & Patterson, C. J. (2008). Individual differences in gender development: Associations with parental sexual orientation, attitudes, and division of labor. *Sex Roles, 58*(5–6), 330–341. https://doi.org/10.1007/s11199-007-9348-4

Fuller, R. L. (1987). The impact of the therapist's pregnancy on the dynamics of the therapeutic process. *Journal of the American Academy of Psychoanalysis, 15*(1), 9–28.

Fullerton, P. M. (2014). *Creating a softening moment in marital conflict authenticity, self-awareness, and connection* (Doctoral Dissertation). Fielding Graduate University.

Furber, C. M., Garrod, D., Maloney, E., Lovell, K., & McGowan, L. (2009). A qualitative study of mild to moderate psychological distress during pregnancy. *International Journal of Nursing Studies, 46*(5), 669–677. https://doi.org/10.1016/j.ijnurstu.2008.12.003

Fursman, L. (2002). Ideologies of motherhood and experiences of work: Pregnant women in management and professional careers. *Working Paper, 34*, 1–10.

Gailey, C. W. (2010). *Blue-ribbon babies and labors of love: Race, class, and gender in U.S. adoption practice.* Austin, TX: University of Texas.

Gates, G. J. (2013). *Same-sex couples in census 2010: Race and ethnicity.* Retrieved from williamsinstitute.law.ucla.edu/wp-content/uploads/Gates-CouplesRaceEthnicity-April-2012.pdf

Gates, G. J., & Cooke, A. M. (2011). *United States census snapshot: 2010.* Los Angeles, CA: UCLA Williams Institute.

Gatrell, C. J. (2011). "I'm a bad mum": Pregnant presenteeism and poor health at work. *Social Science & Medicine, 72*(4), 478–485. https://doi.org/10.1016/j.socscimed.2010.11.020

Gavin, B. (1994). Transference and countertransference in the group's response to the therapist's pregnancy. *Group Analysis, 27*(1), 63–74.

Gerber, J. (2016). *The pregnant therapist: Caring for yourself while working with clients.* Retrieved from http://www.apapracticecentral.org/ce/self-care/pregnancy.aspx

Gerber, J., & Advisory Committee on Colleague Assistance. (2005). *The pregnant therapist: Caring for yourself while working with clients.* Retrieved from http://doi.apa.org/get-pe-doi.cfm?doi=10.1037/e535912011-001

Gerrits, T. (1997). Social and cultural aspects of infertility in Mozambique. *Patient Education and Counseling, 31*(1), 39–48.

Gerson, B. E. (1994). An analyst's pregnancy loss and its effects on treatment disruption and growth. *Psychoanalytic Dialogues, 4*(1), 1–17. https://doi.org/10.1080/10481889409539002

Gerson, B. E. (Ed.). (1996). *The therapist as a person: Life crises, life choices, life experiences, and their effects on treatment.* Hillsdale, NJ: Analytic Press.

Gibb, E. (2004). Reliving abandonment in the face of the therapist's pregnancy. *Psychoanalytic Psychotherapy, 18*(1), 67–85. https://doi.org/10.1080/14749730410001656525

Ginot, E. (2009). The empathic power of enactments: The link between neuropsychological processes and an expanded definition of empathy. *Psychoanalytic Psychology, 26*(3), 290–309. https://doi.org/10.1037/a0016449

Glazer, G. (1989). Anxiety and stressors of expectant fathers. *Western Journal of Nursing Research, 11*(1), 47–59. https://doi.org/10.1177/019394598901100105

Goldberg, A. E. (2010). *Lesbian and gay parents and their children: Research on the family life cycle.* Washington, DC: American Psychological Association. Retrieved from http://content.apa.org/books/12055-000

Goldberg, A. E., & Perry-Jenkins, M. (2007). The division of labor and perceptions of parental roles: Lesbian couples across the transition to parenthood. *Journal of Social and Personal Relationships, 24*(2), 297–318. https://doi.org/10.1177/0265407507075415

Goldberg, A. E., Smith, J. Z., & Perry-Jenkins, M. (2012). The division of labor in lesbian, gay, and heterosexual new adoptive parents. *Journal of Marriage and Family, 74*(4), 812–828. https://doi.org/10.1111/j.1741-3737.2012.00992.x

Goldberger, M. (1991). Pregnancy during analysis—help or hindrance? *Psychoanalytic Quarterly, 60,* 207–226.

Goldberger, M., Gillman, R., Levinson, N., Notman, M., Seelig, B., & Shaw, R. (2003). On supervising the pregnant psychoanalytic candidate. *The Psychoanalytic Quarterly, 72*(2), 439–463. https://doi.org/10.1002/j.2167-4086.2003.tb00137.x

Goldenberg, R. L., Culhane, J. F., Iams, J. D., & Romero, R. (2008). Epidemiology and causes of preterm birth. *The Lancet, 371*(9606), 75–84.

Goldin, C. (2006). *The quiet revolution that transformed women's employment, education, and family.* National Bureau of Economic Research. Retrieved from www.nber.org/papers/w11953

Goldsmith, S. J. Oedipus or Orestes? Homosexual men, their mothers, and other women revisted. *Journal of the American Psychoanalytic Association, 49*(4), 1269–1287.

Golombok, S. (2015). *Modern families: Parents and children in new family forms.* Cambridge: Cambridge University Press. Retrieved from http://ebooks.cambridge.org/ref/id/CBO9781107295377

Gordon, I., Zagoory-Sharon, O., Leckman, J. F., & Feldman, R. (2010). Oxytocin and the development of parenting in humans. *Biological Psychiatry, 68*(4), 377–382. https://doi.org/10.1016/j.biopsych.2010.02.005

Gottlieb, S. (2006). The pregnant therapist. In A. Foster, A. Dickinson, B. Bishop, & J. Klein (Eds.), *Difference: An avoided topic in practice* (pp. 81–99). London, England: Karnac Books.

Gourounti, K. (2016). Psychological stress and adjustment in pregnancy following assisted reproductive technology and spontaneous conception: A systematic review. *Women & Health, 56*(1), 98–118. https://doi.org/10.1080/03630242.2015.1074642

Goz, R., (1973). Women patients and women therapist: Some issues that come up in psychotherapy. *International Journal of Psychoanalytic Psychotherapy,* 298–319.

Granholm, E. L., McQuaid, J. R., & Holden, J. L. (2016). *Cognitive-behavioral social skills training for schizophrenia: A practical treatment guide.* New York: The Guilford Press.

Greenberg, D., Ladge, J., & Clair, J. (2009). Negotiating pregnancy at work: Public and private conflicts. *Negotiation and Conflict Management Research, 2*(1), 42–56. https://doi.org/10.1111/j.1750-4716.2008.00027.x

Greenberg, J. R. (1986). Theoretical models and the analyst's neutrality. *Contemporary Psychoanalysis, 22,* 87–106.

Greil, A. L. (1997). Infertility and psychological distress: A critical review of the literature. *Social Science & Medicine, 45*(11), 1679–1704. https://doi.org/10.1016/S0277-9536(97)00102-0

Grigoriadis, S., & Romans, S. (2006). Postpartum psychiatric disorders: What do we know and where do we go? *Current Psychiatry Reviews, 2*(1), 151–158.

Gross, H., & Pattison, H. (2007). *Sanctioning pregnancy: A psychological perspective on the paradoxes and culture of research.* London: Routledge.

Grossman, H. Y. (1990). The pregnant therapist: Professional and personal worlds intertwine. In H. Y. Grossman and N. L. Chester (Eds.), *The experience and meaning of work in women's lives* (pp. 57–81). Hillsdale, NJ: Lawrence Erlbaum Associates.

Grotevant, H. D., & Kohler, J. K. (1999). Adoptive families. In M. E. Lamb (Ed.), *Parenting and development in nontraditional families* (pp. 161–190). Mahwah, NJ: Lawrence Erlbaum Associates.

Guinjoan, S. M., & Ross, D. R. (2000). Consequences of a male therapist disclosing the birth of his child. *Psychodynamic Psychiatry, 28*(1), 39–50.

Guy, J. D., Guy, M. P., & Liaboe, G. P. (1986). First pregnancy: Therapeutic issues for both female and male psychotherapists. *Psychotherapy: Theory, Research, Practice, Training, 23*(2), 297–302. https://doi.org/10.1037/h0085612

Haber, S. (1992). Women in independent practice: Issues of pregnancy and motherhood. *Psychotherapy in Private Practice, 11*(3), 25–29.

Hackel, L. S., & Ruble, D. N. (1992). Changes in the marital relationship after the first baby is born: Predicting the impact of expectancy disconfirmation. *Journal of Personality and Social Psychology, 62*(6), 944–957. https://doi.org/10.1037/0022-3514.62.6.944

Hajela, S., Prasad, S., Kumaran, A., & Kumar, Y. (2016). Stress and infertility: A review. *International Journal of Reproduction, Contraception, Obstetrics and Gynecology, 5*(4), 940–943. https://doi.org/10.18203/2320-1770.ijrcog20160846

Hall, E. O. C. (1995). From fun and excitement to joy and trouble: An explorative study of three Danish fathers' experiences around birth. *Scandinavian Journal of Caring Sciences, 9*(3), 171–179. https://doi.org/10.1111/j.1471-6712.1995.tb00408.x

Halton, I. H. (2004). Two is too much: The impact of a therapist's successive pregnancies on a female patient. *Psychoanalytic Psychotherapy, 18*(1), 86–98. https://doi.org/10.1080/14749730410001656534

Hamilton, J. G., & Lobel, M. (2008). Types, patterns, and predictors of coping with stress during pregnancy: Examination of the revised prenatal coping inventory in a diverse sample. *Journal of Psychosomatic Obstetrics & Gynecology, 29*(2), 97–104. https://doi.org/10.1080/01674820701690624

Hämmerli, K., Znoj, H., & Berger, T. (2010). What are the issues confronting infertile women? A qualitative and quantitative approach. *The Qualitative Report, 15*(4), 766.

Harmon, A. (2005). Actually, these days, first comes the baby carriage. *New York Times.* Retrieved from www.nytimes.com/2005/10/13/fashion/thursdaystyles/first-comes-the-baby-carriage.html?_r=0

Harris, B. (2002). Postpartum depression. *Psychiatric Annals, 32*(7), 405–415. https://doi.org/10.3928/0048-5713-20020701-08

Hart, R., & McMahon, C. A. (2006). Mood state and psychological adjustment to pregnancy. *Archives of Women's Mental Health, 9*(6), 329–337. https://doi.org/10.1007/s00737-006-0141-0

Hartwell-Walker, M. (2016). Transference or not? Client response to therapist pregnancy. https://pro.psychcentral.com/transference-or-not-client-response-to-therapist-pregnancy/0013622.html

Haviland, B., James, K., Killman, M., & Trbovich, K. (2015). Supporting breastfeeding in the workplace. *Australasian Journal of Early Childhood, 38*(3), 118–119.

Hayes, S. C. (2004). Acceptance and commitment therapy, relational frame theory, and the third wave of behavioral and cognitive therapies. *Behavior Therapy, 35*(4), 639–665.

Hayes, S. C. (2016). Acceptance and commitment therapy, relational frame theory, and the third wave of behavioral and cognitive therapies. *Behavior Therapy, 35*(4), 639–665. https://doi.org/10.1016/j.beth.2016.11.006

Hemp, P. (2004). Presenteeism: At work-but out of it. *Harvard Business Review, 82*(10), 49–58.

Hennekam, S. (2016). Identity transition during pregnancy: The importance of role models. *Human Relations, 69*(9), 1765–1790. https://doi.org/10.1177/0018726716631402

Henretty, J. R., & Levitt, H. M. (2010). The role of therapist self-disclosure in psychotherapy: A qualitative review. *Clinical Psychology Review, 30*(1), 63–77. https://doi.org/10.1016/j.cpr.2009.09.004

Henry, J. D., & Rendell, P. G. (2007). A review of the impact of pregnancy on memory function. *Journal of Clinical and Experimental Neuropsychology, 29*(8), 793–803. https://doi.org/10.1080/13803390701612209

Herek, G. M. (2009). Sexual stigma and sexual prejudice in the United States: A conceptual framework. In A. Hope (Ed.), *Contemporary perspective on lesbian, gay, and bisexual identities* (pp. 65–111). Lincoln, NE: University of Nebraska. Doi: 10.1007/978-0-387-09556-1_4.

Herrin, D. C. (2001, August). *A survey of dance/movement therapists and the effects of pregnancy on their clinical experiences.* Philadelphia, PA: MCP Hahnemann University.

Hersh, L. B., & Jorns, M. S. (1975). Use of 5-deazaFAD to study hydrogen transfer in the D-amino acid oxidase reaction. *The Journal of Biological Chemistry, 250*(22), 8728–8734.

Higgins, C., Duxbury, L., & Johnson, K. L. (2000). Part-time work for women: Does it really help balance work and family? *Human Resource Management, 39*(1), 17–32. https://doi.org/10.1002/(SICI)1099-050X(200021)39:1<17::AID-HRM3>3.0.CO;2-Y

Hiller, D. V. & Philliber, W. W. (1986). The division of labor in contemporary marriage: Expectations, perceptions, and performance. *Social Problems, 33*(3), 191–201.

Hilty, D. M. (2005). A day in the life of a psychiatry resident: A pilot qualitative analysis. *Academic Psychiatry, 29*(4), 405–407. https://doi.org/10.1176/appi.ap.29.4.405

Hilty, D. M., Maynes, S. M., Kellner, M., Clark, M. S., Bourgeois, J. A., & Servis, M. E. (2005). A day in the life of a psychiatry resident: A pilot qualitative analysis. *Academic Psychiatry, 29*(4), 405–407.

Hjalmarsson, H. (2005). Transference opportunities during the therapist's pregnancy: Three case vignettes. *Psychoanalytic Social Work, 12*(1), 1–11. https://doi.org/10.1300/J032v12n01_01

Hochschild, A. R. (1997). *The time bind: When work becomes home and home becomes work*. New York: Henry Holt/Metropolitan Books.

Hochschild, A. (1989). *The second shift: Working parents and the revolution at home*. New York: Viking Press.

Holditch-Davis, D., Sandelowski, M., & Harris, B. G. (1999). Effect of infertility on mothers' and fathers' interactions with young infants. *Journal of Reproductive and Infant Psychology, 17*(2), 159–173. https://doi.org/10.1080/02646839908409095

Hollander, M., & Ford, C. (1990). *Dynamic psychotherapy*. Washington, DC: American Psychiatric Press.

Hollos, M., Larsen, U., Obono, O., & Whitehouse, B. (2009). The problem of infertility in high fertility populations: Meanings, consequences and coping mechanisms in two Nigerian communities. *Social Science & Medicine, 68*(11), 2061–2068. https://doi.org/10.1016/j.socscimed.2009.03.008

Hopkins, S. (2004). Pregnancy: An unthinkable reality. *Psychoanalytic Psychotherapy, 18*(1), 44–66. https://doi.org/10.1080/14749730410001656516

Horner, A. J. (1990). *The primacy of structure: Psychotherapy of underlying character pathology*. Northvale, NJ: Jason Aronson.

Hughes, P., Turton, P., Hoper, E., & Evans, C.D.H. (2002). Assessment of guidelines for good practice in psychosocial care of mothers after stillbirth: A cohort study. *Lancet (London, England), 360*(9327), 114–118.

Humberd, B., Ladge, J. J., & Harrington, B. (2015). The "new" dad: Navigating fathering identity within organizational contexts. *Journal of Business and Psychology, 30*(2), 249–266. https://doi.org/10.1007/s10869-014-9361-x

Hyssälä, L., Hyttinen, M., Rautava, P., & Sillanpää, M. (1993). The Finnish family competence study: The transition to fatherhood. *The Journal of Genetic Psychology, 154*(2), 199–208. https://doi.org/10.1080/00221325.1993.9914733

Iasenza, S. (1997). Working with the enemy? Therapy with a homophobic client. *In the Family, July*, 21–23.

Imber, R. R. (1990). The avoidance of countertransference awareness in a pregnant analyst. *Contemporary Psychoanalysis, 26*, 223–236.

Imber, R. R. (1995). The role of the supervisor and the pregnant analyst. *Psychoanalytic Psychology, 12*(2), 281–296. https://doi.org/10.1037/h0079633

Irhammar, M., & Bengtsson, H. (2004). Attachment in a group of adult international adoptees. *Adoption Quarterly, 8*(2), 1–25.

Isay, R. A. (1996). Psychoanalytic therapy with gay men: Developmental considerations. In R. Cabai & T. Stein (Eds.), *Textbook of homosexuality and mental health* (pp. 451–469). Washington, DC: American Psychiatric Press.

Jackel, M. M. (1966). Interruptions during psychoanalytic treatment and the wish for a child. *Journal of the American Psychoanalytic Association, 14*, 730–735.

Jaffe, J., & Diamond, M. O. (2011a). Developmental tasks of adulthood: Losses of opportunity. In J. Jaffe & M. O. Diamond (Eds.), *Reproductive trauma: Psychotherapy with infertility and pregnancy loss clients* (pp. 31–49). Washington, DC: American Psychological Association. Retrieved from http://content.apa.org/books/12347-002

Jaffe, J., & Diamond, M. O. (2011b). Pregnancy and parenthood after infertility or reproductive loss. In J. Jaffe & M. O. Diamond (Eds.), *Reproductive trauma: Psychotherapy with infertility and pregnancy loss clients* (pp. 215–229). Washington, DC: American Psychological Association. Retrieved from http://content.apa.org/books/12347-011

Jaffe, J., & Diamond, M. O. (2011c). Self-disclosure, transference, and countertransference. In J. Jaffe & M. O. Diamond (Eds.), *Reproductive trauma: Psychotherapy with infertility and pregnancy loss clients* (pp. 159–177). Washington, DC: American Psychological Association. Retrieved from http://content.apa.org/books/12347-008

Johansson, M., Edwardsson, C., & Hildingsson, I. (2015). The "Pregnant Man"—expecting fathers experience pregnancy-related changes: A longitudinal study with a mixed method approach. *Journal of Men's Health, 11*(6), 8–18.

Johnson, S., & O'Connor, E. (2002). *The gay baby boom: The psychology of gay parenthood.* New York, NY: NYU Press.

Jones, S. (2015). The psychological miscarriage: An exploration of women's experience of miscarriage in the light of Winnicott's "Primary Maternal Preoccupation", the process of grief according to Bowlby and Parkes, and Klein's theory of mourning: The psychological miscarriage. *British Journal of Psychotherapy, 31*(4), 433–447. https://doi.org/10.1111/bjp.12172

Kaplan, E., & Granrose, C. S. (1993). Factors influencing women's decision to leave an organization following childbirth. *Employee Responsibilities and Rights Journal, 6*(1), 45–54.

Karterud, S. (2015). *Mentalization-based group therapy (MBT-G): A theoretical, clinical, and research manual.* Oxford: Oxford University Press.

Katz-Bearnot, S. (2010). The internal triangle: New theories of female development, by Lucy Holmes. Jason Aronson, New York, 2008, 149 pp. *The Journal of the American Academy of Psychoanalysis and Dynamic Psychiatry, 38*, 739–740.

Katzman, M. A. (1993). The pregnant therapist and the eating-disordered woman: The challenge of futility. *Eating Disorders, 1*(1), 17–30.

Katz-Wise, S. L., Priess, H. A., & Hyde, J. S. (2010). Gender-role attitudes and behavior across the transition to parenthood. *Developmental Psychology, 46*(1), 18–28. https://doi.org/10.1037/a0017820

Kaufman, G., & Uhlenberg, P. (2000). The influence of parenthood on the work effort of married men and women. *Social Forces, 78*(3), 931–947. https://doi.org/10.1093/sf/78.3.931

Kempke, S., & Luyten, P. (2007). Psychodynamic and cognitive—behavioral approaches of obsessive—compulsive disorder: Is it time to work through our ambivalence? *Bulletin of the Menninger Clinic, 71*(4), 291–311. https://doi.org/10.1521/bumc.2007.71.4.291

Kendall, J. (2014, June 13). Review: *"Do fathers matter?" Attempts to redefine 21st century fatherhood.* LA Times. Retrieved September 7, 2015, from www.latimes.com/books/jacketcopy/la-ca-jc-paul-raeburn-20140615-story.html

Kernberg, P. F. (1994). Mechanisms of defense: Development and research perspectives. *Bulletin of the Menninger Clinic, 58*(1), 55–87.

Kestenberg, J. S. (1982). The inner-genital phase: Prephallic and preoedipal. In D. Mendel (Ed.), *Early female development* (pp. 81–126). New York: S. P. Medical and Scientific Books.

Kibel, H. D. (1981). The rationale for the use of group psychotherapy for borderline patients on a short-term unit. *International Journal of Group Psychotherapy, 28*(3), 339–358.

Killien, M. G. (2005). The role of social support in facilitating postpartum women's return to employment. *Journal of Obstetric, Gynecologic & Neonatal Nursing, 34*(5), 639–646. https://doi.org/10.1177/0884217505280192

Kinsey, C., Baptiste-Roberts, K., Zhu, J., & Kjerulff, K. H. (2015). Effect of previous miscarriage on depressive symptoms during subsequent pregnancy and postpartum in the first baby study. *Maternal and Child Health Journal, 19*(2), 391–400. https://doi.org/10.1007/s10995-014-1521-0

Kirk, H. D. (1981). *Adoptive kinship: A modern institution in need of reforms.* Toronto: Butterworth.

Kiselica, M. S., Benton-Wright, S., & Englar-Carlson, M. (2016). Accentuating positive masculinity: A new foundation for the psychology of boys, men, and masculinity. In Y. J. Wong & S. R. Wester (Eds.), *APA handbook of men and masculinities* (pp. 123–143). Washington, DC: American Psychological Association. Retrieved from http://content.apa.org/books/14594-006

Klein, M. (1975). *Envy and gratitude, and other works, 1946-1963.* London: Hogarth Press and the Institute of Psycho-Analysis.

Klein, M. J., Hyde, J. S., Essex, M. J., & Clark, R. (1998). Maternity leave, role quality, work involvement, and mental health one year after delivery. *Psychology of Women Quarterly, 22*, 239–266.

Klock, S. C. (2009). Psychological issues related to infertility. *The Global Library of Women's Medicine.* Retrieved from https://doi.org/10.3843/GLOWM.10413

Knox, S., & Hill, C. E. (2003). Therapist self-disclosure: Research-based suggestions for practitioners. *Journal of Clinical Psychology, 59*(5), 529–539. https://doi.org/10.1002/jclp.10157

Koestner, R., Franz, C., & Weinberger, J. (1990). The family origins of empathic concern: A 26-year longitudinal study. *Journal of Personality and Social Psychology, 58*(4), 709–717. https://doi.org/10.1037/0022-3514.58.4.709

Kong, G., Chung, T., Lai, B., & Lok, I. (2010). Gender comparison of psychological reaction after miscarriage-a 1-year longitudinal study: Reaction on miscarriage. *BJOG: An International Journal of Obstetrics & Gynaecology, 117*(10), 1211–1219. https://doi.org/10.1111/j.1471-0528.2010.02653.x

Korenis, P., & Billick, S. B. (2014). The pregnant therapist: The effect of a negative pregnancy outcome on a psychotherapy patient. *Psychiatric Quarterly, 85*(3), 377–382. https://doi.org/10.1007/s11126-014-9298-2

Koropeckyj-Cox, T., & Call, V.R.A. (2007). Characteristics of older childless persons and parents: Cross-national comparisons. *Journal of Family Issues, 28*(10), 1362–1414. https://doi.org/10.1177/0192513X07303837

Kriebel, D., & Wentzel, K. (2011). Parenting as a moderator of cumulative risk for behavioral competence in adopted children. *Adoption Quarterly, 14*(1), 37–60. https://doi.org/10.1080/10926755.2011.557945

Kübler-Ross, E. (1969). *On death and dying.* New York, NY: Macmillan.

Kuhman, D., Joyner, K., & Bloomer, R. (2015). Cognitive performance and mood following ingestion of a theacrine-containing dietary supplement, caffeine, or placebo by young men and women. *Nutrients, 7*(12), 9618–9632. https://doi.org/10.3390/nu7115484

Lachance-Grzela, M., & Bouchard, G. (2010). Why do women do the lion's share of housework? A decade of research. *Sex Roles, 63*(11–12), 767–780. https://doi.org/10.1007/s11199-010-9797-z

Ladores, S., & Aroian, K. (2015). The early postpartum experience of previously infertile mothers. *Journal of Obstetric, Gynecologic & Neonatal Nursing, 44*(3), 370–379. https://doi.org/10.1111/1552-6909.12576

Lamb, M. E. (1986). The changing roles of fathers. In M. E. Lamb (Ed.), *The father§s role: Applied perspectives* (pp. 3–27). New York: Wiley.

Lamb, M. E. (Ed.). (2010). *The role of the father in child development* (Fifth edition). Hoboken, NJ: Wiley.

LaMothe, R. (2001). Vitalizing objects and psychoanalytic psychotherapy. *Psychoanalytic Psychology, 18*(2), 320–329.

Langs, R. (1971). *The technique of psychoanalytic psychotherapy* (Volume II). New York: Jason Aronson.

Langs, R. (1975). The therapeutic relationship and deviations in technique. *International Journal of Psychoanalytic Psychotherapy, 4*, 106–141.

LaRossa, R. (1997). *The modernization of fatherhood: a social and political history.* Chicago: University of Chicago Press.

Larson, R., Richards, M. H., & Perry-Jenkins, M. (1994). Divergent worlds: The daily emotional experience of mothers and fathers in the domestic and public spheres. *Journal of Personality and Social Psychology, 67*, 1034–1046.

Lasker, J. N., & Toedter, L. J. (2000). Predicting outcomes after pregnancy loss: Results from studies using the Perinatal Grief Scale. *Illness, Crisis & Loss, 8*(4), 350–372.

Lasky, R. (1990). Catastrophic illness in the analyst and the analyst's emotional reactions to it. *The International Journal of Psycho-Analysis, 71*(Pt 3), 455–473.

Latza, T. E. (2005, July 12). *The use of the therapist's pregnancy in the psychodynamic treatment of a young girl with fears of abandonment* (Doctoral Dissertation). The Chicago School of Professional Psychology, Chicago, IL. Retrieved from UMI Dissertation Publishing. (UMI No. 3215585)

Laughlin, L. (2011). *Maternity leave and employment patterns of first-time mothers: 1961–2008* (Current Population Reports) (pp. 70–128). Retrieved from www.census.gov/prod/2011pubs/p70-128.pdf

Lawrence, E., Nylen, K., & Cobb, R. J. (2007). Prenatal expectations and marital satisfaction over the transition to parenthood. *Journal of Family Psychology, 21*(2), 155–164. https://doi.org/10.1037/0893-3200.21.2.155

Lax, R. (1969). Some considerations about transference and countertransference manifestations evoked by the analyst's pregnancy. *International Journal of Psychoanalysis, 50*, 363–372.

Layne, L. (1996). Never such innocence again: Irony, nature, and technoscience in narratives of pregnancy loss. In R. Cevil (Ed.), *Comparative studies in miscarriage, stillbirth and neonatal death* (pp. 131–152). Oxford: Berg Press.

Lazar, S. G. (1990). Patients' responses to pregnancy and miscarriage in the analyst. In H. J. Schwartz & A.-L. S. Silver (Eds.), *Illness in the analyst: Implications for the treatment relationship* (pp. 199–226). Madison, CT: International Universities Press.

Leahy, R. L., & Tirch, D. D. (2008). Cognitive behavioral therapy for jealousy. *International Journal of Cognitive Therapy, 1*(1), 18–32. https://doi.org/10.1521/ijct.2008.1.1.18

Leahy-Warren, P., & McCarthy, G. (2011). Maternal parental self-efficacy in the postpartum period. *Midwifery, 27*(6), 802–810. https://doi.org/10.1016/j.midw.2010.07.008

Lecours, S., Bouchard, M.-A., & Normandin, L. (1995). Countertransference as the therapist's mental activity: Experience and gender differences among psychoanalytically oriented psychologists. *Psychoanalytic Psychology, 12*(2), 259–279. https://doi.org/10.1037/h0079634

Lederman, R. P. (1996). *Psychosocial adaptation in pregnancy: Assessment of seven dimensions of maternal development* (Second edition). New York: Springer Publishing Company.

Leech, K., Salo, V., Rowe, M., & Cabrera, N. (2013). Father input and child vocabulary development: The importance of *wh* questions and clarification requests. *Seminars in Speech and Language, 34*(4), 249–259. https://doi.org/10.1055/s-0033-1353445

Leibowitz, L. (1996). Reflections of a childless analyst. In B. Gerson (Ed.), *The therapist as a person: Life crises, life choices, life experiences, and their effects on treatment* (pp. 71–89). New York, NY: Routledge.

Leifer, M. (1977). Psychological changes accompanying pregnancy and motherhood. *Genetic Psychology Monographs, 95,* 55–96.

Leifer, M. (1980). *Psychological Effects of Motherhood.* New York: Praeger Scientific.

Leon, I. G. (2009). Psychology of reproduction: Pregnancy, parenthood, and parental ties. *The Global Library of Women's Medicine.* http://www.glowm.com/section_view/item/418

Lester, E. P., & Notman, M. T. (1986). Pregnancy, developmental crisis and object relations: Psychoanalytic considerations. *The International Journal of Psycho-Analysis, 67*(Pt 3), 357–366.

Leve, L. D., Scaramella, L. V., & Fagot, B. I. (2001). Infant temperament, pleasure in parenting, and marital happiness in adoptive families. *Infant Mental Health Journal, 22*(5), 545–558. https://doi.org/10.1002/imhj.1017

Levine, L. (2015). "Generative co-constructions": An exploration of the analyst's influence and desire: Commentary on paper by Richard Almond. *Psychoanalytic Dialogues, 25*(3), 368–377. https://doi.org/10.1080/10481885.2015.1034565

Levy, J. (1998). In the therapy room: Coming out to straight clients. *In the Family, 7,* 22–23.

Lewis, R. J., Derlega, V. J., Griffin, J. L., & Krowinski, A. C. (2003). Stressors for gay men and lesbians: Life stress, gay-related stress, stigma consciousness, and depressive symptoms. *Journal of Social and Clinical Psychology, 22*(6), 716–729.

Lewis, S. N. C., & Cooper, C. L. (1988). The transition to parenthood in dual-earner couples. *Psychological Medicine, 18*(2), 477. https://doi.org/10.1017/S00332917000 08011

Lingiardi, V., & McWilliams, N. (2017) Psychodynamic Diagnostic Manual, Second edition PDM-2. New York, NY: Guilford.

Lingiardi, V., McWilliams, N., Bornstein, R. F., Gazzillo, F., & Gordon, R. M. (2015). The psychodynamic diagnostic manual version 2 (PDM-2): Assessing patients for improved clinical practice and research. *Psychoanalytic Psychology, 32*(1), 94–115. https://doi.org/10.1037/a0038546

Liu, W., & Gong, C. (n.d.). *Traditional Chinese medicine/TCM and infertility 2.* Retrieved August 7, 2016, from www.tcmpage.com/infertlity_2.html

Livingston, G. (2014a). *Fewer than half of U.S. kids today living in a "traditional" family.* Retrieved from www.pewresearch.org/fact-tank/2014/12/22/less-than-half-of-u-s-kids-today-live-in-a-traditional-family/

Livingston, G. (2014b). *Growing number of dads home with the kids: Biggest increase among those caring for family* (Pew Research Center's Social and Demographic Trends Project). Washington, DC: Pew Research Center. Retrieved from www.pewsocial trends.org/files/2014/06/2014-06-05_Stay-at-Home-Dads.pdf

Locker-Forman, A. (2005). *When real meets pretend: An exploration of the impact of the therapist's pregnancy on child psychotherapy* (Doctoral Dissertation). The City University of New York, New York. Retrieved from UMI Dissertation Publishing. (UMI No. 3159230)

Loth, K. A., Bauer, K. W., Wall, M., Berge, J., & Neumark-Sztainer, D. (2011). Body satisfaction during pregnancy. *Body Image, 8*(3), 297–300. https://doi.org/10.1016/j.bodyim.2011.03.002

Lovett, L. L. (2007). *Conceiving the future: Pronatalism, reproduction, and the family in the United States, 1890–1938.* Chapel Hill, SC: University of North Carolina Press. Retrieved from http://northcarolina.universitypressscholarship.com/view/10.5149/9780807868102_lovett/upso-9780807831076

Lubbe, T. (2003). Diagnosing a male hysteric: Don Juan-type. *The International Journal of Psychoanalysis, 84*(4), 1043–1059. https://doi.org/10.1516/002075703768284740

Lyndon, L. G. (2013, May). *Pregnancy, motherhood, and career: Negotiating maternal desires and professional ambition* (Doctoral Dissertation). The Wright Institute Graduate School of Psychology, Berkeley, CA. Retrieved from UMI Dissertation Publishing. (UMI No. 3578746)

Lyness, K. S., Thompson, C. A., Francesco, A. M., & Judiesch, M. K. (1999). Work and pregnancy: Individual and organizational factors influencing organizational commitment, time of maternity leave and return to work. *Sex Roles, 41*(7–8), 485–508. https://doi.org/10.1023/A:1018887119627

McCann, J. T. (1999). Obsessive-compulsive and negativistic personality disorders. In T. Millon, P. H. Blaney, & R. D. Davis (Eds.), *Oxford textbook of psychopathology.* New York: Oxford University Press.

McCarty, T., Schneider-Braus, K., & Goodwin, J. (1986). Use of alternate therapist during pregnancy leave. *Journal of the American Academy of Psychoanalysis, 14*(3), 377–383.

McCluskey, M. C. (2016). The pregnant therapist: A qualitative examination of the client experience. *Clinical Social Work Journal.* http://link.springer.com/10.1007/s10615-016-0599-9

McCoyd, J. L. M. (2009). Discrepant feeling rules and unscripted emotion work: Women coping with termination for fetal anomaly. *American Journal of Orthopsychiatry, 79*(4), 441–451. https://doi.org/10.1037/a0010483

McDaniel, S. H., Doherty, W. J., & Hepworth, J. (2014). Pregnancy loss, infertility, and reproductive technology. In S. H. McDaniel, W. J. Doherty, & J. Hepworth (Eds.), *Medical family therapy and integrated care* (2nd ed., pp. 169–193). Washington, DC: American Psychological Association. Retrieved from http://content.apa.org/books/14256-009

McGarty, M. (1988). The analyst's pregnancy. *Contemporary Psychoanalysis, 24,* 684–692.

McGourty, A. (2013). The pregnant therapist and the psychotic client: A phenomenological understanding of the impact of the therapist's pregnancy on the therapeutic process. *European Journal of Psychotherapy & Counselling, 15*(1), 18–31. https://doi.org/10.1080/13642537.2013.763462

McKay, B. (2015). *Do fathers matter? With Paul Raeburn.* Retrieved from www.artofmanliness.com/2015/06/20/podcast-do-fathers-matter/

McKelley, R. A., & Rochlen, A. B. (2016). Furthering fathering: What we know and what we need to know. In Y. J. Wong & S. R. Wester (Eds.), *APA handbook of men and masculinities* (pp. 525–549). Washington, DC: American Psychological Association. Retrieved from http://content.apa.org/books/14594-024

McLaren, J. L. (2008). The great balancing act: Pregnancy during residency. *American Journal of Psychiatry Resident's Journal, 3*(3), 2.

Maconochie, N., Doyle, P., Prior, S., & Simmons, R. (2007). Risk factors for first trimester miscarriage-results from a UK-population-based case-control study. *BJOG: An International Journal of Obstetrics & Gynaecology, 114*(2), 170–186. https://doi.org/10.1111/j.1471-0528.2006.01193.x

McQuillan, J., Greil, A. L., Shreffler, K. M., & Bedrous, A. V. (2015). The importance of motherhood and fertility intentions among U.S. women. *Sociological Perspectives*, 58(1), 20–35. https://doi.org/10.1177/0731121414534393

McQuillan, J., Greil, A. L., Shreffler, K. M., & Tichenor, V. (2008). The importance of motherhood among women in the contemporary United States. *Gender & Society*, 22(4), 477–496. https://doi.org/10.1177/0891243208319359

McWilliams, N. (1980). Pregnancy in the analyst. *The American Journal of Psychoanalysis*, 40(4), 367–369. https://doi.org/10.1007/BF01253426

McWilliams, N. (2011). *Psychoanalytic diagnosis: Understanding personality structure in the clinical process* (2nd ed.). New York: Guilford Press.

Maloney, R. (1985). Childbirth education classes: expectant parents' expectations. *Journal of Obstetrics, Gynecologic and Neonatal Nursing*, 14(3), 245–248.

Makar, A. B., McMartin, K. E., Palese, M., & Tephly, T. R. (1975). Formate assay in body fluids: Application in methanol poisoning. *Biochemical Medicine*, 13(2), 117–126.

Mango Hurdman, C. (1999). Clinical issues and client reactions arising from the art therapist's pregnancy. *The Arts in Psychotherapy*, 26(4), 233–246. https://doi.org/10.1016/S0197-4556(99)00012-X

Mann, M. (2014). Recent advances in reproductive technology and the increased use of repeated in-vitro fertilization trials, failures, and the repetition compulsion. In M. Mann (Ed.), *Psychoanalytic aspects of assisted reproductive technology* (pp. 3–18). London, England: Karnac Books.

Marche, S. (2014, June 13). *Manifesto of the new fatherhood [Magazine]*. Retrieved September 5, 2015, from www.esquire.com/lifestyle/news/a28987/manifesto-of-the-new-fatherhood-0614/

Mariotti, P. (1993). The analyst's pregnancy: The patient, the analyst, and the space of the unknown. *The International Journal of Psychoanalysis*, 74, 151–164.

Marks, N. F., & McLanahan, S. S. (1993). Gender, family structure, and social support among parents. *Journal of Marriage and the Family*, 55(2), 481–493. https://doi.org/10.2307/352817

Marmarosh, C. L., & Tasca, G. A. (2013). Adult attachment anxiety: Using group therapy to promote change: Attachment anxiety in group therapy. *Journal of Clinical Psychology*, 69(11), 1172–1182. https://doi.org/10.1002/jclp.22044

Martindale, B., & Summers, A. (2013). The psychodynamics of psychosis. *Advances in Psychiatric Treatment*, 19(2), 124–131. https://doi.org/10.1192/apt.bp.111.009126

Martinez, D. (1989). Pains and gains: A study of forced terminations. *Journal of the American Psychoanalytic Association*, 37, 89–115.

Masser, B., Grass, K., & Nesic, M. (2007). "We like you, but we don't want you"—The impact of pregnancy in the workplace. *Sex Roles*, 57(9–10), 703–712. https://doi.org/10.1007/s11199-007-9305-2

Matozzo, L. M. (2000). Impact of the therapist's pregnancy on relationships with clients: A comparative study. Widener University, Institute for Graduate Clinical Psychology, United States—Pennsylvania. Retrieved from http://0-search.proquest.com.libcat.widener.edu/dissertations/docview/304676078/abstract/F60C10CF5E1E457APQ/1

Matthews, A. M., & Matthews, R. (1986). Beyond the mechanics of infertility: Perspectives on the social psychology of infertility and involuntary childlessness. *Family Relations*, 35(4), 479.

Matthews, T., MacDorman, M., & Thoma, M. (2015). *Infant mortality statistics from the 2013 period linked birth/infant death data set* (National Vital Statistics Reports No.

2015–1120). Hyattsville, MD: National Center for Health Statistics. Retrieved from www.cdc.gov/nchs/data/nvsr/nvsr64/nvsr64_09.pdf

May, K. A. (1981). Three phases of father involvement in pregnancy. In R. H. Moos (Ed.), *Coping with life crises* (pp. 115–127). Boston, MA: Springer. Retrieved from http://link.springer.com/10.1007/978-1-4684-7021-5_8

McNary, S. W., & Dies, R. R. (1993). Cotherapist modeling in group psychotherapy: Fact or fantasy? Group, 17(3), 131–142.

Meglich, P., Mihelič, K. K., & Zupan, N. (2016). The outcomes of perceived work-based support for mothers: A conceptual model. *Management: Journal of Contemporary Management Issues, 21*(Special issue), 21–50.

Meléndez Moral, J. C., Fortuna Terrero, F. B., Sales Galán, A., & Mayordomo Rodríguez, T. (2015). Effect of integrative reminiscence therapy on depression, well-being, integrity, self-esteem, and life satisfaction in older adults. *The Journal of Positive Psychology, 10*(3), 240–247. https://doi.org/10.1080/17439760.2014.936968

Meyer, I. H. (2003). Prejudice, social stress, and mental health in lesbian, gay, and bisexual populations: Conceptual issues and research evidence. *Psychological Bulletin, 129*, 674–697. Doi: 10.1037/0033-2909.129.5.674.

Mikulincer, M., & Arad, D. (1999). Attachment working models and cognitive openness in close relationships: A test of chronic and temporary accessibility effects. *Journal of Personality and Social Psychology, 77*(4), 710–725. https://doi.org/10.1037/0022-3514.77.4.710

Miller, J. R. (1992). Play therapy with young children during the pregnancy of a novice therapist. *Psychotherapy: Theory, Research, Practice, Training, 29*(4), 631–634. https://doi.org/10.1037/0033-3204.29.4.631

Miller, S. (1996). Questioning, resisting, acquiescing, balancing: New mothers' career reentry strategies. *Health Care for Women International, 17*, 109–131.

Minnotte, K. L. (2016). Extending the job demands–resources model: Predicting perceived parental success among dual-earners. *Journal of Family Issues, 37*(3), 416–440.

Möller, B., Schreier, H., Li, A., & Romer, G. (2009). Gender identity disorder in children and adolescents. *Current Problems in Pediatric and Adolescent Health Care, 39*(5), 117–143. https://doi.org/10.1016/j.cppeds.2009.02.001

Moore, K. A. (2007). Embryo adoption: The legal and moral challenges. *University of St. Thomas Journal of Law and Public Policy, 1*(1), 101–121.

Morell, C. (2000). Saying no: Women's experiences with reproductive refusal. *Feminism & Psychology, 10*(3), 313–322. https://doi.org/10.1177/0959353500010003002

Morris, J. F., Balsam, K. F., & Rothblum, E. D. (2002). Lesbian and bisexual mothers and nonmothers: Demographics and the coming-out process. *Journal of Family Psychology, 16*(2), 144–156. https://doi.org/10.1037/0893-3200.16.2.144

Morrissey, J., & Tribe, R. (2001). Parallel process in supervision. *Counselling Psychology Quarterly, 14*(2), 103–110. https://doi.org/10.1080/09515070126329

Mothersole, G. (1999). Parallel process: A review. *The Clinical Supervisor, 18*(2), 107–121. https://doi.org/10.1300/J001v18n02_08

Moulder, C. (1994). Towards a preliminary framework for understanding pregnancy loss. *Journal of Reproductive and Infant Psychology, 12*, 65–67.

Munk-Olsen, T., Laursen, T. M., Pedersen, C. B., Lidegaard, Ø., & Mortensen, P. B. (2011). Induced first-trimester abortion and risk of mental disorder. *New England Journal of Medicine, 364*(4), 332–339.

Naparstek, B. (1976). Treatment guidelines for the pregnant therapist. *Psychiatric Opinion, 13*, 20–25.

Napoli, M. (1999). Issues for pregnant therapists: Missed appointments and fee payments. *British Journal of Psychotherapy, 15*(3), 355–357. https://doi.org/10.1111/j.17 52-0118.1999.tb00459.x

Nehring, D., & Alvarado, E. (2009). Intimacy and reproduction: The role of Hispanic groups in American fertility. *Florida Atlantic Comparative Studies Journal, 11*. Retrieved from http://home.fau.edu/peralta/web/facs/hispanicfertility.pdf

Notman, M. T., & Nadelson, C. C. (2004). Gender in the consulting room. *The Journal of the American Academy of Psychoanalysis and Dynamic Psychiatry, 32*(1), 193–200. https://doi.org/10.1521/jaap.32.1.193.28338

Ogden, T. (2001). Reading Winnicott. *Psychoanalytic Quarterly, 70*, 299–323.

O'hara, M. W., & Swain, A. M. (1996). Rates and risk of postpartum depression—a meta-analysis. *International Review of Psychiatry, 8*(1), 37–54. https://doi.org/10.3109/09540269609037816

Okonofua, F. E., Harris, D., Odebiyi, A., Kane, T., & Snow, R. C. (1997). The social meaning of infertility in Southwest Nigeria. *Health Transition Review, 7*, 205–220.

Osofsky, H. (1982). Expectant and new fatherhood as a developmental crisis. *Bulletin of the Menninger Clinic, 46*(3), 209–230.

Pablo, R. Y. (1976). Job satisfaction in a chronic care facility. *Dimensions in Health Service, 53*(1), 36–39.

Pacheco Palha, A., & Lourenco, M. F. (2011). Psychological and cross-cultural aspects of infertility and human sexuality. In *Sexual dysfunction: Beyond the brain-body connection* (Vol. 31, pp. 164–183). Karger Publishers. Retrieved from www.karger.com/Article/Fulltext/328922

Padawer, R. (2009, November 17). *Who knew I was not the father?* [Magazine]. Retrieved September 5, 2015, from www.nytimes.com/2009/11/22/magazine/22Paternity-t.html?pagewanted=all&_r=0

Padovano-Janik, A. K., Brabender, V. M., & Rutter, P. A. (2015). Young adult daughters of lesbian mothers speak: A qualitative study on identity formation. *Journal of GLBT Family Studies, 11*(5), 465–492. https://doi.org/10.1080/1550428X.2015.1009224

Paluszny, M., & Posnanski, E. (1971). Reactions of patients during pregnancy of the psychotherapist. *Child Psychiatry and Human Development, 1*(4), 226–275.

Pancsofar, N., & Vernon-Feagans, L. (2010). Fathers' early contributions to children's language development in families from low-income rural communities. *Early Childhood Research Quarterly, 25*(4), 450–463. https://doi.org/10.1016/j.ecresq.2010.02.001

Parcsi, L., & Curtin, M. (2013). Experiences of occupational therapists returning to work after maternity leave. *Australian Occupational Therapy Journal, 60*(4), 252–259. https://doi.org/10.1111/1440-1630.12051

Parens, H. (1990). On the girl§s psychosexual development: Reconsiderations suggested from direct observation. *Journal of the American Psychoanalytic Association, 38*, 743–772.

Parke, M. (2003). *Are married parents really better for children? What research says about the effects of family structure on child well-being.* Retrieved from http://files.eric.ed.gov/fulltext/ED476114.pdf

Parke, R. D. (2002). Fathers and families. In M. Bornstein (Ed.), *Handbook of parenting* (2nd ed., Vol. 3, pp. 27–73). Mahwah, NJ: Erlbaum.

Parke, R. D. (2013). *Future families: Diverse forms, rich possibilities.* Hoboken, NJ: John Wiley & Sons. Retrieved from http://doi.wiley.com/10.1002/9781118602386

Parker, K., & Wang, W. (2013). *Modern parenthood: Roles of moms and dads converge as they balance work and family.* Pew Research Center.

Pasch, L. A., & Sullivan, K. T. (2017). Stress and coping in couples facing infertility. *Current Opinion in Psychology, 13,* 131–135. https://doi.org/10.1016/j.copsyc.2016.07.004

Patterson, C. J. (2009). Children of lesbian and gay parents: Psychology, law, and policy. *American Psychologist, 64*(8), 727–736. https://doi.org/10.1037/0003-066X.64.8.727

Pattison, H. M., Gross, H., & Cast, C. (1997). Pregnancy and employment: The perceptions and beliefs of fellow workers. *Journal of Reproductive and Infant Psychology, 15*(3–4), 303–313. https://doi.org/10.1080/02646839708404552

Pavao, J. (2007). Variations in clinical issues for children adopted as infants and those adopted as older children. In R. A. Javier, A. L. Baden, F. A. Biafora, & A. Camacho-Gengerich (Eds.), *Handbook of adoption: Implications for researchers, practitioners, and families* (pp. 283–292). Thousand Oaks, CA: Sage Publications, Inc. Retrieved from http://sk.sagepub.com/reference/hdbk_adoption/n18.xml

Penn, L. S. (1986). The pregnant therapist: Transference and countertransference issues In J. L. Alpert (Ed.), *Psychoanalysis and women: Contemporary reappraisals* (pp. 287–315). Hillside, NJ: Analytic.

Perlman, L. (1986). The analyst's pregnancy: Transference and countertransference reactions. *Modern Psychoanalysis, 11,* 89–102.

Perry-Jenkins, M., Seery, B., & Crouter, A. C. (1992). Linkages between women's provider-role attitudes, psychological well-being, and family relationships. *Psychology of Women Quarterly, 16,* 311–329.

Pertman, A. (2011). *Adoption nation: How the adoption revolution is transforming our families—and America* (2nd ed., and updated). Boston, MA: Harvard Common Press.

Pew Research Center. (2013). *How mothers and fathers divide household chores.* Retrieved from www.pewsocialtrends.org/2013/10/08/parents-time-with-kids-more-rewarding-than-paid-work-and-more-exhausting/st-parental-time-use-10-2013-10/

Pew Research Center. (2015). *Raising kids and running a household: How working parents share the load.*

Phelan, S. T. (1988). Pregnancy during residency: II. Obstetric complications. *Obstetrics and Gynecology, 72*(3 Pt 1), 431–436.

Phillips, J., King, R., & Skouteris, H. (2014). The influence of psychological distress during pregnancy on early postpartum weight retention. *Journal of Reproductive and Infant Psychology, 32*(1), 25–40. https://doi.org/10.1080/02646838.2013.845873

Pielack, L. K. (1989). Transference, countertransference, and the mental health counselor's pregnancy. *Journal of Mental Health Counseling, 11,* 155–176.

Pines, D. (1972). Pregnancy and motherhood: Interaction between fantasy and reality. *British Journal of Medical Psychology, 45,* 333–343.

Pines, D. (1982). The relevance of early psychic development to pregnancy and abortion. *International Journal of Psycho-Analysis, 63,* 311–319.

Pleck, E. H., & Pleck, J. H. (1997). Fatherhood ideals in the united states: Historical dimensions. In M. E. Lamb (Ed.), *The role of the father in child development* (Third edition, 33–48). New York: Wiley.

Pong, S., Dronkers, J., & Hampden-Thompson, G. (2003). Family policies and children's school achievement in single-versus two-parent families. *Journal of Marriage and Family*, 65(3), 681–699. https://doi.org/10.1111/j.1741-3737.2003.00681.x

Prevost, M., Zelkowitz, P., Tulandi, T., Hayton, B., Feeley, N., Carter, C. S., & Gold, I. (2014). Oxytocin in pregnancy and the postpartum: Relations to labor and its management. *Frontiers in Public Health*, 2. https://doi.org/10.3389/fpubh.2014.00001

Prince Cooke, L., & Baxter, J. (2010). "Families" in international context: Comparing institutional effects across western societies. *Journal of Marriage and Family*, 72(3), 516–536. https://doi.org/10.1111/j.1741-3737.2010.00716.x

Racker, H. (1972). The meanings and uses of countertransference. *Psychoanalytic Quarterly*, 41, 487–506.

Racker, H. (1982). *Transference and countertransference*. London: Karnac Books. Retrieved from http://site.ebrary.com/id/10497236

Racker, H. (2012). *Transference and countertransference*. London: Karnac Books.

Raeburn, P. (2014a). *Do fathers matter? What science is telling us about the parent we've overlooked*. New York: Scientific American/Farrer, Straus and Giroux.

Raeburn, P. (2014b, May 1). *How dads influence teens' happiness* [Magazine]. Retrieved September 7, 2015, from www.scientificamerican.com/article/how-dads-influence-teens-happiness/

Rainsford, K. D., & Whitehouse, M. W. (1976). Concerning the merits of copper aspirin as a potential anti-inflammatory drug. *The Journal of Pharmacy and Pharmacology*, 28(1), 83–86.

Ramirez, D. (2000). Blood thicker than water? Iconoclastic aspects of adoption one moment in an analysis. *Psychologist Psychoanalyst*, 20(3), 44–46.

Ranjbar, F., Akhondi, M.-M., Borimnejad, L., Ghaffari, S.-R., & Behboodi-Moghadam, Z. (2015). Paradox of modern pregnancy: A phenomenological study of women's lived experiences from assisted pregnancy. *Journal of Pregnancy*, 2015, 1–8. https://doi.org/10.1155/2015/543210

Raphael-Leff, J. (1980). Psychotherapy with pregnant women. In B. L. Blum (Ed.), *Psychological aspects of pregnancy, birthing and bonding* (pp. 174–205). New York: Human Sciences Press.

Raphael-Leff, J. (2004). Unconscious transmissions between patient and pregnant analyst. *Studies in Gender and Sexuality*, 5(3), 317–330. https://doi.org/10.1080/15240650509349253

Ray, R., Gornick, J. C., & Schmitt, J. (2010). Who cares? Assessing generosity and gender equality in parental leave policy designs in 21 countries. *Journal of European Social Policy*, 20(3), 196–216. https://doi.org/10.1177/0958928710364434

Reider, N. (1953). A type of transference to institutions. *Journal of Hillside Hospital*, 2, 23–29.

Reuters. (2011, February 24). U.S. way behind the rest of the world in parental leave policy: Human Rights Watch. *New York Daily News*. Retrieved from www.nydailynews.com/news/national/u-s-behind-world-parental-leave-policy-study-papua-new-guinea-swaziland-u-s-lag-article-1.134271

Reynolds, J. J. (2004). Stillbirth: To hold or not to hold . . . *OMEGA—Journal of Death and Dying*, 48(1), 85–88. https://doi.org/10.2190/L7PR-3744-8GLD-W4CQ

Richards, L. N., & Schmiege, C. J. (1993). Problems and strengths of single-parent families: Implications for practice and policy. *Family Relations*, 42(3), 277. https://doi.org/10.2307/585557

Richardson, P. (1990). Women's experiences of body change during normal pregnancy. *Maternal-Child Nursing Journal, 19*(2), 93–111.

Ridgeway, C. L., & Correll, S. J. (2004). Motherhood as a status characteristic. *Journal of Social Issues, 60*(4), 683–700.

Riggs, D. W. (2013). *Transgender men's self-representations of bearing children post-transition.* Retrieved from http://dspace2.flinders.edu.au/xmlui/handle/2328/35786

Rijk, C.H.A.M., Hoksbergen, R.A.C., ter Laak, J.J.F., van Dijkum, C., & Robbroeckx, L.H.M. (2006). Parents who adopt deprived children have a difficult task. *Adoption Quarterly, 9*(2–3), 37–61. https://doi.org/10.1300/J145v09n02_03

Robbins, (1998). The impact of pregnancy on the psychotherapeutic process. *Therapeutic Presence: Bridging Expression and Form,* 142–152.

Roberts, J. (2005). Transparency and self-disclosure in family therapy: Dangers and possibilities. *Family Process, 44*(1), 45–63.

Robertson E., Cote-Arsenault, D., Tang, W., Glover, V., Evans, J., Golding, J., & O'Connor, T. G. (2011). Previous prenatal loss as a predictor of perinatal depression and anxiety. *The British Journal of Psychiatry, 198*(5), 373–378. https://doi.org/10.11 92/bjp.bp.110.083105

Robertson, S. (2015, October 21). *Infertility social impact.* Retrieved August 7, 2016, from www.news-medical.net/health/Infertility-Social-Impact.aspx

Robinson, G. E. (2011). Dilemmas related to pregnancy loss. *The Journal of Nervous and Mental Disease, 199*(8), 571–574. https://doi.org/10.1097/NMD.0b013e318225f31e

Robinson, G. E. (2014). Pregnancy loss. *Best Practice & Research Clinical Obstetrics & Gynaecology, 28*(1), 169–178. https://doi.org/10.1016/j.bpobgyn.2013.08.012

Rochebrochard, E. de La, & Thonneau, P. (2002). Paternal age and maternal age are risk factors for miscarriage; results of a multicentre European study. *Human Reproduction, 17*(6), 1649–1656.

Rogers, C. (1994). The group and the group analyst's pregnancies. *Group Analysis, 27,* 51–61.

Rojjanasrirat, W. (2004). Working women's breastfeeding experiences. *MCN: The American Journal of Maternal/Child Nursing, 29*(4), 222–227.

Rosen, P. (1989). The pregnant therapist: A matter of style and emphasis. *Journal of College Student Psychotherapy, 4*(1), 23–26.

Rosenberg, E. B. (1992). *The adoption life cycle: The children and their families through the years.* New York: Free Press.

Rothblum, E. D., & Factor, R. (2001). Lesbians and their sisters as a control group: Demographic and mental health factors. *Psychological Science, 12*(1), 63–69. https://doi. org/10.1111/1467-9280.00311

Rothstein, A. (1999). Some implications of the analyst feeling disturbed while working with disturbed patients. *Psychoanalytic Quarterly, 68,* 541–558.

Rotundo, E. A. (1985). American fatherhood: A historical perspective. *American Behavioral Scientist, 29,* 7–25.

Roy, R. N., Schumm, W. R., & Britt, S. L. (2014). *Transition to parenthood.* New York: Springer. Retrieved from http://link.springer.com/10.1007/978-1-4614-7768-6

Rubin, B. M. (2012, April 18). *Age affects fertility, say Yale researchers.* Retrieved October 3, 2016, from http://articles.chicagotribune.com/2012-04-18/health/ct-x-0418-expert-patrizio-20120418_1_gestational-diabetes-fertility-and-sterility-pregnancies

Rubin, C. (1980). Notes from a pregnant therapist. *Social Work, 5,* 210–215.

Rubenstein, C. (1998). *The sacrificial mother: Escaping the trap of self denial.* New York: Hyperion.

Rubinstein, R. L. (1996). Childlessness, legacy, and generativity. *Generations, 20,* 58–60.

Ryding, E. L., Lukasse, M., Parys, A.-S. V., Wangel, A.-M., Karro, H., Kristjansdottir, H., ... Bidens Group. (2015). Fear of childbirth and risk of cesarean delivery: A cohort study in six European countries. *Birth (Berkeley, Calif.), 42*(1), 48–55. https://doi.org/10.1111/birt.12147

Saakvitne, K. W. (2000, April). *Your children are not your children: Therapist as adoptive and transferential mother.* Paper presented at the 20th Annual Meeting of the Division of Psychoanalysis, American Psychological Association, San Francisco, CA.

Salihu, H. M., Myers, J., & August, E. M. (2012). Pregnancy in the workplace. *Occupational Medicine, 62*(2), 88–97. https://doi.org/10.1093/occmed/kqr198

Sarkadi, A., Kristiansson, R., Oberklaid, F., & Bremberg, S. (2008). Fathers' involvement and children's developmental outcomes: A systematic review of longitudinal studies. *Acta Paediatrica, 97*(2), 153–158. https://doi.org/10.1111/j.1651-2227.2007.00572.x

Sayer, L. C., Bianchi, S. M., & Robinson, J. P. (2004). Are parents investing less in children? Trends in mothers' and fathers' time with children. *American Journal of Sociology, 110*(1), 1–43. https://doi.org/10.1086/386270

Schachner, D. A., Shaver, P. R., & Mikulincer, M. (2003). Adult attachment theory, psychodynamics, and couple relationships. In S. M. Johnson & V. E. Whiffen (Eds.), *Attachment processes in couple and family therapy* (pp. 18–42). New York: Guilford Press.

Schmidt, F.M.D., Fiorini, G. P., & Röhnelt Ramires, V. R. (2015). Psychoanalytic psychotherapy and the pregnant therapist: A literature review. *Research in Psychotherapy: Psychopathology, Process and Outcome, 18*(2), 50–61. https://doi.org/10.741/RP.2015.107

Schneider-Braus, K., & Goodwin, J. (1985). Group supervision for psychiatric residents during pregnancy and lactation. *Journal of Psychiatric Education, 9,* 88–98.

Schuchts, R. A., & Witkin, S. L. (1989). Assessing marital change during the transition to parenthood. *Social Casework, 70*(2), 67–75.

Schut, M., & Stroebe, H. (1999). The dual process model of coping with bereavement: Rationale and description. *Death Studies, 23*(3), 197–224.

Schwartz, F. N. (1989). Management women and the new facts of life. *Harvard Business Review,* January-February, 65–76.

Searles, H. F. (1955). The informational value of the supervisor's emotional experiences. *Psychiatry, 18,* 135–146. https://doi.org/10.1080/00332747.2015.1069638

Sell-Smith, J. A., & Lax, W. (2013). A journey of pregnancy loss: From positivism to autoethnography. *The Qualitative Report, 18*(46), 1.

Shapiro, J. L. (1987). The expectant father. *Psychology Today, 21*(1), 36–42. https://doi.org/10.1037/e400792009-002

Shapiro, S. L., Brown, K. W., & Biegel, G. M. (2007). Teaching self-care to caregivers: Effects of mindfulness-based stress reduction on the mental health of therapists in training. *Training and Education in Professional Psychology, 1*(2), 105–115. https://doi.org/10.1037/1931-3918.1.2.105

Shaw, E., & Breckenridge, J. (2014). How being pregnant and becoming a mother impacts the therapy relationship. In P. Bueskens (Ed.), *Mothering and psychoanalysis: Clinical, sociological and feminist perspectives* (pp. 139–157). Bradford, ON: Demeter Press.

Shek, D.T.L. (1996). Hong Kong parents' attitudes about marital quality and children. *The Journal of Genetic Psychology, 157*(2), 125–135. https://doi.org/10.1080/0022132 5.1996.9914851

Sherwen, L. N. (1986). Third trimester fantasies of first-time expectant fathers. *Maternal-Child Nursing Journal, 15*(3), 153–170.

Shorey, H. S., Nath, S. R., & Carter, M. (2013). Using research to inform best practices in working with adoptive families. In V. M. Brabender, A. E. Fallon, V. M. Brabender, & A. E. Fallon (Eds.), *Working with adoptive parents: Research, theory, and therapeutic interventions* (pp. 45–60). Hoboken, NJ: Wiley.

Shrier, D., & Mahmood, F. (1988). Issues in supervision of the pregnant psychiatric resident. *Journal of Psychiatric Education, 12*, 117–124.

Siebold, C. (2005). Commentary on "Transference opportunities during the therapist's pregnancy: Three case vignettes." *Psychoanalytic Social Work, 12*(1), 13–18. https://doi.org/10.1300/J032v12n01_02

Silver, R. M., Varner, M. W., Reddy, U., Goldenberg, R., Pinar, H., Conway, D., . . . Stoll, B. (2007). Work-up of stillbirth: A review of the evidence. *American Journal of Obstetrics and Gynecology, 196*(5), 433–444. https://doi.org/10.1016/j.ajog.2006.11.041

Silverman, S. (2001). Inevitable disclosure: Countertransference dilemmas and the pregnant lesbian therapist. *Journal of Gay & Lesbian Psychotherapy, 4*(3–4), 45–61. https://doi.org/10.1300/J236v04n03_04

Silverstein, L. B., & Auerbach, C. F. (1999). Deconstructing the essential father. *American Psychologist, 54*(6), 397.

Simmel, C. (2007). Risk and protective factors contributing to the longitudinal psychosocial well-being of adopted foster children. *Journal of Emotional and Behavioral Disorders, 15*(4), 237–249. https://doi.org/10.1177/10634266070150040501

Simone, D. H., McCarthy, P., & Skay, C. L. (1998). An investigation of client and counselor variables that influence likelihood of counselor self-disclosure. *Journal of Counseling and Development: JCD, 76*(2), 174.

Simonis-Gayed, D., & Levin, L. A. (1994). The therapist's pregnancy: Children's transference and countertransference reactions. *Psychotherapy: Theory, Research, Practice, Training, 31*(1), 196–200. https://doi.org/10.1037/0033-3204.31.1.196

Sit, D., Rothschild, A. J., & Wisner, K. L. (2006). A Review of Postpartum Psychosis. *Journal of Women's Health (2002), 15*(4), 352–368. http://doi.org/10.1089/jwh.2006.15.352

Sives, A. (2014). *Breaking the silence: Exploring the impact of pregnancy loss on women who delayed childbirth and remain childless* (Master's Thesis). University of Chester.

Skaife, S. (2012). The pregnant art therapist's countertransference. In S. Hogan (Ed.), *Revisiting feminist approaches to art therapy* (pp. 237–254). New York, NY: Berghahn Books.

Skouteris, H., Carr, R., Wertheim, E. H., Paxton, S. J., & Duncombe, D. (2005). A prospective study of factors that lead to body dissatisfaction during pregnancy. *Body Image, 2*(4), 347–361. https://doi.org/10.1016/j.bodyim.2005.09.002

Slade, P. (1994). Predicting the psychological impact of miscarriage. *Journal of Reproductive and Infant Psychology, 12*(1), 5–16. https://doi.org/10.1080/02646839408 408862

Slama, R. (2005). Influence of paternal age on the risk of spontaneous abortion. *American Journal of Epidemiology*, *161*(9), 816–823. https://doi.org/10.1093/aje/kwi097

Sneed, T. (2015, March 25). *Supreme Court rules against UPS in pregnancy discrimination case*. Retrieved from www.usnews.com/news/articles/2015/03/25/supreme-court-rules-against-ups-in-pregnancy-discrimination-case

Snyder, D. K., Castellani, A. M., & Whisman, M. A. (2006). Current status and future directions in couple therapy. *Annual Review of Psychology*, *57*(1), 317–344. https://doi.org/10.1146/annurev.psych.56.091103.070154

Spence, D. (1973). Tracing a thought stream by computer. In B. Rubenstein (Ed.), *Psychoanalysis and contemporary science* (Vol. 2). New York: MacMillan.

Spillius, E. B. (1993). Varieties of envious experiences. *International Journal of Psychoanalysis*, *24*, 1199–1212.

Spinelli, M., Frigerio, A., Montali, L., Fasolo, M., Spada, M. S., & Mangili, G. (2016). "I still have difficulties feeling like a mother": The transition to motherhood of preterm infants mothers. *Psychology & Health*, *31*(2), 184–204. https://doi.org/10.1080/08870446.2015.1088015

Stacey, J. (2004). Cruising to familyland: Gay hypergamy and rainbow Kinship. *Current Sociology*, *52*(2), 181–197. https://doi.org/10.1177/0011392104041807

Staehelin, K., Bertea, P. C., & Stutz, E. Z. (2007). Length of maternity leave and health of mother and child—a review. *International Journal of Public Health*, *52*(4), 202–209. https://doi.org/10.1007/s00038-007-5122-1

Steinberg, G., & Hall, B. (2000). *Inside transracial adoption: Strength-based, culture-sensitizing parenting strategies for inter-county or domestic adoptive families that don't match*. Indianapolis, IN: Perspectives Press.

Steiner, J. (2004). Foreword. *Psychoanalytic Psychotherapy*, *18*(1), 1–4. https://doi.org/10.1080/14749730410001656471

Stern, D. N. (1998). *The motherhood constellation: a unified view of parent-infant psychotherapy*. London: Karnac Books.

Sternke, E. A., & Abrahamson, K. (2015). Perceptions of women with infertility on stigma and disability. *Sexuality and Disability*, *33*(1), 3–17. https://doi.org/10.1007/s11195-014-9348-6

Stevens, D., Kiger, G., & Riley, P. J. (2001). Working hard and hardly working: Domestic labor and marital satisfaction among dual-earner couples. *Journal of Marriage and Family*, *63*(2), 514–526. https://doi.org/10.1111/j.1741-3737.2001.00514.x

Stockman, A. F., & Green-Emrich, A. (1994). Impact of therapist pregnancy on the process of counseling and psychotherapy. *Psychotherapy: Theory, Research, Practice, Training*, *31*(3), 456–462. https://doi.org/10.1037/0033-3204.31.3.456

Storesund, A., & Helle, K. B. (1975). Practolol, caffeine and calcium in the regulation of mechanical activity of the cardiac ventricle in *Myxine glutinosa* (L.). *Comparative Biochemistry and Physiology. C: Comparative Pharmacology*, *52*(1), 17–22.

Storey, A. E., Walsh, C. J., Quinton, R. L., & Wynne-Edwards, K. E. (2000). Hormonal correlates of paternal responsiveness in new and expectant fathers. *Evolution and Human Behavior*, *21*(2), 79–95. https://doi.org/10.1016/S1090-5138(99)00042-2

Strang, V. R., & Sullivan, P. L. (1985). Body image attitudes during pregnancy and the postpartum period. *Journal of Obstetric, Gynecologic, and Neonatal Nursing: JOGNN*, *14*(4), 332–337.

Strickland, O. L. (1987). The occurrence of symptoms in expectant fathers. *Nursing Research*, *36*(3), 184–188. https://doi.org/10.1097/00006199-198705000-00015

Strobeck, L. N. (2005, June). *The impact of the therapist's pregnancy on the eating disorder patient: Implications for object relations and self psychological treatment* (Doctoral Dissertation). Widener University, Chester, PA. Retrieved from UMI Dissertation Publishing. (UMI No. 3179441)

Stuart, J. J. (1997). Pregnancy in the therapist: Consequences of a gradually discernible physical change. *Psychoanalytic Psychology, 14*(3), 347–364. https://doi.org/10.1037/h0079730

Sugarman, A. (2007). Whatever happened to neurosis? Who are we analyzing? And how? The importance of mental organization. *Psychoanalytic Psychology, 24*(3), 409–428. https://doi.org/10.1037/0736-9735.24.3.409

Sumra, M. K., & Schillaci, M. A. (2015). Stress and the multiple-role woman: Taking a closer look at the "Superwoman." *PLOS ONE, 10*(3), e0120952. https://doi.org/10.1371/journal.pone.0120952

Surkan, P. J., Rådestad, I., Cnattingius, S., Steineck, G., & Dickman, P. W. (2008). Events after stillbirth in relation to maternal depressive symptoms: A brief report. *Birth, 35*(2), 153–157.

Sutherland, S. M. (1997, July). *Pregnancy: A social construction.* Thunder Bay, Ontario: Lakehead University.

Suyes, K., Abrahams, S. W., & Labbok, M. H. (2008). Breastfeeding in the workplace: Other employees' attitudes towards services for lactating mothers. *International Breastfeeding Journal, 3*(1), 25. https://doi.org/10.1186/1746-4358-3-25

Swanson, K. M. (1999). Effects of caring, measurement, and time on miscarriage impact and women's well-being. *Nursing Research, 48*(6). Retrieved from http://journals.lww.com/nursingresearchonline/Fulltext/1999/11000/Effects_of_Caring,_Measurement,_and_Time_on.4.aspx

Swartz, A., Brabender, V., Fallon, A., & Shorey, H. S. (2012). The maternal bonding trajectory for mothers who adopt young, international children: A qualitative analysis. *Journal of Social Distress and the Homeless, 21*(3–4), 138–167.

Szymanski, D. M., & Chung, Y. B. (2003). Feminist attitudes and coping resources as correlates of lesbian internalized heterosexism. *Feminism & Psychology, 13*(3), 369–389.

Tabong, P. T.-N., & Adongo, P. B. (2013). Understanding the social meaning of infertility and childbearing: A qualitative study of the perception of childbearing and childlessness in Northern Ghana. *PLoS ONE, 8*(1), e54429. https://doi.org/10.1371/journal.pone.0054429

Tasker, F., & Wood, S. (2016). The transition into adoptive parenthood: Adoption as a process of continued unsafe uncertainty when family scripts collide. *Clinical Child Psychology and Psychiatry, 21*(4), 520–535. https://doi.org/10.1177/1359104516638911

Taubman-Ben-Ari, O., Shlomo, S. B., Sivan, E., & Dolizki, M. (2009). The transition to motherhood-A time for growth. *Journal of Social and Clinical Psychology, 28*(8), 943.

Taylor, P., & Passel, D.J.S. (2011). For millennials, parenthood trumps marriage. *Pew Social & Demographic Trends.* Retrieved from www.pewsocialtrends.org/files/2011/03/millennials-marriage.pdf

Thoma, M. E., Boulet, S., Martin, J. A., & Kissin, D. (2014). National vital statistics reports. *National Vital Statistics Reports, 63*(8), 1–12. Retrieved from http://citeseerx.ist.psu.edu/viewdoc/download?doi=10.1.1.699.626&rep=rep1&type=pdf

Thompson, L., & Walker, A. J. (1989). Gender in families: Women and men in marriage, work and parenthood. *Journal of Marriage and the Family, 51*, 845–871.

Tinsley, J. A. (2000). Pregnancy of the early-career psychiatrist. *Psychiatric Services*, *51*(1), 105–110. https://doi.org/10.1176/ps.51.1.105

Tinsley, J. A., & Mellman, L. A. (2003). Patient reactions to a psychiatrist's pregnancy. *American Journal of Psychiatry*, *160*(1), 27–31. https://doi.org/10.1176/appi. ajp.160.1.27

Tither, J. M., & Ellis, B. J. (2008). Impact of fathers on daughters' age at menarche: A genetically and environmentally controlled sibling study. *Developmental Psychology*, *44*(5), 1409–1420. https://doi.org/10.1037/a0013065

Toffol, E., Koponen, P., & Partonen, T. (2013). Miscarriage and mental health: Results of two population-based studies. *Psychiatry Research*, *205*(1–2), 151–158. https://doi. org/10.1016/j.psychres.2012.08.029

Tomlinson, P. S., & Irwin, B. (1993). Qualitative study of women's reports of family adaptation pattern four years following transition to parenthood. *Issues in Mental Health Nursing*, *14*(2), 119–138. https://doi.org/10.3109/01612849309031612

Tong, S., Kaur, A., Walker, S. P., Bryant, V., Onwude, J. L., & Permezel, M. (2008). Miscarriage risk for asymptomatic women after a normal first-trimester prenatal visit: *Obstetrics & Gynecology*, *111*(3), 710–714. https://doi.org/10.1097/AOG.0b013e318163747c

Tonon, C. B., Romani, P. F., & Grossi, R. (2012). The therapist's pregnancy and its consequences on the psychotherapeutic process. *Psicologia: Teoria E Pesquisa*, *28*(1), 87–92.

Toomey, J. (2011). *Breaking boundaries: An exploration of the experience of the pregnant trainee therapist*. Dublin Business School.

Trad, P. V. (1990). Emergence and resolution of ambivalence in expectant mothers. *American Journal of Psychotherapy*, *44*, 577–589.

Trad, P. V. (1991). Adaptation to developmental transformations during various phases of motherhood. *Journal of the American Academy of Psycho-Analysis*, *19*, 403–421.

Trinidad, D. R., Gilpin, E. A., White, M. M., & Pierce, J. P. (2005). Why does adult African-American smoking prevalence in California remain higher than for non-Hispanic whites? *Ethnicity and Disease*, *15*(3), 505.

Troilo, J. (2015). Stay tuned: Portrayals of fatherhood to come. *Psychology of Popular Media Culture*, *6*, 82–94. https://doi.org/10.1037/ppm0000086

Trotzer, J. P. (2004). Conducting a group: Guidelines for choosing and using activities. In J. DeLucia-Waack, D. Gerrity, C. Kalodner, & M. Riva (Eds.), *Handbook of group counseling and psychotherapy* (pp. 76–90). Thousand Oaks, CA: Sage Publications, Inc. Retrieved from http://sk.sagepub.com/reference/handbook-of-group-counseling-and-psychotherapy/n6.xml

Tudiver, F., & Tudiver, J. (1982). Pregnancy and psychological preparation for parenthood. *Canadian Family Physician*, *28*, 1564–1568.

Turkel, A. R. (1993). Clinical issues of pregnant psychoanalyst. *Journal of the American Academy of Psychoanalysis*, *21*(1), 117–131.

Turton, P., Evans, C., & Hughes, P. (2009). Long-term psychosocial sequelae of stillbirth: Phase II of a nested case-control cohort study. *Archives of Women's Mental Health*, *12*(1), 35–41. https://doi.org/10.1007/s00737-008-0040-7

Twenge, J. M., Campbell, W. K., & Foster, C. A. (2003). Parenthood and marital satisfaction: A meta-analytic review. *Journal of Marriage & Family*, *65*(3), 574–583.

Ulanov, A. B. (1973). Birth and rebirth: The effect of an analyst's pregnancy on the transferences of three patients. *Journal of Analytic Psychology*, *18*, 146–164.

Ulman, K. H. (2001). Unwitting exposure of the therapist: Transferential and countertransferential dilemmas. *Journal of Psychotherapy Practice and Research*, *10*, 14–22.

Ulrich, M., & Weatherall, A. (2000). Motherhood and infertility: Viewing motherhood through the lens of infertility. *Feminism & Psychology, 10*(3), 323–336.

Underwood, M. M., & Underwood, E. D. (1976). Clinical observations of a pregnant therapist. *Social Work, 21,* 512–514.

United States Bureau of Labor Statistics. (2015). *Household data annual averages: Employed persons by occupation, sex, and age* (Annual average data) (p. 1). Washington, DC: U.S. Department of Labor. Retrieved from www.bls.gov/cps/cpsaat09.pdf

United States Census Bureau. (2015). *Quick facts: United States.* Retrieved from www.census.gov/quickfacts/table/PST045215/00

United States Department of Commerce. (2009). *Community facts.* Retrieved from http://factfinder.census.gov/faces/nav/jsf/pages/index.xhtml

United States Department of Commerce. (2010). *America's family and living arrangements.* Retrieved from www.census.gov/population/www/socdemo/hh-fam/cps2010. html.

United States Department of Labor. Fair Labor Standards Act, Pub. L. No. 29 U.S.C. 207, § 7(r) (2010). Retrieved from www.dol.gov/whd/nursingmothers/Sec7rFLSA_btnm. htm

Uyehara, L. A., Austrian, S., Upton, L., Warner, R. H., & Williamson, R. C. A. (1995). Telling about the analyst's pregnancy. *Journal of the American Psychoanalytic Association, 43*(1), 113–135.

Vandereycken, W., & DeKerf, A. (2010). Eating-disordered patients' perception of pregnancy in important others and therapists. *Eating and Weight Disorders—Studies on Anorexia, Bulimia and Obesity, 15*(1–2), 98–99.

Vanier, A. (2001). Some remarks on adolescence with particular reference to Winnicott and Lacan. *The Psychoanalytic Quarterly, 70*(3), 579–597.

Van Niel, M. S. (1993). Pregnancy: The obvious and evoactive real event in a therapist's life. In J. H. Gold & J. C. Nemiah (Eds.), *Beyond transference: When the therapist's real life intrudes.* Washington, DC: American Psychiatric Press.

von Bertanlanffy, L. (1966). General system theory and psychiatry. In S. Arieti (Ed.), *American handbook of psychiatry* (Vol. 3, pp. 705–721). New York: Basic Books.

Wagner, H., Häberle, H., Maier, V., & Lang, R. E. (1978). Transmitter mediated arginine vasopressin release from superfused hypothalamus and pituitary gland. *Journal of Endocrinological Investigation, 1*(3), 215–220. https://doi.org/10.1007/BF03350383

Wagner, L. B. (2000). *The adoptive journey: identity changes in the analytic therapist.* Presented at the 20th Annual Meeting of the Division of Psychoanalysis, American Psychological Association, San Francisco, CA.

Waldman, J. (2003). New mother/old therapist: Transference and countertransference challenges in the return to work. *American Journal of Psychotherapy, 57*(1), 52–63.

Walker, K. F., & Thornton, J. G. (in press, 2016). Advanced maternal age. *Obstetrics, Gynecology & Reproductive Medicine.* https://doi.org/10.1016/j.ogrm.2016.09.005

Walker, P. (2015, June 16). Fathers need support to spend more time on children and chores— report. *The Guardian.* Retrieved from www.theguardian.com/lifeandstyle/2015/ jun/16/fathers-need-support-to-spend-more-time-on-children-and-chores-report

Walks, M. (2013). *Gender identity and in/fertility* (Doctoral Dissertation). University of British Columbia.

Walls, F. K. (2002, September 18). *Transference and countertransference in the psychotherapy of a mid-life man with schizoaffective disorder during the therapist's pregnancy:*

A case study (Doctoral Dissertation). The Chicago School of Professional Psychology, Chicago, IL. Retrieved from UMI Dissertation Publishing. (UMI No. 3093614)

Walsh, A., Gold, M., Jensen, P., & Jedrzkiewicz, M. (2005). Motherhood during residency training: challenges and strategies. *Canadian Family Physician, 51*(7), 990–991.

Wang, L., Wu, T., Anderson, J. L., & Florence, J. E. (2011). Prevalence and risk factors of maternal depression during the first three years of child rearing. *Journal of Women's Health, 20*(5), 711–718. https://doi.org/10.1089/jwh.2010.2232

Wang, W. (2013). *Parents' Time with kids more rewarding than paid work—and more exhausting* (Social & Demographic Trends). Pew Research Center.

Wang, W., Parker, K., & Taylor, P. (2013). Breadwinner moms. *Pew Research Center.* Washington, DC. Retrieved from www.pewsocialtrends.org/2013/05/29/breadwinner-moms/4/

Warren, C. S., Crowley, M. E., Olivardia, R., & Schoen, A. (2008). Treating patients with eating disorders: An examination of treatment providers' experiences. *Eating Disorders, 17*(1), 27–45. https://doi.org/10.1080/10640260802570098

Watkins, C. E. (2012). Psychotherapy supervision in the new millennium: Competency-based, evidence-based, particularized, and energized. *Journal of Contemporary Psychotherapy, 42*(3), 193–203. https://doi.org/10.1007/s10879-011-9202-4

Watson, W. J., Watson, L., Wetzel, W., Bader, E., & Talbot, Y. (1995). Transition to parenthood. What about fathers? *Canadian Family Physician, 41*, 807.

Wedderkopp, A. (1990). The therapist's pregnancy: Evocative intrusion. *Psychoanalytic Psychotherapy, 5*(1), 37–58. https://doi.org/10.1080/02668739000700041

Wegar, K. (1997). *Adoption, identity and kinship: The debate over sealed birth records.* New Haven, CT: Yale University Press.

Weiner, I. B., & Bornstein, R. F. (2009). *Principles of psychotherapy: Promoting evidence-based psychodynamic practice.* Hoboken, NJ: John Wiley & Sons.

Weir, K. N. (2003). Adoptive family "leap-frogging" patterns. *Adoption Quarterly, 7*(1), 27–41. https://doi.org/10.1300/J145v07n01_03

Weisman, O., Zagoory-Sharon, O., & Feldman, R. (2014). Oxytocin administration, salivary testosterone, and father—infant social behavior. *Progress in Neuro-Psychopharmacology and Biological Psychiatry, 49*, 47–52. https://doi.org/10.1016/j.pnpbp.2013.11.006

Wellendorf, F. (1986). Supervision als Institutions analyse [Supervision as institutional analysis]. In H. Pühl & W. Schmidbauer (Eds.), *Supervision und Psychoanalyse: Selbstreflexion der Helfenden Berufe* [Supervision and psychoanalysis: Self-reflections in the helping professions] (pp. 49–65). München, Germany: Kösel-Verlag.

Wellenkamp, J. (1995). Cultural similarities and differences regarding emotional disclosure: Some examples from Indonesia and the Pacific. In J. W. Pennebaker (Ed.), *Emotion, disclosure, and health* (pp. 293–311). Washington, DC: American Pscyhological Association.

Westin, M., Källén, K., Saltvedt, S., Almström, H., Grunewald, C., & Valentin, L. (2007). Miscarriage after a normal scan at 12–14 gestational weeks in women at low risk of carrying a fetus with chromosomal anomaly according to nuchal translucency screening. *Ultrasound in Obstetrics and Gynecology, 30*(5), 728–736. https://doi.org/10.1002/uog.5138

Whitaker, K. M., Wilcox, S., Liu, J., Blair, S. N., & Pate, R. R. (2016). Patient and provider perceptions of weight gain, physical activity, and nutrition counseling during pregnancy: A qualitative study. *Women's Health Issues, 26*(1), 116–122. https://doi. org/10.1016/j.whi.2015.10.007

Whyte, N. (2004a). The analyst's pregnancy: A non-negotiable fact: The challenge to existing object relations. *Psychoanalytic Psychotherapy, 18*(1), 27–43. https://doi.org/1 0.1080/14749730410001656507

Whyte, N. (2004b). Bibliography. *Psychoanalytic Psychotherapy, 18*(1), 139–139. https:// doi.org/10.1080/14749730410001656570

Whyte, N. (2004c). Introduction. *Psychoanalytic Psychotherapy, 18*(1), 5–14. https://doi. org/10.1080/14749730410001656480

Whyte, N. (2004d). Review of the literature. *Psychoanalytic Psychotherapy, 18*(1), 15–26. https://doi.org/10.1080/14749730410001656499

Widseth, J. C. (1989). Commentary: Recollections and reflections from my pregnancies. *Journal of college Student Psychotherapy, 4*(1), 17–21.

Wiese, B. S., & Heidemeier, H. (2012). Successful return to work after maternity leave: Self-regulatory and contextual influences. *Research in Human Development, 9*(4), 317–336. https://doi.org/10.1080/15427609.2012.729913

Wiese, B. S., & Ritter, J. O. (2012). Timing matters: Length of leave and working mothers' daily reentry regrets. *Developmental Psychology, 48*(6), 1797–1807. https://doi. org/10.1037/a0026211

Wiesenthal, S. (2008). Pregnancy and the psychiatry resident: Implications for psychotherapy and supervision. *Residents' Journal—The American Journal of Psychiatry, 3*(7), 1–2.

Williams, M. (2013, January 6). *40% of fathers do not to take paternity leave | Guardian Careers | The Guardian* [Newspaper]. Retrieved March 7, 2016, from www.the guardian.com/careers/fathers-choose-not-to-take-paternity-leave

Wilson, M. (2015). Commentary on "Patients' pregnancies during treatment: The influence of the analyst's psychology" by Richard Almond. *Psychoanalytic Dialogues, 25*(3), 359–367. https://doi.org/10.1080/10481885.2015.1034561

Winnicott, D. W. (1945). Primitive emotional development. In *Through pediatrics to psychoanalysis* (pp. 145–156). New York: Basic Books.

Winnicott, D. W. (1956). *Collected Papers: Through pediatrics to Psycho-analysis.* New York: Basic Books.

Winnicott, D. W. (1965). *The maturational process and the facilitating environment.* New York: International Universities Press.

Wingzinger, M., Fallon, A., & Brabender, V. (2016). Mothers' experiences in creating an emotional connection with their adopted children: A qualitative study. In S. Akhtar (Ed.), *The new motherhoods: Patterns of early child care in contemporary culture* (pp. 81–105). Lanham, MD: Rowman & Littlefield.

Wolfe, E. H. (2013). *The therapist's pregnancy and the client-therapist relationship: An exploratory study* (Doctoral Dissertation).

Wollheim, I. (1999). *Therapist pregnancy: A phenomenological exploration of the therapist's experience* (Doctoral Dissertation). California School of Professional Psychology, Fresno, CA. Retrieved from UMI Dissertation Publishing. (UMI No. 9988379)

Wurzer, R. (2005, August). *The changing roles and expectations of fathers through three generations.* Menomonie, WI: University of Wisconsin-Stout. Retrieved from http:// www2.uwstout.edu/content/lib/thesis/2005/2005wurzerr.pdf

Wynne-Edwards, K. E. (2004, June 28). *Why do some men experience pregnancy symptoms such as vomiting and nausea when their wives are pregnant?* Retrieved March 8, 2016, from www.scientificamerican.com/article/why-do-some-men-experienc/

Yang, Y., & Morgan, P. A. (2003). How big are educational and racial fertility differentials in the U.S.? *Social Biology, 50*(3–4), 167–187.

Zackson, J. (2012). *The impact of primary maternal preoccupation on therapists' ability to work with patients* (Doctoral Dissertation). The City University of New York, New York. Retrieved from UMI Dissertation Publishing. (UMI No. 3508739)

Zalusky, S. (2000). Infertility in the age of technology. *Journal of the American Psychoanalytic Association, 48*(4), 1541–1562.

Zargham-Boroujeni, A., Jafarzadeh-Kenarsari, F., Ghahiri, A., & Habibi, M. (2014). Empowerment and sense of adequacy in infertile couples: A fundamental need in treatment process of infertility-a qualitative study. *The Qualitative Report, 19*(6), 1.

Zheng, A. (2014). The dilemma of receiving support from in-laws: A study of the discourse of online pregnancy and childbirth support groups. *China Media Research, 10*(3), 32–43.

Zucker, J. (2014, October 15). *Saying it loudly: I had a miscarriage.* Retrieved August 7, 2016, from http://parenting.blogs.nytimes.com/2014/10/15/saying-it-loudly-i-had-a-miscarriage/

Zucker, J. (2015, April 28). The pregnant therapist. *The New York Times.* Retrieved from http://opinionator.blogs.nytimes.com/2015/04/28/the-pregnant-therapist/?_r=0

Index

421